SKIN CANCERS – RISK FACTORS, PREVENTION AND THERAPY

Edited by **Caterina AM La Porta**

Skin Cancers – Risk Factors, Prevention and Therapy
Edited by Caterina AM La Porta

Published by InTech
Janeza Trdine 9, 51000 Rijeka, Croatia

Publishing Process Manager Tajana Jevtic

Technical Editor Teodora Smiljanic

Cover Designer InTech Design Team

Additional hard copies can be obtained from orders@intechopen.com

Skin Cancers – Risk Factors, Prevention and Therapy, Edited by Caterina AM La Porta
p. cm.
ISBN 978-953-307-722-2

For EU product safety concerns:
IN TECH d.o.o., Prolaz Marije Krucifikse Kozulić 3, 51000 Rijeka, Croatia,
info@intechopen.com or visit our website at intechopen.com.

Meet the editor

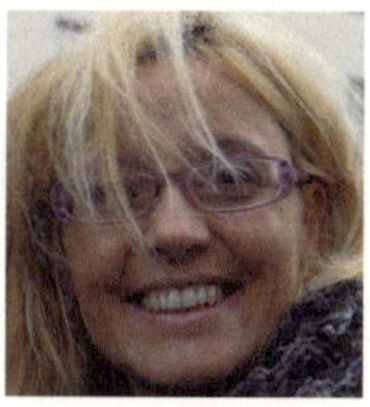

Research associate professor of General Pathology at University of Milan, visiting scientist in many universities and institutes, she is a member of many international societies, referee of many international journals and member of editorial boards of many international journals. She collaborates with many international institutions, mainly in USA. Her research is devoted mainly to melanoma and in this filed recently her group identified a more aggressive subpopulation expressing CXCR6.

Contents

Preface

Skin cancers are the fastest growing type of cancer in the United States and represent the most commonly diagnosed malignancy, surpassing lung, breast, colorectal and prostate cancer. In Europe, the British Isles have been the highest rates of skin cancer in children and adolescents. The most common types of skin cancer are basal cell carcinoma (BCC) and squamous cell carcinoma (SCC). In particular BCC of the skin is the most prevalent type of cancer affecting Caucasians. However, the most dangerous type of skin cancer is malignant melanoma. This form of skin cancer can be fatal if it is not treated early but comprises only a small proportion of all skin cancers.

This book discusses the most interesting and new aspects related to skin cancer focusing on three main issues: 1) risk factors, including extrinsic factors (i.e., indoor tanning which plays in west society an important social function, or UV and virus) and intrinsic factors (i.e., genetic predisposition, intracellular signaling, inflammation); 2) new diagnostic tools for prevention (i.e. optical imaging); 3) a more clear and scientific explanation of the strategies for prevention and treatment of skin cancer using natural compounds or nano-particle drug delivery and photodynamic therapy.

The overall idea of the book is to provide the reader with up to date information on the possible tools to use for prevention, diagnosis and treatment of skin cancer.

The impact of indoor tanning is discussed in *Chapter 1*, which is a quite common practice in USA and Western countries. The chapter contains an interesting historical description and psychological motivations are also discussed. The authors report a robust literature documenting a strong link between indoor tanning and incidence of skin cancer. Policy and regulations are also discussed.

The molecular mechanisms triggered by UV radiation are discussed in *Chapter 2*. In particular, the effect of UV radiation on the immunosystem is discussed in depth. In fact, UV inducing immunosuppression, seems to contribute to the development and progression of skin tumor. The immunosurveillance of tumor is actually an important and crucial aspect as anti-tumor activity.

Chapter 3 focuses on cutaneous squamous carcinoma and genetic abnormalities closely associated with it. A number of familial cancer syndromes, recessive dystrophic epidermolysis bullosa appear to be associated with an increased risk of developing cutaneous squamous carcinoma as well as hereditary skin disorders. The molecular mechanisms involved are not completely understood but an important and interesting aspect seems to be the microenvironment.

Chapter 4 focuses on RAS-RAF-MEK pathway in melanoma as chemotherapeutic target. However, an important aspect to further investigate is the toxicity of these drugs.

The involvement of Merkel cell polyomavirus in Merkel cell carcinoma is presented in *Chapter 5*. Interesting perspectives and new development of the research are discussed. For instance, integration sites, route of infection, cell tropism etc. are not clarified yet. Further studies are needed in this filed.

Chapter 6 discusses the accelerating effect of over-expression of macrophage migration inhibitor factor (MIF) on photocarcinogenesis in the skin. Chronic exposure to UV irradiation is involved in the early-onset skin carcinogenesis. Many cytokines like as MIF, seem to be related to the induction of UV-induced skin cancer. This chapter points out the pivotal role of inflammation process.

Chapter 7 focused on COX-2 as potential target for anti-tumor activity in non melanoma skin cancer. The possible use of pharmacological and natural compounds acting on COX-2 are discussed in view of a chemo-prevention treatment.

Several optical modalities are under study to improve cancer diagnosis. *Chapter 8* review this aspect, discussing the efficacy of the optical techniques based on its specificity and sensitivity rates.

Finally the last three chapters discuss chemoprevention and new therapeutic strategies. *Chapter 9* discusses the possible use of natural compounds for chemoprevention in skin cancer and their intracellular mechanisms.

Chapter 10 is focused on photodynamic therapy in skin cancer. A critical discussion of the literature is reported. *Chapter 11* discusses the use of topical administration of anticancer drugs and, in particular, nanoparticulate drugs to overcome the skin barrier and to improve the efficacy of topical skin cancer therapy.

In each chapter there is the *state of the art* and a critical discussion of the literature with the aim to give to the reader a useful tool for his/her future research.

Caterina AM La Porta, PhD
Department of Biomolecular Science and Biotechnology,
University of Milan, Milan,
Italy

Part 1

Risk Factors for Skin Cancer

1

Indoor Tanning: A Bio-Behavioral Risk Factor for Skin Cancer

Carolyn J. Heckman[1] and Sharon L. Manne[2]
[1]*Fox Chase Cancer Center*
[2]*University of Medicine and Dentistry of New Jersey*
Cancer Institute of New Jersey
USA

1. Introduction

Despite attempts to regulate the tanning industry, indoor tanning is a relatively common practice, particularly in the USA and other Western countries. Young women who tan to enhance their appearance are the most common patrons of tanning salons. Indoor tanning has been linked to the development of melanoma and non-melanoma skin cancers, and a disturbing increase in the incidence of melanoma among young adult women has been observed recently. This chapter will provide a review of the literature concerning some of the key facts about indoor tanning including the prevalence of indoor tanning around the world, evidence supporting the association of indoor tanning with skin cancers, the historical context of indoor tanning, psychological motivations for indoor tanning including tanning dependence, and attempts to regulate the tanning industry. The following terms will be used to describe tanning, tanning devices, and tanning establishments: indoor tanning, artificial ultraviolet (UV) tanning, tanning beds, tanning booths, sunbeds, sunlamps, tanning salons, tanning parlors, and solaria.

2. Prevalence of indoor tanning

Indoor tanning prevalence rates vary depending on the country and the population under study (See systematic review by Schneider & Kramer, 2010). Much of the research on indoor tanning has been conducted in the US. The prevalence of indoor tanning in the past year among US adults is approximately 5-16% (Choi et al., 2010; Coups, Manne, & Heckman, 2008; Heckman, Coups, & Manne, 2008; Stryker et al., 2007). Among US college students, the past year prevalence of indoor tanning is higher, with estimates ranging from 33 to 60% (Bagdasarov et al., 2008; Hillhouse, Turrisi, & Shields, 2007). Past year indoor tanning rates among US adolescents range from 3 to 26% (Cokkinides et al., 2009; Hoerster et al., 2007; Lazovich et al., 2004; Ma et al., 2007; Mayer et al., 2011). Approximately 30% of US adolescents have engaged in indoor tanning in their lifetime (Zeller et al., 2006).

Sunbed use is also common in Northern European countries, particularly in Nordic countries. A 2001 study of Swedish young adults found that 44% had ever used sunbeds

(Branstrom, Ullen, & Brandberg, 2004). One 1993 study of high school students found that about three-quarters (75%) of Norwegian girls and 65% of Norwegian boys had used a sunbed during the past year (Wichstrom, 1994). The prevalence of indoor tanning in the past year among Danish adults is approximately 30% (Koster et al., 2009). Indoor tanning rates among Danish adolescents are also high. Forty-three percent of adolescents between the ages of 15 and 18 have indoor tanned in the past year, 13% of 12 to 14 year old adolescents have indoor tanned in the past year and 2% of 8 to11 year olds have indoor tanned in the past year (Krarup et al., 2011). Rates of skin cancer correspond with these high rates of indoor tanning: after Australia and New Zealand, Denmark has the highest incidence of melanoma skin cancer (Krarup et al., 2011). Between 2004 and 2007, 26% of the Icelandic population had used a sunbed in the last year (Hery et al., 2010). As of 2008, 50% of adolescent girls and 30% of boys reported using a sunbed in the last year (Hery et al., 2010).

Rates of sunbed use vary across Western Europe. An analysis of French data from 1994-95 found that 15% of adults reported sunbed use, with its being significantly more common in the north (13%) than in the south (10%) of France (Ezzedine et al., 2008). Two recent studies found that between 29% and 47% of German adults have ever used a sunbed (Diehl et al., 2010; Dissel et al., 2009). The prevalence of indoor tanning in the past year among German adults is 21% (Diehl et al., 2010; Schneider et al., 2009). Rates in Spain are significantly lower, with only 4% of Spanish adults reporting sunbed use in the last year (Galan et al., 2011).

Compared to European countries, sunbed use is significantly lower in the UK, Canada, and Australia. However, sunbed use varies across geographical regions within the UK. On average, ever use is about 7% among children, adolescents, and adults alike (Canadian Cancer Society, 2009; Thomson et al., 2010). Sunbed use among adolescents has been found to be more common in Northwest England (Liverpool 20%, Merseyside 43%) than in Southeast England (Southhampton 6.2%; (Canadian Cancer Society, 2009; Mackay, Lowe, Edwards et al., 2007). In a recent study from Northern Ireland, 20% of adults reported ever having used a sunbed in 2008, and 1% reported indoor tanning in the past year (Boyle et al., 2010). The lifetime rate of indoor tanning is 22% among adolescents in Wales (Roberts & Foley, 2009).

With regard to Canadian sunbed use, approximately 20% of Canadian adults and 10-15% of adolescents report having ever indoor tanned (Canadian Cancer Society, 2006; Gordon & Guenther, 2009). According to recent data, 11% of Canadian adults had indoor tanned in the past 12 months (Canadian Cancer Society, 2006; Gordon & Guenther, 2009). At-home sunbeds have been common in Canada as in parts of Western Europe (Autier et al., 1994).

Sunbed use in Australia is much lower compared to most European countries or Canada, likely due to the sunny warm weather, high proportion of individuals with very UV-sensitive skin, and their long-running and successful skin cancer prevention campaigns. Nine percent of Australian adults report ever using a sunbed, and less than 1% report indoor tanning in the last year (Lawler et al., 2006). Three percent of Australian adolescents report ever having used a sunbed (Francis et al., 2010).

In summary, indoor tanning is quite common in the USA, Nordic countries, and Northern Europe. Sunbed use in the UK, Canada, and Australia is more modest. There is little data on sunbed use in southern (e.g., Italy) and eastern European countries (e.g., Poland). We are not aware of any English language literature on indoor tanning in Asian countries, perhaps because traditional Asian cultures tend to value fair skin.

3. Association between indoor tanning and skin cancer

UV radiation induces DNA damage in the skin that leads to pigmentation/tanning and can lead to carcinogenesis. Indoor tanning devices such as tanning beds and booths emit approximately 95% UVA (315-400 nm) and 5% UVB (280-315 nm), similar to the sun (Woo & Eide, 2010). UVA tends to penetrate into the dermis and cause tanning, and UVB causes burning of the epidermis (Mouret et al., 2006). More recent high-pressure tanning bulbs emit as much as 99-100% UVA radiation in order to increase the intensity and duration of tans while decreasing the likelihood of some negative effects of UVB such as skin burning and dryness (Woo & Eide, 2010). The skin cancers linked with indoor tanning are melanoma and non-melanoma skin cancers (basal cell carcinoma and squamous cell carcinoma). We will review the evidence linking indoor tanning to each.

In 2006, the International Agency for Research on Cancer (IARC), part of the World Health Organization (WHO) conducted a systematic review of 19 studies investigating the association between melanoma and indoor tanning (IARC, 2006). Individuals who had ever indoor tanned had a 1.15 relative risk of developing melanoma (IARC, 2006). In other words, individuals who had ever indoor tanned had a 15% greater chance of developing melanoma compared to individuals who had never indoor tanned. Individuals who had indoor tanned before age 35 had a relative risk of 1.75 (IARC, 2006), which translates to a 75% greater chance of developing melanoma compared to those who had not indoor tanned. There was no correlation between melanoma risk and year of publication among the articles reviewed, indicating that newer tanning devices were not safer than older ones.

Chronic UV exposure has been found to be directly related to squamous cell carcinomas (SCC), whereas intermittent exposure is more closely related to basal cell carcinoma (BCC) (Lim et al., 2011). As they did for melanoma, the IARC conducted a review of nine studies that investigated the association between SCC and BCC and indoor tanning. The review revealed that individuals who had ever used a tanning bed had a 2.25 relative risk for SCC but a 1.03 relative risk for BCC when compared to those who had never indoor tanned (IARC, 2006). However, a review by Karagas and colleagues found that the risk for both cancers increased significantly with indoor tanning (Karagas et al., 2002). The authors also found that the association with non-melanomas was inversely related to the age of indoor tanning initiation.

In 2009, the IARC reclassified UV radiation as a group 1 carcinogen or "carcinogenic to humans", rather than the previous classification of "probably carcinogenic" (El Ghissassi et al., 2009; Mogensen & Jemec, 2010). Additional studies investigating the association of sunbeds and melanoma have been published since then. For example, in a recent study of Minnesota melanoma cases and controls, 63% of cases and 51% of controls had tanned indoors (adjusted OR 1.74) (Lazovich et al., 2010). A dose response was noted in terms of years, hours, or sessions of indoor tanning. Dose was found to be more closely associated with melanoma development than age of initiation. Among US women, Fears and colleagues (Fears et al., 2011) also found a dose response relationship with melanoma risk increasing with increasing session time and frequency of sessions. The authors estimated that 5-min indoor tanning sessions would increase melanoma risk by 19% for frequent users (10+ sessions) and by 3% for occasional users (1-9 sessions). For men, measures of sunbed use were not significantly associated with melanoma risk.

Whereas most cancers strike older individuals, melanoma has become the most common cancer among 25-29 year old women in the USA, and the second most common cancer among 15-29 year old women (Herzog et al., 2007). With regard to studies conducted outside the USA, a study of the English population also found that 25% of melanomas among young women can be attributed to indoor tanning (Diffey, 2007). Sunbed use among Australians was found to be associated with increased risk of early-onset melanoma, with risk increasing with greater use, an earlier age at first use, or for earlier onset disease (Cust et al., 2011). Among individuals who were diagnosed with melanoma between 18 and 29 years of age, three quarters (76%) of melanomas were attributable to sunbed use (Cust et al., 2011). Melanoma risk has also been found to be significantly higher among Norwegian/Swedish individuals who indoor tanned than those who had not (Veierod et al., 2010).

In addition to skin cancers, UV radiation can cause immunosuppression, photo-aging, photodermatoses, pruritis, cataracts, and photokeratitis, among others (Lim et al., 2011). One of the main reasons for tanning promoted by the tanning industry is the health benefit of vitamin D (e.g., bone health, colon cancer prevention), which is produced by the skin after UV exposure (Gilchrest, 2007). However, like the sun under varying conditions, tanning beds differ as to the amount of vitamin D produced (Sayre, Dowdy, & Shepherd, 2010). In particular, modern high pressure tanning units that filter out most UVB result in the production of insignificant levels of vitamin D (Sayre et al., 2010) since UVA is not effective for vitamin D photosynthesis. In other words, the more vitamin D produced, the greater the risk of sunburn. Likewise, vitamin D production plateaus after a few indoor tanning sessions, whereas DNA damage does not (Lim et al., 2011). Additionally, vitamin D is readily available as an oral supplement, and the high prevalence of vitamin D deficiency and claimed health benefits of high vitamin D levels are not well-established (Gilchrest 2007). There has been a great deal of recent interest and controversy surrounding vitamin D deficiency and whether one should seek UV exposure to enhance vitamin D levels. Lim and colleagues refer to the latter as a "pseudo-controversy" (Lim et al., 2011). Most dermatologists and scientists agree that for most people, it is not necessary to risk skin cancer in order to protect themselves from other diseases by intentionally seeking UV radiation for its vitamin D producing properties.

Regarding indoor tanning, Weinstock and Fisher (Weinstock & Fisher, 2010) state that at this point, "The link between this form of UV exposure and both melanoma and non-melanoma skin cancers has been clarified through multiple lines of evidence from epidemiology and laboratory science reflected in recent reports by multiple prestigious bodies." A dose response relationship has been found in many studies, indicating that the greater the UV exposure, the greater the risk for melanoma.

4. Attitudes toward tanning throughout history

4.1 Pre-industrial revolution

Not only has the understanding of UV and skin cancer changed over time, but the societal meaning of skin color also has varied across history and geography. Depending on these factors, both darker and lighter skin colors have been associated with social status.

Many ancient cultures including the Aztecs, Inca, Egyptians, Romans, and Greeks worshipped the sun and valued sun exposure (Randle, 1997). However, for much of human history, pale skin has been highly preferred, being associated with positive personal qualities including purity, cleanliness, and flawlessness. For example, pale skin was valued by ancient Asian cultures, the Bible, renaissance art, classical literature by Homer, Dante, and Goethe, European court poets, and fairy tales such as "Snow White" (Holubar, 1998; Holubar & Schmidt, 1998).

In Europe and the USA prior to the 1900s, pale skin was associated with a higher social stature. The upper classes protected themselves from the sun using clothing, gloves, wide-brimmed hats, parasols, and heavy drapes, and bleached their skin to achieve a pale appearance (Albert & Ostheimer, 2002; Segrave, 2005). Only the lower and working classes were forced to work outside and therefore had darker appearing skin. In the early 1900s, the sun was viewed as unhealthy, being associated with tropical diseases (Carter, 2007).

4.2 Post-industrialization

Since industrialization and urbanization of the Western workforce, tanned skin has been perceived increasingly as attractive and fashionable among naturally light-skinned individuals. This attitude has been attributed to the fact that initially the lower classes worked in factories and lived in polluted, crowded, unsanitary slum areas where tuberculosis and rickets were common (Carter, 2007; Randle, 1997; Stradling, 1999). Pale skin was viewed as unhealthy and even associated with mental illness and alcoholism (Carter, 2007; Randle, 1997; Stradling, 1999). Only the upper classes had the time and money to take beach vacations and engage in outdoor hobbies; fashions such as bathing suits mirrored these trends.

In the late 1800s, the health benefits of UV were realized with the treatment of tuberculosis by the bactericidal properties of sun exposure or heliotherapy in sanitaria (Albert & Ostheimer, 2002). In 1903, Danish physician Niels Finsen won the Nobel Prize for curing cutaneous tuberculosis by developing the first artificial sunlamp (Randle, 1997). Around this time, it was discovered that childhood rickets could be prevented and treated with artificial phototherapy or heliotherapy (Albert & Ostheimer, 2003; Holick, 2008). During World War I, heliotherapy was used throughout Europe to treat infected wounds (Lim, Honigsman, & Hawk, 2007). Preventive medicine and public health professionals promoted sunlight for adults and sunbaths and even sunburns for babies and children (Albert & Ostheimer, 2003; Randle, 1997; Segrave, 2005).

The aesthetic benefits of the tan were popularized in 1929 when the fashion designer Coco Chanel was pictured with a tan in *Vogue* magazine after returning from a vacation in the French Riviera (Chapman, Marks, & King, 1992). The popularity of sunlamps peaked in the 1930s and 40s with the help of ads in *Vogue*, ads by General Electric, use in office buildings such as the US House Office Building, and prescription by physicians (Chapman et al., 1992; Martin et al., 2009; Segrave, 2005).

4.3 Modern America

Several economic and social trends in the mid twentieth century led to greater value being placed on a tanned appearance. In the 1950s and 60s, middle-class Americans were able to afford more travel including beach vacations, during which sun exposure is the norm (Lencek & Bosker, 1999; Pendergast & Pendergast, 2000; Randle, 1997). In the 1960s, beach party movies became popular in Hollywood (Lencek & Bosker, 1999), and technical advances were seen with the development of first-generation tanning beds and booths (Diffey, 1995; Spencer & Amonette, 1995). Together, these trends were associated with both outdoor and indoor tanning becoming more appealing to a greater portion of the American population. Through the 1970s, most sun care products were tan enhancers with minimal sunscreens, further increasing the level of skin cancer risk conferred by tanning.

The first tanning salon, Tantrific, opened in Arkansas in 1978 (Segrave, 2005). By 1980, there were 1,000 tanning salons in the USA and many individual tanning units in health- and fitness-related establishments (Segrave, 2005). In the early to mid 1980s, many of the 18,000 tanning salons began to increase the UVA and decrease the UVB levels emitted from their beds in order to market a "safer" tan with a lower likelihood of burning (Kwon et al., 2002; Segrave, 2005).

4.4 Current America

In two studies during the 1980s and 90s, clear evidence for the link between indoor tanning and melanoma was not found (Osterlind et al., 1988; Swerdlow & Weinstock, 1998). The tanning industry purchased advertising space in conspicuous venues such as *The New York Times* presenting these findings. The advertisement contained a message that indoor tanning was not proven to cause melanoma and that there were health benefits such as vitamin D production which would be missed if people avoided exposure.

Despite the current widespread knowledge regarding skin cancer etiology, media representations of tanning have continued to be primarily positive. For example, an analysis of articles in eight American magazines targeting girls and women from 1997 to 2006 found that the amount of coverage of negative consequences of indoor tanning was less than 50% of the amount of coverage of tanning benefits (Cho et al., 2010).

Indoor tanning is now a $5 billion per year industry in the US with more than 40,000 indoor tanning establishments (Looking Fit, 2009-2010). Thirty million Americans indoor tan each year, and one million tan indoors each day (Fisher & James, 2010). In a recent report, Hoerster and colleagues found more indoor tanning facilities in each of 116 large US cities than the number of Starbucks coffee shops and McDonald's restaurants in those cities (Hoerster et al., 2009). US and international regulation of indoor tanning has begun to increase. Future research will be able to provide insight into the effects of these recent and upcoming changes.

5. Psychosocial issues in indoor tanning and tanning dependence

5.1 Correlates of and motives for indoor tanning

Indoor tanners are more likely than non-tanners to be Caucasian, female, adolescents and young adults, and live in northerly climates (e.g., Heckman, Coups et al., 2008). Indoor tanners are also more likely to sunbathe, not wear protective clothing, use sunless tanners, and have low to moderate skin sensitivity to the sun (e.g., Heckman et al., 2008). Other correlates of indoor tanning include knowing other people who tan indoors, and greater use of alcohol, cigarettes, and other substances (Mosher & Danoff-Burg, 2010b).

The fact that many individuals indoor tan despite awareness of the link between UV radiation exposure and skin cancer suggests that there are important psychosocial motivations to tan that sometimes outweigh an individual's concern for his or her health. Appearance enhancement is the most commonly-cited reason given for intentional indoor tanning (Amir et al., 2000; Beasley & Kittel, 1997; Boldeman et al., 1997; Brandberg et al., 1998; Cafri, Thompson, & Jacobsen, 2006; Cafri et al., 2006; Rhainds, De Guire, & Claveau, 1999; Sjöberg et al., 2004; Young & Walker, 1998). For example, one study involving qualitative interviews with college male and female indoor tanners found that they were often told they look "good", "sexy", "beautiful", "young", "healthy" because of their tanned appearance and that these reactions were important to their self-image (Vannini & McCright, 2004). Additionally, tanning and body dysmorphic disorder are common co-occurrences, and many individuals with body dysmorphic disorder focus on perceived skin imperfections such as paleness (Phillips et al., 2006; Phillips et al., 2000).

Direct emotional effects such as relaxation, enhanced mood, stress relief, and improved energy comprise the second most often-cited category of motivations for indoor tanning (Beasley & Kittel, 1997; Boldeman et al., 1997; Feldman et al., 2004; Kourosh, Harrington, & Adinoff, 2010; Mawn & Fleischer, 1993; Zeller et al., 2006). For example, Danoff-Burg and Mosher (Danoff-Burg & Mosher, 2006) found that stress-relief and social alternatives to indoor tanning were significantly negatively related to indoor tanning behavior among young adults, whereas appearance-related alternatives were not. In terms of mood, Hillhouse and Turrisi (Hillhouse, Stapleton, & Turrisi, 2005) found a subset of frequent tanners who have seasonal affective disorder (SAD). These individuals may be using tanning, particularly during the winter, for self-medication purposes. However, the artificial light that is effective for SAD treatment must penetrate the eyes and does not contain UV, whereas individuals often close their eyes or wear goggles when indoor tanning.

Indoor tanning behavior is heavily influenced by the normative behavior of others. Several studies have found associations between adolescents' and young adults' indoor tanning and perceived indoor tanning behavior of their friends and peers (Bagdasarov et al., 2008; Hoerster et al., 2007; Lazovich et al., 2004). Likewise, studies have found associations between parental and adolescent indoor tanning, particularly among girls and their mothers (Cokkinides et al., 2009; Cokkinides et al., 2002; Hoerster et al., 2007; Stryker et al., 2004). For example, a recent study found that adolescent women who had initiated indoor tanning accompanied by their mothers were more likely to become frequent, habitual indoor tanners by young adulthood (Baker, Hillhouse, & Liu, 2010). Additionally, Cafri and colleagues (Cafri et al., 2009) found associations between indoor tanning behavior and perceptions of peer, family, significant other, and celebrity attitudes towards tanning.

Indoor tanning behavior is also influenced by beliefs about its effects on the skin in terms of skin cancer and other skin damage such as photo-aging. Some studies have found higher perceived skin damage susceptibility to be associated with greater indoor tanning behavior (Cafri, Thompson, Roehrig et al., 2006; Coups et al., 2008; Greene & Brinn, 2003; Heckman, Coups et al., 2008), some have found higher perceived threat of or susceptibility to skin harm to be associated with lower indoor tanning intentions (Cafri, Thompson, & Jacobsen, 2006; Cafri, Thompson, Roehrig et al., 2006; Greene & Brinn, 2003), and at least one has found no association (Hillhouse, Stair, & Adler, 1996). Differences in measurement may account for such varied results.

Several studies by Hillhouse and colleagues have found that together, combinations of variables from the aforementioned domains can account for high proportions of variance in indoor tanning attitudes, intentions, and behaviors (Cafri et al., 2009).

5.2 Tanning dependence

An additional reason for frequent tanning is tanning dependence or addiction, colloquially referred to as "tanorexia" (Heckman, 2011). A number of studies have provided evidence for the phenomenon of tanning dependence, with plausible biologic underpinnings that are primarily related to the opioid system. Tanning dependent individuals may tan frequently and put themselves at even great risk of skin cancer than other tanners.

While tanning dependence in not an official disorder according to the American Psychiatric Association's Diagnostic and Statistical Manual-IV (DSM-IV), tanning dependence has been defined based on traditional substance dependence criteria and measures. Several approaches to measuring tanning dependence have been taken. Warthan and colleagues (Warthan, Uchida, & Wagner, 2005) modified the substance dependence criteria from the DSM-IV and those of the four-item CAGE scale, traditionally used to screen for potential problems with alcohol use. The modified seven-item DSM-IV criteria include tolerance, withdrawal, and engaging in the behavior despite negative consequences, key criteria for the diagnosis of substance dependence. More recently, Hillhouse and colleagues (Hillhouse et al., 2010) developed the Tanning Pathology Scale (TAPAS) based on empirical data from indoor tanners. The four factors of the scale are: perceiving tanning as a problem, opiate-like reactions to tanning, evidence of tolerance to tanning, and dissatisfaction with skin tone. The TAPAS is an improvement over the modified DSM-IV and CAGE scales because its psychometric properties have been assessed and been found to be adequate, and it was developed empirically with the population of interest rather than simply being modified from existing alcohol and substance use measures (Heckman, 2011).

There is accumulating evidence supporting the phenomenon of tanning dependence (Heckman, 2011). Behavioral studies of adolescents and young adults have found addictive tendencies among indoor tanners including higher rates of other substance use (Mosher & Danoff-Burg, 2010a) and anticipated difficulty quitting indoor tanning (Lazovich et al., 2004). The prevalence of tanning dependence varies by population and measurement strategy. Among tanning salon patrons in the US, tanning dependence rates range from 33-41% (Harrington et al., 2010). Among beachgoers, rates range from 26-53% (Warthan et al., 2005). Rates are 22-45% among undergraduate indoor tanners (Heckman, Egleston et al., 2008; Mosher & Danoff-Burg, 2010a, 2010b; Poorsattar & Hornung, 2007). Among general college student samples in the USA, rates range from 12-27% (Heckman, Egleston et al., 2008; Mosher & Danoff-Burg, 2010a, 2010b; Poorsattar & Hornung, 2007).

5.2.1 Proposed mechanism of tanning dependence

The putative mechanism of tanning dependence involves UV exposure causing the up-regulation of the tumor suppressor gene p53 in skin cells, which leads to the release of beta-endorphin, a natural opioid analgesic involved in the brain's pleasure center (Cui et al., 2007). Beta-endorphin released into the blood during tanning may reach the brain in sufficient concentration to induce feelings of relaxation. However, we do not yet know how well beta-endorphin levels in the skin correlate with beta-endorphin levels in the blood or brain. Some individuals may find the feelings of relaxation, euphoria, and/or analgesic effects of beta-endorphin particularly rewarding and be more likely to tan repeatedly in order to continue to achieve these feelings (Heckman, 2011). If an individual tans frequently, his/her body may compensate for the effects of tanning, thus producing symptoms of tolerance and withdrawal, which may make discontinuing tanning aversive (Heckman, 2011).

There is biological evidence for this proposed mechanism involving beta-endorphin production during UV exposure. Expression of beta-endorphin in the epidermis of mice and human skin cells has been found to be induced by UV exposure (Wintzen et al., 2001). Human keratinocyte skin cell cultures produce proopiomelanocortin (POMC), β-lipotropic hormone, and beta-endorphin, with significant increases subsequent to UV exposure (Wintzen & Gilchrest, 1996). POMC plays a role in the regulation of skin pigmentation, stress, sleep, and energy homeostasis. One study found that keratinocytes express a *u*-opiate receptor and down-regulate it in the presence of beta-endorphin or the opioid antagonist naloxone (Bigliardi et al., 1998). The evidence for UV's ability to induce increased levels of serum endorphin is somewhat conflicting, however. While both the in vitro and in vivo release of endorphins after UV exposure have been reported, other studies have failed to confirm these findings. For example, a small, double-blind, placebo-controlled, randomized trial of three frequent and three non-frequent indoor tanners did not detect an increase in plasma beta-endorphin levels after UV exposure (Kaur et al., 2006).

There is also clinical evidence for tanning dependence. In a small single-blinded study, frequent tanners almost always chose to tan in a UV-light-emitting rather than a non-UV bed, reporting relaxation and lowered tension as reasons for their choice (Feldman et al., 2004). In a follow-up study, opioid blockade by the opioid antagonist naltrexone was shown to reduce this preference for the UV bed among indoor tanners and, at higher doses, induce withdrawal-like symptoms such as nausea, fatigue, and poor concentration (Kaur et al., 2006). Finally, in a small study of patients with fibromyalgia, participants reported a greater short-term decrease in pain after exposure to UV compared to non-UV exposure (Taylor et al., 2009).

Recently Lim and colleagues stated that "the addictive nature of indoor tanning is well-established"(Lim et al., 2011). However, our knowledge of tanning dependence is still in its infancy, and there is great potential for development in the field that could be modeled after traditional substance use research. This research could include cue response, brain imaging, and interventional investigations. For example, a recent single photon emission tomography (SPECT) imaging study showed increased striatal activation and decreased tanning desire when tanning dependent indoor tanners were exposed to a UV tanning canopy compared to a sham (non-UV) canopy (Harrington et al., 2011).

In addition to tanning dependence, alternative conceptualizations could classify frequent tanning as a disorder of body image, anxiety, mood, or impulse control (e.g., pathological gambling disorder) given its association with these problems (Heckman, 2011). Serotonin may represent another potential physiologic mechanism underlying tanning dependence, but it has not been well-established in the literature (Heckman, 2011). However, it is unclear whether the association between tanning/tanning dependence and related psychiatric problems is correlative or causative.

5.3 Psychosocial interventions to reduce indoor tanning

Most of the interventions that have been successful in changing indoor tanning behavior have focused on appearance issues as at least one component of the intervention (Dodd & Forshaw, 2010). One intervention that has been found to be successful is the "Appearance Booklet" by Hillhouse and colleagues. This booklet focuses on normative influences such as recent fashion trends toward natural skin tones, and also includes material about the history of tanning, UV radiation and its contribution to skin cancer and photo-aging, harm-reduction strategies to reduce or stop indoor tanning including use of sunless tanners, and appearance-enhancing alternatives to tanning including exercise, apparel, and sunless tanning products (Hillhouse & Turrisi, 2002). A randomized controlled trial of college female indoor tanners showed the intervention to reduce indoor tanning by half at two-month follow up (Hillhouse & Turrisi, 2002). A second study with a larger sample and using more objective outcome measures by the same group found that the intervention reduced indoor tanning relative to no treatment controls by over 35% at nine-month follow up (Hillhouse et al., 2008). Additional analyses found that the intervention was most effective for high frequency or low-knowledge tanners (Abar et al., 2010; Stapleton et al., 2010).

A second successful intervention focusing on appearance issues is showing participants UV-filtered photos illustrating current damage to facial skin in combination with information about UV exposure, focusing on appearance consequences. Two randomized controlled studies of college students found significant reductions in indoor tanning behavior at four-week follow up (Gibbons et al., 2005).

Another intervention to reduce indoor tanning used 30-minutes of a combination of motivational interviewing (MI) counseling, cognitive behavioral training, and written personalized feedback provided by undergraduate peers. Female undergraduate indoor tanners were randomized into an MI plus feedback, mailed feedback, or a no treatment control group. Participants in the MI group reported significantly fewer indoor tanning episodes at the three-month follow-up than both of the other groups (Turrisi et al., 2008).

Finally, two studies focusing on skin cancer risk and mortality demonstrated some success. Green and Brinn (Greene & Brinn, 2003) found that participants in both a statistical information about skin cancer condition and a personal narrative skin cancer case study condition reduced their indoor tanning at six months. Another study using the Mortality Salience approach also demonstrated reduced interest in indoor tanning (Routledge, Arndt, & Goldenberg, 2004). In this study mortality salience was increased by having participants answer questions intended to increase thoughts about death. Participants in the mortality salience condition reported less interest in indoor tanning compared to controls.

The literature on interventions to reduce indoor tanning is growing, and more rigorous research including more longitudinal trials is needed. Interventions for frequent tanners and tanning dependent individuals will likely need to be more intensive and focus on additional emotional and addiction issues beyond appearance and skin cancer risk.

6. Policies and regulations

Another similarity between tanning and other addictions is that policy level interventions have been particularly effective in reducing tobacco use and limiting youth access to tobacco products, and therefore, may be useful strategies for effective reduction of indoor tanning. The two industries use four primary marketing strategies: "mitigating health concerns, appealing to a sense of social acceptance, emphasizing psychotropic effects, and targeting specific population segments" (Greenman & Jones, 2010). UV definitively increases skin cancer risk; however, there are other issues related to indoor tanning that may contribute to even greater levels of risk: many children and adolescents tan, leading to high levels of lifetime UV exposure; very fair-skinned individuals at high risk for burning are often permitted to tan; salon proprietors sometimes do not know what type or how much UV is emitted from their devices; many tanning devices are not monitored; and/or UV-related regulations are not enforced.

6.1 US state regulations

All US states except Louisiana require parental consent for medical UV treatments for minors (Dellavalle, Parker et al., 2003; Dellavalle, Schilling et al., 2003; National Conference of State Legislatures, 2010). Currently, at least 32 US states regulate cosmetic tanning by children, nine states ban access to children under age 14, and two states ban access to children under 16 or 16.5 (Elwood & Gallagher, 2010). In states in which cosmetic indoor tanning is permitted for minors, several require parental consent. States with regulations related to cosmetic indoor tanning among minors have maintained adolescent indoor tanning levels, while states without these regulations have experienced increases over time.

One reason for the limited success of efforts to reduce indoor tanning may be that tanning regulations are not enforced. In 2007, less than 50% of the cities in each state gave citations for indoor tanning facility violations, 32% did not perform inspections and 32% did not perform yearly inspections (Mayer et al., 2008). Even in the states that have clear regulations for tanning bed sanitation, these regulations are rarely enforced. The New York State Department of Health 2008 regulations state that all salons are required to provide "adequate antimicrobial treatment by a disinfectant determined to be capable of destroying pathogenic organisms on treated surfaces" (Russak & Rigel, 2010). However, in a recent study of tanning salons in Manhattan, microbes that have been associated with serious skin infections were found in all ten salons (Russak & Rigel, 2010). Other studies have found human papillomavirus, the virus responsible for warts as well as cervical and other cancers (Russak & Rigel, 2010).

In 2004, the American Association of Dermatology (AAD), the American Society of Photobiology, and the FDA agreed the highest priority with regard to indoor tanning was restricting access of minors from indoor tanning facilities (Lim et al., 2004). In a study investigating the barriers to banning indoor tanning among minors, Obayan and colleagues (Obayan et al., 2010) conducted in-depth surveys with anti-tanning advocates in 10 states and legislators in 5 states (a 60% response rate). Advocates reported that the major barriers to legislation were strong lobbying from the tanning industry, proceedings after the bill was filed, and obtaining support from other organizations. For legislators, the biggest barrier was raising awareness of the health effects of indoor tanning among their colleagues (Obayan et al., 2010).

6.2 US federal regulations

The US Food and Drug Administration (USFDA) is responsible for insuring the safety and efficacy of medical devices, cosmetics, and products that emit radiation. Cosmetic tanning units are not considered medical devices; thus, the FDA is limited to regulating their emissions. However, the FDA does not regulate the relative proportion of UVA versus UVB that is emitted (Hornung et al., 2003). Thus, the proportions vary from bed to bed and salon to salon, and patrons may be burned when switching to a new tanning bed or salon. There are FDA-mandated requirements for tanning device specifications, posting of warning labels, and provision of appropriate eye protection (US Department of Health and Human Services-Food and Drug Administration, 1985; US Department of Health and Human Services, 1986). However, most of the FDA's regulation of tanning beds is based on tanning equipment manufacturer product reports, periodic inspections of manufacturers, and infrequent FDA inspections of tanning salons.

The FDA recommends that UV exposure should be restricted to "no more than 0.75 minimal erythemal dose (MED), three times during the first week" of exposure, gradually increasing the exposure thereafter (United States Department of Health and Human Services, 1988; United States Department of Health and Human Services, 1986). Numerous studies conducted throughout the USA have found widespread noncompliance with these FDA recommendations (Fairchild & Gemson, 1992; Hornung et al., 2003; Kwon et al., 2002; Pichon et al., 2009). Many beds have been found to emit 2-4 times the UV radiation as the summer sun at noon (Hornung et al., 2003). In a study of tanning facilities in 116 large US cities, confederates were granted permission to tan daily by a significant proportion of staff (Pichon et al., 2009). This same study found that living in a state with youth-access laws had no relationship to indoor tanning behavior among minors, suggesting that enforcement is inadequate (Mayer et al., 2011). Over a third of indoor tanning injury reports filed with the FDA and Consumer Product Safety Commission occur during episodes of non-compliance with FDA recommendations (Dowdy, Sayre, & Shepherd, 2009).

In 2007 the FDA Tanning Accountability and Notification (TAN) Act (HR 4767) was signed (US Food and Drug Administration, 2009). This amendment requires that the FDA conduct consumer testing of the warning statements on tanning devices to determine whether they provide adequate information about the risks of indoor tanning (US Food and Drug Administration, 2007). The Federal Trade Commission (FTC) regulates US advertising and prohibits false and deceptive statements. After a campaign by the AAD, the FTC charged the tanning industry with making false health and safety claims about indoor tanning (FTC, 2010). On January 26, 2010, the Indoor Tanning Association agreed to a settlement (FTC, 2010). In the future, ads that make claims about the health and safety benefits of tanning devices including vitamin D production are required to clearly and prominently make this disclosure: "**NOTICE:** You do not need to become tan for your skin to make vitamin D. Exposure to ultraviolet radiation may increase the likelihood of developing skin cancer and can cause serious eye injury" (Poole, 2010). Again, enforcement has been problematic. For example, during the spring of 2010, of all the tanning facilities in New York City, more than one-third of the tanning devices observed in half of the facilities visited did not have health risk warning signs posted, and signs were difficult to see in many others (Brouse, Basch, & Neugut, 2011).

On March 23, 2010, the US President Barrack Obama signed into law the Patient Protection and Affordable Care Act, which includes a 10% federal tax on indoor tanning services (Cable News Network, 2010). This tax may be a particularly effective deterrent for adolescents, who are more affected by smaller market fluctuations than adults. Also, at a specially-convened task force meeting on March 25, 2010, an FDA panel unanimously recommended reclassifying tanning beds from class I to class II devices (US Food and Drug Administration, 2010). Class I denotes minimal potential for harm such as tongue depressors, bedpans, and elastic bandages (Lim et al., 2011). Tanning devices are currently exempt from design controls and premarket notification to demonstrate safety and efficacy. Class II devices include X-ray machines, wheelchairs, UV and laser devices for dermatologic procedures, and even tampons. The proposed reclassification of tanning beds would mean that they would require additional labeling, inspections, calibration, and monitoring (Lim et al., 2011). The panel also recommended increased restrictions on the use of tanning beds for minors. At the time of publication of this book, it remains to be seen what position the FDA will ultimately take and what effect this may have on the use of tanning beds in the USA.

6.3 Regulations outside of the US

As in the US, regulation of indoor tanning has been increasing around the world. Consistent with the WHO recommendations (World Health Organization, 2005), the following countries have now banned indoor tanning among minors: France, Scotland (Elwood & Gallagher, 2010), Austria, Finland, Germany, and Great Britain (Fisher & James, 2010). Some Canadian Provinces have prohibited indoor tanning among minors as well (Salomone et al., 2009). In 2009, a law was passed in Brazil banning all cosmetic tanning (Teich, August 2009).

While some countries have developed specific rules for sunbed installation, operation, and use, there is no standardized regulation across the European Union. Unfortunately, in the Netherlands and parts of Canada and the UK, such recommendations have been developed with the indoor tanning industry itself (Autier, 2004, 2005). Sunbed users across a number of countries report that they receive little to no instruction on avoiding sunburns or how to protect their eyes using goggles (Boldeman et al., 2003; Dissel et al., 2009; Schneider et al., 2009; Szepietowski et al., 2002).

A study of the majority of tanning salons in Ireland in 2007 obtained several interesting results (Gavin et al., 2010). The UV type in machines was unknown by staff in 71% of the salons, while 16% reported using type 4 high-dose UV devices; 36% of premises did not service sunbeds regularly, or staff were unsure of the service schedule (Gavin et al., 2010). Unsupervised sunbed use was reported in 9% of salons (Gavin et al., 2010). Eye protection was available in 98% of salons, but 35% charged for the service, and only 80% sanitized goggles between uses (Gavin et al., 2010). The 16% of the sample who were members of the Sunbed Association were more likely to keep maintenance records and operating manuals but were also more likely to provide a home sunbed service (Gavin et al., 2010).

In 2008, 78 tanning facilities throughout Norway containing municipalities with and without local salon inspections were assessed (Nilsen et al., 2011). Ninety percent of the tanning facilities were unattended by staff. Irradiances varied among solaria: UVB and UVA irradiances were 0.5-3.7 and 3-26 times, respectively, higher than those of the Oslo summer sun (Nilsen et al., 2011). Solaria in municipalities with local inspections were more compliant with regulations than solaria in other areas; however, irradiances were also significantly higher in municipalities with inspections.

Australia's voluntary indoor tanning code prohibits tanning by minors and individuals with type 1 (very fair) skin. However, one study found that 90% of salons permitted tanning by adults with type 1 skin, 75% reassured patrons about the benefits of indoor tanning, more than 50% permitted 16-year-olds to tan, and 14% offered inadequate or no eye protection (Dobbinson et al., 2008). Of 20 solaria examined in detail by an Australian radiation safety agency, only one had emissions of intensity less than UV Index 12, typical of mid-latitude summer sunlight, 15 units emitted more than UV Index 20, while three units emitted at intensities above UV Index 36 (Gies et al., 2010). UVA emissions were found to be as high as more than six times the UVA content of mid-latitude summer sunshine.

Numerous state, federal, and international regulations focus on age restrictions, parental consent requirements, UV radiation exposure amount and frequency, warning labeling on the devices, and taxation. Although the tanning industry is becoming increasingly regulated, the lack of enforcement and poor communication between the salons and their patrons regarding the recommended use of sunbeds has been documented widely.

7. Conclusion

Indoor tanning is common in the Western world and may still be gaining popularity in some countries. Indoor tanning is now known to be a definitive risk factor for skin cancers. Several studies have demonstrated a dose response relationship between indoor tanning and skin cancer. Like tobacco, indoor tanning has been marketed aggressively and appeals to adolescents and young adults, putting these populations at risk for high levels of long-term exposure to UV radiation. Appearance enhancement is the primary motivation for indoor tanning, particularly among young Caucasian women. However, there are several other compelling reasons cited for the behavior, including tanning dependence, which may also lead to high levels of lifetime UV exposures. Behavioral interventions have been little-studied and have not demonstrated strong and durable effects. Recent regulations around the world have been shown to have some effect on indoor tanning rates; however, increased regulation and stronger enforcement are needed. As new regulations are enacted, additional longitudinal and population-based research will be necessary to track indoor tanning patterns, enforcement of regulations, and skin cancer incidence around the world.

8. Acknowledgment

Some of this chapter is based on material from Heckman, C.J. & Manne, S.L. (Eds.). (in press with expected publication date of October, 2011). *Shedding Light on Indoor Tanning.* Netherlands: Springer. We would like to acknowledge the chapter authors of that book.

9. References

Abar, B. W., Turrisi, R., Hillhouse, J., Loken, E., Stapleton, J., & Gunn, H. (2010). Preventing skin cancer in college females: Heterogeneous effects over time. *Health Psychol.* doi: 2010-21226-001 [pii] 10.1037/a0021236

Albert, M. R., & Ostheimer, K. G. (2002). The evolution of current medical and popular attitudes toward ultraviolet light exposure: part 1. *J Am Acad Dermatol, 47*(6), 930-937. doi: 10.1067/mjd.2002.127254 S0190962202003250 [pii]

Albert, M. R., & Ostheimer, K. G. (2003). The evolution of current medical and popular attitudes toward ultraviolet light exposure: part 2. *J Am Acad Dermatol, 48*(6), 909-918. doi: 10.1067/mjd.2003.272 S0190962203003414 [pii]

Amir, Z., Wright, A., Kernohan, E. E., & Hart, G. (2000). Attitudes, beliefs and behaviour regarding the use of sunbeds amongst healthcare workers in Bradford. *Eur J Cancer Care (Engl), 9*(2), 76-79.

Autier, P. (2004). Perspectives in melanoma prevention: the case of sunbeds. *Eur J Cancer, 40*(16), 2367-2376. doi: S0959-8049(04)00602-1 [pii] 10.1016/j.ejca.2004.07.018

Autier, P. (2005). Cutaneous malignant melanoma: facts about sunbeds and sunscreen. *Expert Rev Anticancer Ther, 5*(5), 821-833. doi: 10.1586/14737140.5.5.821

Autier, P., Dore, J. F., Lejeune, F., Koelmel, K. F., Geffeler, O., Hille, P., et al. (1994). Cutaneous malignant melanoma and exposure to sunlamps or sunbeds: an EORTC multicenter case-control study in Belgium, France and Germany. EORTC Melanoma Cooperative Group. *Int J Cancer, 58*(6), 809-813.

Bagdasarov, Z., Banerjee, S., Greene, K., & Campo, S. (2008). Indoor tanning and problem behavior. *J Am Coll Health, 56*(5), 555-561. doi: 0411401743618456 [pii] 10.3200/JACH.56.5.555-562

Baker, M. K., Hillhouse, J. J., & Liu, X. (2010). The effect of initial indoor tanning with mother on current tanning patterns. *Arch Dermatol, 146*(12), 1427-1428.

Beasley, T. M., & Kittel, B. S. (1997). Factors that influence health risk behaviors among tanning salon patrons. *Eval Health Prof, 20*(4), 371-388.

Bigliardi, P. L., Bigliardi-Qi, M., Buechner, S., & Rufli, T. (1998). Expression of mu-opiate receptor in human epidermis and keratinocytes. *J Invest Dermatol, 111*(2), 297-301. doi: 10.1046/j.1523-1747.1998.00259.x

Boldeman, C., Jansson, B., Dal, H., & Ullen, H. (2003). Sunbed use among Swedish adolescents in the 1990s: a decline with an unchanged relationship to health risk behaviors. *Scand J Public Health, 31*(3), 233-237.

Boldeman, C., Jansson, B., Nilsson, B., & Ullen, H. (1997). Sunbed use in Swedish urban adolescents related to behavioral characteristics. *Prev Med, 26*(1), 114-119.

Boyle, R., O'Hagan, A. H., Donnelly, D., Donnelly, C., Gordon, S., McElwee, G., & Gavin, A. (2010). Trends in reported sun bed use, sunburn, and sun care knowledge and attitudes in a U.K. region: results of a survey of the Northern Ireland population. *Br J Dermatol, 163*(6), 1269-1275. doi: BJD9977 [pii] 10.1111/j.1365-2133.2010.09977.x

Brandberg, Y., Ullen, H., Sjoberg, L., & Holm, L. E. (1998). Sunbathing and sunbed use related to self-image in a randomized sample of Swedish adolescents. *Eur J Cancer Prev, 7*(4), 321-329.

Branstrom, R., Ullen, H., & Brandberg, Y. (2004). Attitudes, subjective norms and perception of behavioural control as predictors of sun-related behaviour in Swedish adults. *Prev Med, 39*(5), 992-999. doi: S0091743504002063 [pii] 10.1016/j.ypmed.2004.04.004

Brouse, C. H., Basch, C. E., & Neugut, A. I. (2011). Warning signs observed in tanning salons in new york city: implications for skin cancer prevention. *Prev Chronic Dis, 8*(4), A88. doi: A88 [pii]

Cafri, G., Thompson, J. K., & Jacobsen, P. B. (2006). Appearance reasons for tanning mediate the relationship between media influence and UV exposure and sun protection. *Arch Dermatol, 142*(8), 1067-1069. doi: 142/8/1067 [pii] 10.1001/archderm.142.8.1067

Cafri, G., Thompson, J. K., Jacobsen, P. B., & Hillhouse, J. (2009). Investigating the role of appearance-based factors in predicting sunbathing and tanning salon use. *J Behav Med. doi*: 10.1007/s10865-009-9224-5

Cafri, G., Thompson, J. K., Roehrig, M., van den Berg, P., Jacobsen, P. B., & Stark, S. (2006). An investigation of appearance motives for tanning: The development and evaluation of the Physical Appearance Reasons For Tanning Scale (PARTS) and its relation to sunbathing and indoor tanning intentions. *Body Image, 3*(3), 199-209. doi: S1740-1445(06)00055-6 [pii] 10.1016/j.bodyim.2006.05.002

Canadian Cancer Society. (2006). Sun bed usage and attitudes among students in Ontario grades 7-12 *Youthography-summary results.*

Canadian Cancer Society. (2009). Sunbeds *Cancer Research UK Policy Statement.*

Carter, S. (2007). *Rise and shine:Sunlight, technology, and health.* Oxford: Berg.

Chapman, S., Marks, R., & King, M. (1992). Trends in tans and skin protection in Australian fashion magazines, 1982 through 1991. *Am J Public Health, 82*(12), 1677-1680.

Cho, H., Hall, J. G., Kosmoski, C., Fox, R. L., & Mastin, T. (2010). Tanning, skin cancer risk, and prevention: a content analysis of eight popular magazines that target female readers, 1997-2006. *Health Commun, 25*(1), 1-10. doi: 10.1080/10410230903265938

Choi, K., Lazovich, D., Southwell, B., Forster, J., Rolnick, S. J., & Jackson, J. (2010). Prevalence and characteristics of indoor tanning use among men and women in the US. *Arch Dermatol, 146*(12), 1356-1361. doi: 146/12/1356 [pii] 10.1001/archdermatol.2010.355

Cable News Network (CNN). (2010). Obama signs health care bill; Senate takes up House changes., from http://articles.cnn.com/2010-03-23/politics/health.care.main_1_health-care-obama-and-democratic-leaders-health-insurance?_s=PM:POLITICS

Cokkinides, V., Weinstock, M., Lazovich, D., Ward, E., & Thun, M. (2009). Indoor tanning use among adolescents in the US, 1998 to 2004. *Cancer, 115*(1), 190-198. doi: 10.1002/cncr.24010

Cokkinides, V. E., Weinstock, M. A., O'Connell, M. C., & Thun, M. J. (2002). Use of indoor tanning sunlamps by US youth, ages 11-18 years, and by their parent or guardian caregivers: prevalence and correlates. *Pediatrics, 109*(6), 1124-1130.

Coups, E. J., Manne, S. L., & Heckman, C. J. (2008). Multiple skin cancer risk behaviors in the U.S. population. *Am J Prev Med, 34*(2), 87-93. doi: S0749-3797(07)00655-1 [pii] 10.1016/j.amepre.2007.09.032

Cui, R., Widlund, H. R., Feige, E., Lin, J. Y., Wilensky, D. L., Igras, V. E., . . . Fisher, D. E. (2007). Central role of p53 in the suntan response and pathologic hyperpigmentation. *Cell, 128*(5), 853-864.

Cust, A. E., Armstrong, B. K., Goumas, C., Jenkins, M. A., Schmid, H., Hopper, J. L., . . . Mann, G. J. (2011). Sunbed use during adolescence and early adulthood is associated with increased risk of early-onset melanoma. *Int J Cancer.* doi: 10.1002/ijc.25576

Danoff-Burg, S., & Mosher, C. E. (2006). Predictors of tanning salon use: behavioral alternatives for enhancing appearance, relaxing and socializing. *J Health Psychol, 11*(3), 511-518.

Dellavalle, R. P., Parker, E. R., Cersonsky, N., Hester, E. J., Hemme, B., Burkhardt, D. L., . . . Schilling, L. M. (2003). Youth access laws: in the dark at the tanning parlor? *Arch Dermatol, 139*(4), 443-448. doi: 10.1001/archderm.139.4.443 139/4/443 [pii]

Dellavalle, R. P., Schilling, L. M., Chen, A. K., & Hester, E. J. (2003). Teenagers in the UV tanning booth? Tax the tan. *Arch Pediatr Adolesc Med, 157*(9), 845-846. doi: 10.1001/archpedi.157.9.845 157/9/845 [pii]

Diehl, K., Litaker, D. G., Greinert, R., Zimmermann, S., Breitbart, E. W., & Schneider, S. (2010). The prevalence of current sunbed use and user characteristics: the SUN-Study 2008. *Int J Public Health, 55*(5), 513-516. doi: 10.1007/s00038-009-0100-4

Diffey, B. (2007). Sunbeds, beauty and melanoma. *Br J Dermatol, 157*(2), 215-216. doi: BJD7960 [pii] 10.1111/j.1365-2133.2007.07960.x

Diffey, B. L. (1995). Cosmetic tanning and human skin cancer. In H. Mukhtar (Ed.), *Skin cancer: Mechanisms and human relevance*. Boca Raton: CRC Press

Dissel, M., Rotterdam, S., Altmeyer, P., & Gambichler, T. (2009). Indoor tanning in North Rhine-Westphalia Germany: a self-reported survey. *Photodermatol Photoimmunol Photomed, 25*(2), 94-100. doi: PPP417 [pii] 10.1111/j.1600-0781.2009.00417.x

Dobbinson, S., Wakefield, M., Hill, D., Girgis, A., Aitken, J. F., Beckmann, K., . . . Bowles, K. A. (2008). Prevalence and determinants of Australian adolescents' and adults' weekend sun protection and sunburn, summer 2003-2004. *J Am Acad Dermatol, 59*(4), 602-614. doi: S0190-9622(08)00733-0 [pii] 10.1016/j.jaad.2008.06.011

Dodd, L. J., & Forshaw, M. J. (2010). Assessing the efficacy of appearance-focused interventions to prevent skin cancer: a systemic review of the literature. *Health Psychol Rev.*

Dowdy, J. C., Sayre, R. M., & Shepherd, J. G. (2009). Indoor tanning injuries: an evaluation of FDA adverse event reporting data. *Photodermatology, Photodermatol Photoimmunol Photomed, 25*(4), 216-220. doi: PPP440 [pii] 10.1111/j.1600-0781.2009.00440.x

El Ghissassi, F., Baan, R., Straif, K., Grosse, Y., Secretan, B., Bouvard, V., Group, W. I. A. f. R. o. C. M. W. (2009). A review of human carcinogens--part D: radiation. *Lancet Oncol, 10*(8), 751-752.

Elwood, J. M., & Gallagher, R. P. (2010). Reducing sunbed use in young people. *BMJ, 340*, c990.

Ezzedine, K., Malvy, D., Mauger, E., Nageotte, O., Galan, P., Hercberg, S., & Guinot, C. (2008). Artificial and natural ultraviolet radiation exposure: beliefs and behaviour of 7200 French adults. *J Eur Acad Dermatol Venereol, 22*(2), 186-194. doi: JDV2367 [pii] 10.1111/j.1468-3083.2007.02367.x

Fairchild, A. L., & Gemson, D. H. (1992). Safety information provided to customers of New York City suntanning salons. *Am J Prev Med, 8*(6), 381-383.

Fears, T. R., Sagebiel, R. W., Halpern, A., Elder, D. E., Holly, E. A., Guerry, D. t., & Tucker, M. A. (2011). Sunbeds and sunlamps: who used them and their risk for melanoma. *Pigment Cell Melanoma Res, 24*(3), 574-581. doi: 10.1111/j.1755-148X.2011.00842.x

Feldman, S. R., Liguori, A., Kucenic, M., Rapp, S. R., Fleischer, A. B., Jr., Lang, W., & Kaur, M. (2004). Ultraviolet exposure is a reinforcing stimulus in frequent indoor tanners. *J Am Acad Dermatol, 51*(1), 45-51.

Fisher, D. E., & James, W. D. (2010). Indoor tanning--science, behavior, and policy. *N Engl J Med, 363*(10), 901-903. doi: 10.1056/NEJMp1005999

Francis, K., Dobbinson, S., Wakefield, M., & Girgis, A. (2010). Solarium use in Australia, recent trends and context. *Aust N Z J Public Health, 34*(4), 427-430. doi: AZPH578 [pii] 10.1111/j.1753-6405.2010.00578.x

Federal Trade Commission. (2010). Indoor Tanning Association Settles FTC Charges That It Deceived Consumers About Skin Cancer Risks From Tanning Retrieved July 19, 2011, from http://www.ftc.gov/opa/2010/01/tanning.shtm

Galan, I., Rodriguez-Laso, A., Diez-Ganan, L., & Camara, E. (2011). Prevalence and correlates of skin cancer risk behaviors in Madrid (Spain). *Gac Sanit, 25*(1), 44-49. doi: S0213-9111(10)00289-X [pii] 10.1016/j.gaceta.2010.07.013

Gavin, A., Donnelly, C., Devlin, A., Devereux, C., O'Callaghan, G., McElwee, G., . . . O'Hagan, A. H. (2010). Public at risk: a survey of sunbed parlour operating practices in Northern Ireland. *Br J Dermatol, 162*(3), 627-632. doi: BJD9591 [pii] 10.1111/j.1365-2133.2009.09591.x

Gibbons, F. X., Gerrard, M., Lane, D. J., Mahler, H. I., & Kulik, J. A. (2005). Using UV photography to reduce use of tanning booths: a test of cognitive mediation. *Health Psychol, 24*(4), 358-363.

Gies, P., Javorniczky, J., Henderson, S., McLennan, A., Roy, C., Lock, J., . . . Gordon, L. (2010). UVR Emissions from Solaria in Australia and Implications for the Regulation Process. *Photochem Photobiol.* doi: 10.1111/j.1751-1097.2010.00835.x

Gordon, D., & Guenther, L. (2009). Tanning behavior of London-area youth. *J Cutan Med Surg, 13*(1), 22-32.

Greene, K., & Brinn, L. S. (2003). Messages influencing college women's tanning bed use: statistical versus narrative evidence format and a self-assessment to increase perceived susceptibility. *J Health Commun, 8*(5), 443-461.

Greenman, J., & Jones, D. A. (2010). Comparison of advertising strategies between the indoor tanning and tobacco industries. *J Am Acad Dermatol, 62*(4), 685 e681-618. doi: S0190-9622(09)00360-0 [pii] 10.1016/j.jaad.2009.02.045

Harrington, C. R., Beswick, T. C., Graves, M., Jacobe, H. T., Harris, T. S., Kourosh, S., . . . Adinoff, B. (2011). Activation of the mesostriatal reward pathway with exposure to ultraviolet radiation (UVR) vs. sham UVR in frequent tanners: a pilot study. *Addict Biol.* doi: 10.1111/j.1369-1600.2010.00312.x

Harrington, C. R., Beswick, T. C., Leitenberger, J., Minhajuddin, A., Jacobe, H. T., & Adinoff, B. (2010). Addictive-like behaviours to ultraviolet light among frequent indoor tanners. *Clin Exp Dermatol,* 1-6. doi: CED3882 [pii] 10.1111/j.1365-2230.2010.03882.x

Heckman, C. J. (2011). Indoor tanning: Tanning dependence and other health risks. *Household and Personal Care Today, 1,* 20-22.

Heckman, C. J., Coups, E. J., & Manne, S. L. (2008). Prevalence and correlates of indoor tanning among US adults. *J Am Acad Dermatol, 58*(5), 769-780. doi: S0190-9622(08)00132-1 [pii] 10.1016/j.jaad.2008.01.020

Heckman, C. J., Egleston, B. L., Wilson, D. B., & Ingersoll, K. S. (2008). A preliminary investigation of the predictors of tanning dependence. *Am J Health Behav, 32*(5), 451-464. doi: 10.5555/ajhb.2008.32.5.451

Hery, C., Tryggvadottir, L., Sigurdsson, T., Olafsdottir, E., Sigurgeirsson, B., Jonasson, J. G., Autier, P. (2010). A melanoma epidemic in Iceland: possible influence of sunbed use. *Am J Epidemiol, 172*(7), 762-767. doi: kwq238 [pii] 10.1093/aje/kwq238

Herzog, C., Pappo, A. S., Bondy, M. L., Bleyer, A., & Kirkwood, J. (2007). Chapter 5: Malignant melanoma. In A. Bleyer, M. O'Leary & L. A. G. Ries (Eds.), *Cancer epidemiology in older adolescents and young adults 15 to 29 years of age,* (National Cancer Institute, NIH Pub. No. 06-5767, pp. 53-63). Bethesda, MD: US Department of Health and Human Services,.

Hillhouse, J., Stapleton, J., & Turrisi, R. (2005). Association of frequent indoor UV tanning with seasonal affective disorder. *Arch Dermatol, 141*(11).

Hillhouse, J., Turrisi, R., & Shields, A. L. (2007). Patterns of indoor tanning use: implications for clinical interventions. *Arch Dermatol, 143*(12), 1530-1535. doi: 143/12/1530 [pii] 10.1001/archderm.143.12.1530

Hillhouse, J., Turrisi, R., Stapleton, J., & Robinson, J. (2008). A randomized controlled trial of an appearance-focused intervention to prevent skin cancer. *Cancer, 113*(11), 3257-3266. doi: 10.1002/cncr.23922

Hillhouse, J., Turrisi, R., Stapleton, J., & Robinson, J. (2010). Effect of seasonal affective disorder and pathological tanning motives on efficacy of an appearance-focused intervention to prevent skin cancer. *Arch Dermatol, 146*(5), 485-491. doi: 146/5/485 [pii] 10.1001/archdermatol.2010.85

Hillhouse, J. J., Stair, A. W., 3rd, & Adler, C. M. (1996). Predictors of sunbathing and sunscreen use in college undergraduates. *J Behav Med, 19*(6), 543-561.

Hillhouse, J. J., & Turrisi, R. (2002). Examination of the efficacy of an appearance-focused intervention to reduce UV exposure. *J Behav Med, 25*(4), 395-409.

Hoerster, K. D., Garrow, R. L., Mayer, J. A., Clapp, E. J., Weeks, J. R., Woodruff, S. I., . . . Sybert, S. A. (2009). Density of indoor tanning facilities in 116 large U.S. cities. *Am J Prev Med, 36*(3), 243-246.

Hoerster, K. D., Mayer, J. A., Woodruff, S. I., Malcarne, V., Roesch, S. C., & Clapp, E. (2007). The influence of parents and peers on adolescent indoor tanning behavior: findings from a multi-city sample. *J Am Acad Dermatol, 57*(6), 990-997. doi: S0190-9622(07)01025-0 [pii] 10.1016/j.jaad.2007.06.007

Holick, M. (2008). Sunlight, UV-radiation, Vitamin D and skin cancer: How much sunlight do we need? . In J. Reichrath (Ed.), *Sunlight, vitamin D and skin cancer*. USA: Landes Bioscience.

Holubar, K. (1998). Photodamage: an historical perspective. *J Investig Dermatol Symp Proc, 3*(1), 45-46.

Holubar, K., & Schmidt, C. (1998). Historical, anthropological, and biological aspects of sun and the skin. *Clin Dermatol, 16*(1), 19-22. doi: S0738081X97001673 [pii]

Hornung, R. L., Magee, K. H., Lee, W. J., Hansen, L. A., & Hsieh, Y. C. (2003). Tanning facility use: are we exceeding Food and Drug Administration limits? *J Am Acad Dermatol, 49*(4), 655-661. doi: S019096220301586X [pii]

International Agency for Research on Cancer (IARC). (2006). The association of use of sunbeds with cutaneous malignant melanoma and other skin cancers: a systematic review. *Int J Cancer, 120* 1116-1120.

Karagas, M. R., Stannard, V. A., Mott, L. A., Slattery, M. J., Spencer, S. K., & Weinstock, M. A. (2002). Use of tanning devices and risk of basal cell and squamous cell skin cancers. *J Natl Cancer Inst, 94*(3), 224-226.

Kaur, M., Liguori, A., Fleischer, A. B., Jr., & Feldman, S. R. (2006). Plasma beta-endorphin levels in frequent and infrequent tanners before and after UV and non-ultraviolet stimuli. *J Am Acad Dermatol, 54*(5), 919-920. doi: S0190-9622(06)00321-5 [pii] 10.1016/j.jaad.2006.01.062

Kaur, M., Liguori, A., Lang, W., Rapp, S. R., Fleischer, A. B., Jr., & Feldman, S. R. (2006). Induction of withdrawal-like symptoms in a small randomized, controlled trial of opioid blockade in frequent tanners. *J Am Acad Dermatol, 54*(4), 709-711.

Koster, B., Thorgaard, C., Clemmensen, I. H., & Philip, A. (2009). Sunbed use in the Danish population in 2007: a cross-sectional study. *Prev Med, 48*(3), 288-290. doi: S0091-7435(08)00669-5 [pii] 10.1016/j.ypmed.2008.12.012

Kourosh, A. S., Harrington, C. R., & Adinoff, B. (2010). Tanning as a behavioral addiction. *Am J Drug Alcohol Abuse, 36*(5), 284-290. doi: 10.3109/00952990.2010.491883

Krarup, A. F., Koster, B., Thorgaard, C., Philip, A., & Clemmensen, I. H. (2011). Sunbed use by children aged 8-18 years in Denmark in 2008: a cross-sectional study. *Br J Dermatol*. doi: 10.1111/j.1365-2133.2011.10352.x

Kwon, H. T., Mayer, J. A., Walker, K. K., Yu, H., Lewis, E. C., & Belch, G. E. (2002). Promotion of frequent tanning sessions by indoor tanning facilities: two studies. *J Am Acad Dermatol, 46*(5), 700-705.

Lawler, S. P., Kvaskoff, M., DiSipio, T., Whiteman, D., Eakin, E., Aitken, J., & Fritschi, L. (2006). Solaria use in Queensland, Australia. *Aust N Z J Public Health, 30*(5), 479-482.

Lazovich, D., Forster, J., Sorensen, G., Emmons, K., Stryker, J., Demierre, M. F., . . . Remba, N. (2004). Characteristics associated with use or intention to use indoor tanning among adolescents. *Arch Pediatr Adolesc Med, 158*(9), 918-924.

Lazovich, D., Vogel, R. I., Berwick, M., Weinstock, M., Anderson, K. E., & Warshaw, E. M. (2010). Indoor tanning and risk of melanoma: A case-control study in a highly exposed population. *Cancer Epidemiol Biomarkers Prev, 19*(6), 1557-1568.

Lencek, L., & Bosker, G. (1999). *The beach: History of paradise on earth*. USA: Penguin.

Lim, H., Honigsman, H., & Hawk, J. (Eds.). (2007). *Photodermatology*. USA: Informa Healthcare.

Lim, H. W., Cyr, W. H., DeFabo, E., Robinson, J., Weinstock, M. A., Beer, J. Z., . . . Spencer, J. M. (2004). Scientific and regulatory issues related to indoor tanning. *J Am Acad Dermatol, 51*(5), 781-784.

Lim, H. W., James, W. D., Rigel, D. S., Maloney, M. E., Spencer, J. M., & Bhushan, R. (2011). Adverse effects of UV radiation from the use of indoor tanning equipment: Time to ban the tan. *J Am Acad Dermatol, 64*(5), 893-902. doi: S0190-9622(11)00349-5 [pii] 10.1016/j.jaad.2011.03.007

Looking Fit. (2009-2010). Indoor tanning fact book Retrieved Accessed May 4, 2010, from http://www.lookingfit.com/articles/looking-fit-fact-book-2009-2010.html

Ma, F., Collado-Mesa, F., Hu, S., & Kirsner, R. S. (2007). Skin cancer awareness and sun protection behaviors in white Hispanic and white non-Hispanic high school students in Miami, Florida. *Arch Dermatol, 143*(8), 983-988. doi: 143/8/983 [pii] 10.1001/archderm.143.8.983

Mackay, H., Lowe, D., Edwards, D. J., & al., e. (2007). A survey of 14 to 16 year olds as to their attitude toward and use of sunbeds. *Health Educ J, 66*, 141-152.

Martin, J. M., Ghaferi, J. M., Cummins, D. L., Mamelak, A. J., Schmults, C. D., Parikh, M., . . . Liegeois, N. J. (2009). Changes in skin tanning attitudes. Fashion articles and advertisements in the early 20th century. *Am J Public Health, 99*(12), 2140-2146. doi: AJPH.2008.144352 [pii] 10.2105/AJPH.2008.144352

Mawn, V. B., & Fleischer, A. B., Jr. (1993). A survey of attitudes, beliefs, and behavior regarding tanning bed use, sunbathing, and sunscreen use. *J Am Acad Dermatol, 29*(6), 959-962.

Mayer, J. A., Hoerster, K. D., Pichon, L. C., Rubio, D. A., Woodruff, S. I., & Forster, J. L. (2008). Enforcement of state indoor tanning laws in the United States. *Prev. Chronic Dis., 5*(4), A125. doi: A125 [pii]

Mayer, J. A., Woodruff, S. I., Slymen, D. J., Sallis, J. F., Forster, J. L., Clapp, E. J., . . . Gilmer, T. (2011). Adolescents' use of indoor tanning: a large-scale evaluation of psychosocial, environmental, and policy-level correlates. *Am J Public Health, 101*(5), 930-938. doi: AJPH.2010.300079 [pii] 10.2105/AJPH.2010.300079

Mogensen, M., & Jemec, G. B. (2010). The potential carcinogenic risk of tanning beds: clinical guidelines and patient safety advice. *Cancer Manag Res, 2*, 277-282. doi: 10.2147/CMR.S7403

Mosher, C. E., & Danoff-Burg, S. (2010a). Addiction to indoor tanning: relation to anxiety, depression, and substance use. *Arch Dermatol, 146*(4), 412-417. doi: 146/4/412 [pii] 10.1001/archdermatol.2009.385

Mosher, C. E., & Danoff-Burg, S. (2010b). Indoor tanning, mental health, and substance use among college students: The significance of gender. *J Health Psychol.* doi: 1359105309357091 [pii] 10.1177/1359105309357091

Mouret, S., Baudouin, C., Charveron, M., Favier, A., Cadet, J., & Douki, T. (2006). Cyclobutane pyrimidine dimers are predominant DNA lesions in whole human skin exposed to UVA radiation. *Proc Natl Acad Sci USA, 103*(37), 13765-13770. doi: 0604213103 [pii] 10.1073/pnas.0604213103

National Conference of State Legislatures. (2010, 2010). Tanning restrictions for minors. A state-by-state comparison, 2010, from http://www.ncsl.org/programs/health/tanningrestrictions.htm

Nilsen, L. T., Aalerud, T. N., Hannevik, M., & Veierod, M. B. (2011). UVB and UVA irradiances from indoor tanning devices. *Photochem Photobiol Sci.* doi: 10.1039/c1pp05029j

Obayan, B., Geller, A. C., Resnick, E. A., & Demierre, M. F. (2010). Enacting legislation to restrict youth access to tanning beds: a survey of advocates and sponsoring legislators. *J Am Acad Dermatol, 63*(1), 63-70. doi: S0190-9622(09)01214-6 [pii] 10.1016/j.jaad.2009.09.019

Osterlind, A., Tucker, M. A., Stone, B. J., & Jensen, O. M. (1988). The Danish case-control study of cutaneous malignant melanoma. II. Importance of UV-light exposure. *Int J Cancer, 42*(3), 319-324.

Pendergast, T., & Pendergast, S. (2000). *St. James encyclopedia of pop culture*. Detroit: St. James Press.

Phillips, K. A., Conroy, M., Dufresne, R. G., Menard, W., Didie, E. R., Hunter-Yates, J., . . . Pagano, M. (2006). Tanning in body dysmorphic disorder. *Psychiatr Q, 77*(2), 129-138.

Phillips, K. A., Dufresne, R. G., Jr., Wilkel, C. S., & Vittorio, C. C. (2000). Rate of body dysmorphic disorder in dermatology patients. *J Am Acad Dermatol, 42*(3), 436-441. doi: S0190-9622(00)90215-9 [pii]

Pichon, L. C., Mayer, J. A., Hoerster, K. D., Woodruff, S. I., Slymen, D. J., Belch, G. E., . . . Weinstock, M. A. (2009). Youth access to artificial UV radiation exposure: practices of 3647 US indoor tanning facilities. *Arch Dermatol, 145*(9), 997-1002. doi: 145/9/997 [pii] 10.1001/archdermatol.2009.85

Poole, C. (2010, 1/30/2010). Federal Trade Commission Finally Nails the Indoor Tanning Association Retrieved July 15, 2011, from http://forum.melanomaintl.org/toastforums/toast.asp?sub=show&action=posts&fid=3&tid=9422

Poorsattar, S. P., & Hornung, R. L. (2007). UV light abuse and high-risk tanning behavior among undergraduate college students. *J Am Acad Dermatol, 56*(3), 375-379.

Randle, H. W. (1997). Suntanning: differences in perceptions throughout history. *Mayo Clin Proc, 72*(5), 461-466.

Rhainds, M., De Guire, L., & Claveau, J. (1999). A population-based survey on the use of artificial tanning devices in the Province of Quebec, Canada. *J Am Acad Dermatol, 40*(4), 572-576. doi: S0190-9622(99)70439-1 [pii]

Roberts, D. L., & Foley, K. (2009). Sunbed use in children-time for new legislation? *Br J Dermatol, 161*(1), 193-194. doi: BJD9159 [pii] 10.1111/j.1365-2133.2009.09159.x

Routledge, C., Arndt, J., & Goldenberg, J. L. (2004). A time to tan: proximal and distal effects of mortality salience on sun exposure intentions. *Pers Soc Psychol Bull 30*(10), 1347-1358.

Russak, J. E., & Rigel, D. S. (2010). Tanning bed hygiene: microbes found on tanning beds present a potential health risk. *J Am Acad Dermatol, 62*(1), 155-157. doi: S0190-9622(09)00665-3 [pii] 10.1016/j.jaad.2009.05.034

Salomone, C., Majerson, D., Molgo, M., de Santa Maria, M. L., & Romero, W. (2009). Tanning salons in Santiago, Chile: the knowledge of the staff in charge and the quality of information provided to potential clients before and after a new regulatory law. *Photodermatol Photoimmunol Photomed, 25*(2), 86-89. doi: PPP412 [pii] 10.1111/j.1600-0781.2009.00412.x

Schneider, S., & Kramer, H. (2010). Who uses sunbeds? A systematic literature review of risk groups in developed countries. *J Eur Acad Dermatol Venereol, 24*(6), 639-648. doi: JDV3509 [pii] 10.1111/j.1468-3083.2009.03509.x

Schneider, S., Zimmerman, S., Diehl, K., Breitbart, E. W., & Greinert, R. (2009). Sunbed use in German adults: Risk awareness does not correlate with behaviour. *Acta Derm Venereol, 89*(5), 470-475.

Schneider, S., Zimmermann, S., Diehl, K., Breitbart, E. W., & Greinert, R. (2009). Sunbed use in German adults: risk awareness does not correlate with behaviour. *Acta Derm Venereol, 89*(5), 470-475. doi: 10.2340/00015555-0689

Segrave, K. (2005). *Suntanning in 20th century America.* Jefferson, NC: McFarland & Co., Inc.

Sjöberg, L., Holm, L. E., Ullen, H., & Brandberg, Y. (2004). Tanning and risk perception in adolescents. *Health, Risk & Society, 6*(1), 81-94.

Spencer, J. M., & Amonette, R. A. (1995). Indoor tanning: risks, benefits, and future trends. *J Am Acad Dermatol, 33*(2 Pt 1), 288-298.

Stapleton, J., Turrisi, R., Hillhouse, J., Robinson, J. K., & Abar, B. (2010). A comparison of the efficacy of an appearance-focused skin cancer intervention within indoor tanner subgroups identified by latent profile analysis. *J Behav Med, 33*(3), 181-190. doi: 10.1007/s10865-009-9246-z

Stradling, D. (1999). *Smokestacks and progressives: Environmentalists, engineers, and air quality in America, 1881-1951.* Baltimore, MD: Johns Hopkins University Press.

Stryker, J. E., Lazovich, D., Forster, J. L., Emmons, K. M., Sorensen, G., & Demierre, M. F. (2004). Maternal/female caregiver influences on adolescent indoor tanning. *J Adolesc Health, 35*(6), 528 e521-529.

Stryker, J. E., Yaroch, A. L., Moser, R. P., Atienza, A., & Glanz, K. (2007). Prevalence of sunless tanning product use and related behaviors among adults in the United States: results from a national survey. *J Am Acad Dermatol, 56*(3), 387-390. doi: S0190-9622(06)02349-8 [pii] 10.1016/j.jaad.2006.08.051

Swerdlow, A. J., & Weinstock, M. A. (1998). Do tanning lamps cause melanoma? An epidemiologic assessment. *J Am Acad Dermatol, 38*(1), 89-98. doi: S0190-9622(98)70544-4 [pii]

Szepietowski, J. C., Nowicka, D., Soter, K., Strzelecka, E., Kozera, M., & Salomon, J. (2002). Tanning salons in southwest Poland: a survey of safety standards and professional knowledge of the staff. *Photodermatol Photoimmunol Photomed, 18*(4), 179-182. doi: 0699 [pii]

Taylor, S. L., Kaur, M., LoSicco, K., Willard, J., Camacho, F., O'Rourke, K. S., & Feldman, S. R. (2009). Pilot study of the effect of ultraviolet light on pain and mood in fibromyalgia syndrome. *J Altern Complement Med, 15*(1), 15-23. doi: 10.1089/acm.2008.0167

Teich, M. (August 2009). Nations unite against tanning: The impact of the IARC report: Skin Cancer Foundation.

Thomson, C. S., Woolnough, S., Wickenden, M., Hiom, S., & Twelves, C. J. (2010). Sunbed use in children aged 11-17 in England: face to face quota sampling surveys in the National Prevalence Study and Six Cities Study. *BMJ, 340*, c877.

Turrisi, R., Mastroleo, N. R., Stapleton, J., & Mallett, K. (2008). A comparison of 2 brief intervention approaches to reduce indoor tanning behavior in young women who indoor tan very frequently. *Arch Dermatol, 144*(11), 1521-1524. doi: 144/11/1521 [pii] 10.1001/archderm.144.11.1521

US Department of Health and Human Services. (1988). *Quality control guide for sunlamp products*. Rockville, MD.

US Food and Drug Administration. (2010). Executive summary: The potential risks and benefits of tanning lamps. General and plastic surgery devices panel meeting. Retrieved Accessed July 30, 2010, from http://www.fda.gov/downloads/AdvisoryCommittees/CommitteesMeetingMaterials/MedicalDevices/MedicalDevicesAdvisoryCommittee/GeneralandPlasticSurgeryDevicesPanel/UCM205687.pdf.

US Department of Health and Human Services-Food and Drug Administration. (1985). *Sunlamp products perfomance standard; final rule*. Rockville, MD.

US Department of Health and Human Services. (1986). *Policy on maximum timer interval and exposure for sunlamp products*. Rockville, MD.

US Food and Drug Administration. (2007). Tanning Accountability and Notification (TAN) Act. 110-085

US Food and Drug Administration. (2009). Tanning: Radiation-emitting products. Radiation-emitting products: Sunlamps and sunlamp products (tanning beds/booths) Retrieved Accessed March 21, 2010, from http://www.fda.gov/radiation-emittingproducts/radiationemittingproductsandprocedures/tanning/default.htm

Vannini, P., & McCright, A. M. (2004 Summer). To die for: the semiotic seductive power of the tanned body. *Symbolic Interaction, 27*(3), 309-332.

Veierod, M. B., Adami, H. O., Lund, E., Armstrong, B. K., & Weiderpass, E. (2010). Sun and solarium exposure and melanoma risk: effects of age, pigmentary characteristics, and nevi. *Cancer Epidemiol Biomarkers Prev, 19*(1), 111-120. doi: 19/1/111 [pii] 10.1158/1055-9965.EPI-09-0567

Warthan, M. M., Uchida, T., & Wagner, R. F., Jr. (2005). UV light tanning as a type of substance-related disorder. *Arch Dermatol, 141*(8), 963-966.

Weinstock, M. A., & Fisher, D. E. (2010). Indoor ultraviolet tanning: what the data do and do not show regarding risk of melanoma and keratinocyte malignancies. *J Natl Compr Canc Netw, 8*(8), 867-873. doi: 8/8/867 [pii]

Wichstrom, L. (1994). Predictors of Norwegian adolescents' sunbathing and use of sunscreen. *Health Psychol, 13*(5), 412-420.

Wintzen, M., de Winter, S., Out-Luiting, J. J., van Duinen, S. G., & Vermeer, B. J. (2001). Presence of immunoreactive beta-endorphin in human skin. *Exp Dermatol, 10*(5), 305-311.

Wintzen, M., & Gilchrest, B. A. (1996). Proopiomelanocortin, its derived peptides, and the skin. *J Invest Dermatol, 106*(1), 3-10.

Woo, D. K., & Eide, M. J. (2010). Tanning beds, skin cancer, and vitamin D: An examination of the scientific evidence and public health implications. *Dermatol Ther, 23*(1), 61-71. doi: DTH1291 [pii] 10.1111/j.1529-8019.2009.01291.x

World Health Organization. (2005). The World Health Organization recommends that under 18s should not use a sunbed. *J Adv Nursing, 51*(6), 662.

Young, J. C., & Walker, R. (1998). Understanding students' indoor tanning practices and beliefs to reduce skin cancer risks. *Am J Health Studies, 14*, 120–126.

Zeller, S., Lazovich, D., Forster, J., & Widome, R. (2006). Do adolescent indoor tanners exhibit dependency? *J Am Acad Dermatol, 54*(4), 589-596.

2

UV-Induced Immune Suppression that Promotes Skin Cancer Development and Progression

Takuma Kato and Linan Wang
Department of Cellular and Molecular Immunology
Department of Immuno-Gene Therapy
Mie University Graduate School of Medicine
Japan

1. Introduction

Arguably, UV irradiation is one of the most relevant risk factors for the development of skin cancer, including basal and squamous cell carcinoma (SCC), and melanoma (Rigel, 2008). UV-induced DNA damage triggers specific genetic mutations in oncosuppressor genes and/or oncogenes that initiate downstream events for carcinogenesis (de Gruijl & Rebel, 2008). It is increasingly clear that immunity plays a protective role in the detection and elimination of nascent tumors. This process termed "cancer immunosurveillance" has undergone a renaissance with the aid of elegant studies of cancer development in genetically engineered (targeting and/or transgenic) animals, and turned into the refined hypothesis termed "cancer immunoediting" (Vesely et al., 2011). UV radiation suppresses a variety of immune responses that contribute to carcinogenesis. The immunosuppressive effects of UV radiation may be involved in skin cancer development by impairing the antitumor immune responses that can destroy developing skin tumors. Moreover, UV radiation induces antigen-specific immune tolerance, which is largely mediated by regulatory T cells that specifically suppress immune responses against antigens expressed on emerging tumors (Katiyar, 2007). The temporal relationship between UV radiation and carcinogenesis revealed that UV radiation initiates tumor formation followed by suppression of immune responses specific to emerging tumors. Thus, the experiments documenting the immune suppressive effects of UV were conducted using naïve animals exposed to UV radiation prior to immunization. Accordingly, the prevailing notion of UV-induced immune suppression places a supportive role of UV radiation for the initiation of tumor development. However, it is equally important to explore the possibility that UV radiation induces antigen-specific immune suppression in hosts that have established immunity toward corresponding antigen, since UV radiation may suppress anti-tumor immune responses against emerging skin tumors wherein UV radiation may play no causative roles but contributes to tumor progression. This notion of UV-induced immunosuppression contributing to the progression of already emerged tumors, has received less attention and is not well corroborated experimentally. It is important to note that some melanomas arise at sites such as palms, soles, and buttocks, which do not have obvious exposure to UV radiation. There is increasing concern for the decreasing stratospheric ozone levels that leads increase in exposure to short wave length UV-B radiation on the terrestrial surface (Urbach, 1991). Therefore, it is incumbent upon us to gain a better understanding of the mechanisms of UV-induced immunosuppression involved in not only cancers wherein UV radiation plays a carcinogenic role but also those wherein it does not play an obvious causative role.

Based on wavelength, UV light can be divided into three bands: UV-A (λ = 320–400 nm), UV-B (λ = 280–320 nm) and UV-C (λ = 200–280 nm) (Tyrrell, 1994). The stratospheric ozone layer absorbs UV-C and most of UV-B, resulting in the UV component of sunlight reaching terrestrial biosphere consists primarily of UV-A (95%) and UV-B (5%) (Diffey, 2002). The energy carried by each UV component is inversely related to its wavelength and thus UV-B has been historically deemed to be the major UV component in sunlight affecting human health. However, UV-A is the most abundant UV component in sunlight and penetrates deep into the skin, thus quantitatively equally effective in affecting human health. Therefore carcinogenic and immunosuppressive properties of UV-A and UV-B can be dealt without distiction.

This chapter, in addition to presenting a comprehensive review of recent advances in the understanding of the causative roles of UV radiation in skin cancer development in the context of tumor immunology and the underlying cellular and molecular mechanisms involved, will also emphasize the notions of UV-induced immunosuppression contributing to the progression of already emerged tumors.

2. UV-induced DNA damage results in the mutation of critical genes and the dysregulation of microRNA expression leading to malignant transformation

Genome integrity in all living organisms is constantly threatened by endogenous and exogenous agents that modify the chemical integrity of DNA, collectively termed DNA damage, and in turn degenerate its informational contents (Wogan et al., 2004). If DNA damage is left unrepaired it can cause transcriptional silencing, proliferative arrest, and induce apoptosis (Hoeijmakers, 2001; Jackson & Bartek, 2009). To combat threats posed by DNA damage, cells are equipped with numerous mechanisms to detect and repair DNA lesions (Harper & Elledge, 2007; Harrison & Haber, 2006; Wood et al., 2005). Notwithstanding, some lesions remain in DNA during replication and are replicated in an error-prone manner resulting in mutations that enhance cancer risk (Jacinto & Esteller, 2007; Livneh, 2006). The most pervasive environmental DNA-damaging agent is UV radiation, and this is the primary basis for the carcinogenic properties of UV radiation. The International Agency for Research on Cancer published a monograph providing evidence for the carcinogenic properties of UV radiation in sunlight in 1992 (IARC, 1992) and now classifies UV radiation as a human carcinogen (http://monographs.iarc.fr/ENG/Classification/index.php). UV-induced DNA damage initiates a chain of events leading to carcinogenesis, collectively termed as "photocarcinogenesis". This process involves the formation of mutations at sites of DNA damage and, ultimately, results in malignant transformation after the accumulation of a sufficient number of mutations in critical genes (Runger, 2007). These mutations can occur in tumor suppressor genes such as *p53* (Brash et al., 1991; Hussein et al., 2003; Rees, 1994; Ziegler et al., 1994; Ziegler et al., 1993), *CDKN2/p16* (Holly et al., 1995; Saridaki et al., 2003; Soufir et al., 1999; Sparrow et al., 1998), and *PTCH* (D'Errico et al., 2000; Daya-Grosjean & Sarasin, 2000; de Gruijl et al., 2001; Ping et al., 2001; Zhang et al., 2001) as well as proto-oncogenes such as *RAS* (Chan et al., 2002; Kreimer-Erlacher et al., 2001; Spencer et al., 1995; van der Schroeff et al., 1990) and *RAF* (Besaratinia & Pfeifer, 2008; Gaddameedhi et al., 2010). UV-induced DNA damage also induces transcriptional activation of proto-oncogene c-*fos* (Ghosh et al., 1993).

2.1 DNA damage

The heterocyclic bases of DNA efficiently absorb energy in the UV that results in DNA lesions through a photochemical reaction (Ely & Ross, 1949). Thus the efficiency and the type of DNA lesion formation depends on the wavelength, peaking between 260 nm and 265 nm within the UV-B region (Markovitsi et al., 2010). The predominant form of DNA lesions are cyclobutane pyrimidine dimers (CPDs) and pyrimidine 6-4 pyrimidone photoproducts (6-4PPs), which constitute 65% and 35% of UV-B-induced DNA lesions, respectively (Lippke et al., 1981; Mitchell et al., 1992). Although direct absorption of photon energy by DNA is extremely low at the UV-A region, recent studies show that UV-A also triggers DNA-damage via formation of CPDs (Mouret et al., 2006; Rochette et al., 2003). Furthermore, UV-A induces conversion of 6-4PPs into an isomeric secondary product, Dewar valence isomer (Douki et al., 2003; Perdiz et al., 2000). It has been estimated that strong sunlight can induce approximately 100,000 lesions per cell exposed per hour (Jackson & Bartek, 2009). CPDs, 6-4PPs and Dewar valence isomers are induced by natural sunlight in normal human mononuclear cells (Clingen et al., 1995), and result in UV-specific mutations. These photolesions are highly mutagenic because of error-prone repair that results in thymidine substitutions. Although the contribution of 6-4PPs to UV-induced carcinogenesis has been elusive (Jans et al., 2006), the causative role of CPDs in UV-induced carcinogenesis was substantiated by specific removal of these DNA lesions through DNA repair enzymes leading to significantly reduced risk of UV-induced skin cancer in mice (Jans et al., 2005) and human (Yarosh et al., 1992; Yarosh et al., 2001). Besides the formation of DNA-lesions, cis-urocanic acid (cis-UCA) is formed from its isomer trans-UCA, which is abundant in skin exposed to UV radiation. A recent study showed direct evidence that cis-UCA induces reactive oxygen species (ROS) (Sreevidya et al., 2010) that leads the oxidative base modifications, predominantly at guanine base, and to the generation of the mutagenic DNA lesion, 8-oxo-7,8-dihydor-2′-deoxyguanosine (8-oxo-dG) (Douki et al., 1999; Kielbassa et al., 1997; Zhang et al., 1997). All these lesions are assumed to contribute to the generation of p53 mutations in SCC (Brash et al., 1991; Ziegler et al., 1994), Ras mutations in melanoma (Jiveskog et al., 1998), and p16 in actinic keratosis (Kanellou et al., 2008).

2.2 microRNAs

Recent studies implicate a small non-coding RNA species, microRNA, as a new player in the field of UV-induced carcinogenesis. microRNAs have important regulatory roles in diverse cellular pathways through their association with 3′-untranslated region of target mRNAs (Bartel, 2004). Increasing evidence indicates that DNA damage induced by UV irradiation provokes profound changes in expression of microRNAs (Pothof et al., 2009). Enlightening findings on the microRNA expression profile have been obtained in mouse fibroblast cell line NIH3T3 irradiated with UV-B. UV-B irradiation resulted in robust changes in the microRNA expression profile including the upregulation of let-7a, miR-21, and miR-24 and the downregulation of miR-465 (Guo et al., 2009). Subsequent work on microRNA expression in primary human keratinocytes exposed to UV-A or UV-B radiation revealed that UV-A induces miR-21, miR-203, and miR-205, whereas UV-B moderately induces miR-203, reduces miR-205 and had no effect on miR-21 (Dziunycz et al., 2010). Of particular interest is the observation that UV-A, but not UV-B, increased the expression of miR-21, since UV-A is responsible for SCC formation to a much higher extent than UV-B (Dziunycz et al., 2010). miR-21 is one of the most studied microRNAs and has potent carcinogenic properties (Selcuklu et al., 2009). It is currently well recognized that UVR induces aberrant microRNA expression in response to DNA damage. As aberrant microRNA expression has been observed in a variety of cancers (Catto et al., 2011; Selcuklu et al., 2009), the carcinogenic property of UV through DNA-lesion formation may also involve microRNA misexpression. Therefore, UV-induced DNA-lesion that directly causes mutations in critical oncogenes, tumor suppressor genes, or transcriptional regulatory regions of these genes, and UV-mediated modification of microRNA expression may collaboratively induce malignant transformation.

Arguably, cells are equipped with a variety of intrinsic tumor-suppressor mechanisms that attempt to repair genetic mutations and trigger senescence or apoptosis in order to prevent transformation. Normal cells can be transformed into tumor cells by the combination of genetic mutation and failed intrinsic tumor-suppressor mechanisms. However, emerging transformed cells and precancerous cells are usually kept in check by the host immune system, which acts as an extrinsic tumor suppressor mechanism that senses the presence of cancerous cells and restricts their growth. In the following section, the concept of tumor immunosurveillance and its updated hypothesis of tumor immunoediting, as well as the mechanisms by which UV irradiation interferes with these processes to promote tumorigenesis will be explored.

3. UV radiation suppresses the host immune system ability to eliminate emerging transformed cells

3.1 Cancer immunoediting

The relative contribution of the immune system to the control of cancer development and growth has been debated for many years. It was not until 2010 that Hanahan and Weinberg reviewed "immunity" as an emerging hallmark of cancer (Hanahan & Weinberg, 2011) expanded beyond their previous landmark review (Hanahan & Weinberg, 2000), from which immunity was notably absent. Now, there is ample evidence supporting a protective role for immunity in the detection and elimination of nascent tumors. This process called "cancer immunosurveillance", originally conceived in 1909 by Paul Ehrlich and later hypothesized by Burnet and Thomas in the late 1950s, has undergone a renaissance with elegant studies of cancer development in genetically engineered (targeting and/or transgenic) animals, which have helped spawn the notion of "cancer immunoediting". Cancer immunoediting proposes that cancer development and growth are controlled by three sequential phases: elimination, equilibrium, and escape. The elimination phase of cancer immunoediting is equivalent to the process described in the original hypothesis of immunosurveillance, whereby innate and adaptive immunity collaborate to detect and eliminate tumor cells that have developed as a result of failed intrinsic tumor suppressor mechanisms mentioned previously. In instances in which tumor cell destruction goes to completion, the elimination phase represents an endpoint of cancer immunoediting. However, rare tumor cell variants may survive in the elimination phase, leading to an equilibrium state between host immune system and developing tumors. In this equilibrium phase, the host immune system controls net tumor cell outgrowth, which results in the tumor cells remaining functionally dormant, but also sculpts the immunogenicity of the tumor cells. During this phase, T cell-mediated adaptive immunity exerts potent and relentless selection pressure on the tumor cells that is enough to contain but not fully extinguish the tumor bed containing many genetically unstable and mutating tumor cells, which can be viewed as a crucible of Darwinian selection. This phase can last for the life of the host, in which case the host does not develop any clinical manifestations and the equilibrium phase represents the second stable endpoint of cancer immunoediting. However, the constant immune selection pressure placed on genetically unstable tumor cells may lead to the emergence of tumor cell variants with any of the following characteristics: (i) invisible to adaptive immunity (variants with antigen loss or defect in antigen processing or presentation), (ii) insensitive to immune effector mechanisms, and (iii) ability to induce an immunosuppressive state within the tumor microenvironment, collectively referred low-immunogenic tumor variants. Therefore, although many of the original tumor cells that have survived in the elimination phase are destroyed, new variants arise that carry different mutations and altered gene expression profiles which endow them with the means to subvert immune-mediated recognition and destruction. Moreover, the growth of the selected variants is no longer controlled by immune system, leading to the appearance of overt cancer in the escape phase. In the escape phase, tumor cells that have acquired the ability to circumvent immune recognition or destruction emerge as progressively growing tumors and induce various clinical manifestations.

Evidence in support of the process of immunoediting comes mainly from mouse studies comparing the properties of tumors induced by chemical carcinogens in animals that are either immunocompetent or immunodeficient; however, increasing clinical observations have also provided evidence supporting the notion of tumor immunoediting in humans. In mice, immunodeficient mice develop more tumors, more rapidly, and at lower chemical carcinogen doses than wild-type immunocompetent mice (Dighe et al., 1994; Kaplan et al., 1998; Shankaran et al., 2001; Smyth et al., 2001; Street et al., 2001; Street et al., 2002). Immunodeficient mice also display an increased incidence of disseminated lymphomas or spontaneous lung adenocarcinomas, depending on mouse strains. Furthermore, tumors cell lines derived from immunocompetent mice survive well in both immunocompetent and immunodeficient mice upon transplantation, whereas those derived from immunodeficient mice survive only in immunodeficient mice and are easily rejected in immunocompetent mice, indicating that tumors developed in immunocompetent mice are edited to be less immunogenic. In humans, patients with AIDS and organ transplantation recipients that have received immunosuppressants have increased frequencies of malignancies. Although virus-associated malignancies predominate and thus an argument can be made that the increased frequency of virus-associated cancers reflects a breakdown in antiviral immunity rather than reduced immunosurveillance of cancer, these is also an increased risks for the development of noninfectious cancers (Boshoff & Weiss, 2002; Chaturvedi et al., 2007; Frisch et al., 2001; Vajdic et al., 2006). In relation to skin cancer, a 200-fold increased risk of nonmelanoma skin cancers and 2- to 10-fold increased frequency of melanomas have been reported in renal transplant patients (Moloney et al., 2006). Patients with liver transplants also manifest a greater preponderance of nonmelanoma skin cancers (Aberg et al., 2008). Furthermore, there is a direct correlation between the duration of immunosuppressant administration and the incidence of cancer development (Loeffelbein et al., 2009), supporting the existence of human cancer immunosurveillance.

Most of the observations that the immunosuppressive status of the host may promote tumor development and growth largely recapitulate the studies conducted in UV-irradiated mice, in which the pioneering work of Fisher and Kripke established the field of photoimmunology, involving elements of photobiology, immunology, and oncology (Fisher & Kripke, 1977). In the following sections, we will deal with UV-induced immune suppression that supports tumor development and progression.

3.2 UV radiation suppresses anti-tumor immunity and promotes tumor development

The first clear evidence that UV irradiation can affect immune responses emanated from the seminal work of Margaret Kripke and her colleagues in the 1970's, who demonstrated that skin tumors induced by chronic exposure to UV radiation were highly immunogenic, as they were rejected when transplanted into age- and sex-matched healthy syngeneic mice. In hindsight, the tumors developed in UV-irradiated hosts were not edited. They further showed that prior exposure of recipient mice to subcarcinogenic doses of UV-B resulted in the acceptance of the transplanted tumors, clearly indicating that UV systemically suppresses host immunity against tumors (DeFabo & Kripke, 1979; Fisher & Kripke, 1977; Kripke, 1974). Tumors were accepted even when transplanted into sites not directly exposed to UV radiation, indicating that UV radiation exerts systemic immunosuppression (DeFabo & Kripke, 1979; Fisher & Kripke, 1977). The effect of UV on the acceptance of the transplanted tumors was shown to be UV dose-dependent. In another study in primary tumor development model using UV independently as an immunosuppressant and a tumor initiator, de Gruijl et al. demonstrated the immunosuppressive effect of UV via the inhibition of cancer immunosurveillance leading to the acceleration of tumorigenesis (de Gruiji & van der Leun, 1982; de Gruijl & Van Der Leun, 1983). In these studies, hairless mice were pre-irradiated with UV radiation while certain skin areas of the animals were shielded from the radiation. Pre-irradiation was carried out to the point where tumors started to appear in the pre-irradiation skin areas (13 weeks). Then, the initially shielded skin areas were chronically exposed to UV radiation, which resulted in the development of tumors in these skin areas. They demonstrated that the formation of tumors in the initially shielded skin areas was enhanced by the pre-irradiation of the other skin areas. Subsequently, they also showed that the formation of tumors in initially shielded skin areas was still enhanced even when the pre-irradiation was discontinued long before the appearance of tumor in pre-irradiated skin areas. These earlier studies revealed that UV irradiation disturbs cancer immunosurveillance, leading to the accelerated development of tumors and the emergence of highly immunogenic (non-edited) tumors. Collectively, these results indicate that UV-B radiation has a dual effect on skin carcinogenesis, not only as an inducer, but also as a promoter. Subsequent studies utilizing models of contact hypersensitivity (CHS), wherein mice were sensitized by epicutaneous application of contact allergens induced an ear swelling response, recapitulated the immunosuppressive features of UV radiation seen in skin carcinogenesis (Noonan et al., 1981; Toews et al., 1980). In these studies, mice sensitized with a hapten to the skin that had been exposed to UV-defected CHS responses (Toews et al., 1980). Furthermore, these mice exhibited systemic and long-term unresponsiveness to the same hapten, since the mice could not be re-sensitized against the same hapten at a later time point even when the hapten was applied to skin not previously exposed to UV. This unresponsiveness was antigen-specific, since the mice exhibited normal CHS responses against other unrelated haptens. These studies unravel important features of UV-induced immunosuppression, particularly long-lasting and antigen specific immune responses.

3.3 Regulatory T cells are responsible for the UV-induced suppression of anti-tumor immunity

Early work on UV-induced immunosuppression by Kripke and colleagues revealed that UV-B induced immunosuppression was transferable by adoptive transfer of lymphocytes from irradiated mice into non-irradiated mice (Fisher & Kripke, 1977; Hostetler et al., 1989; Kripke & Fisher, 1976; Kripke et al., 1977; Kripke et al., 1979; Roberts et al., 1982; Spellman &

Daynes, 1977; Spellman & Daynes, 1984; Spellman et al., 1977; Ullrich & Kripke, 1984). In these studies, recipient mice infused with T cells from UV-irradiated mice were unable to reject UV-induced tumors (Fisher & Kripke, 1977; Kripke & Fisher, 1976; Kripke et al., 1977; Spellman & Daynes, 1977; Spellman et al., 1977), but not non-UV-induced tumors such as tumors induced by chemical carcinogen (Hostetler et al., 1989; Kripke et al., 1979; Roberts et al., 1982; Spellman & Daynes, 1984; Ullrich & Kripke, 1984), suggesting some degree of antigen-specificity. Subsequent studies using a CHS model further delineated antigen-specific immune suppression by T cells from UV-irradiated hosts. Upon adoptive transfer with T cells obtained from mice that had been treated with a hapten onto UV-exposed skin, the recipient mice were no-longer responsive to the very same hapten; however, these recipient mice could respond normally to other unrelated haptens (Elmets et al., 1983). These results convincingly demonstrated that T cells mediate UV-induced immunosuppression in an antigen-specific manner. Consequently, these T cells were designated as suppressor T cells, and have since been renamed regulatory T cells (Beissert et al., 2006). Even then these early experiments suggested that variations in these regulatory T cell populations might exist depending on the experimental systems used to induce and examine the UV-induced immunosuppression. Although the lack of clear markers that define a specific subset of T cells still impedes the attempts to fully characterize UV-induced regulatory T cells, recent studies have demonstrated that UV-induced regulatory T cells include $CD3^{+}DX5^{+}$ NKT cells (Moodycliffe et al., 2000); $CD4^{+}CD25^{+}$ T cells co-expressing CTLA-4, GITR, and neuropilin-1 (Maeda et al., 2008); $CD4^{+}Foxp3^{+}$ T cells (Ghoreishi & Dutz, 2006; Loser et al., 2006); and type 1 regulatory T cells (Hori et al., 2008; Toda et al., 2010; Wang et al., 2010; Wang et al., 2008).

NK-T cells. The CD1d molecules are structurally similar to MHC class I molecules that presents lipid antigens to NKT cells (Brigl & Brenner, 2004). Moodycliffe et al. have demonstrated that CD1d-deficient mice are resistant to UV-induced immune suppression (Moodycliffe et al., 2000). Adoptive transfer of a purified population of $CD3^{+}DX5^{+}$ NKT cells from UV-irradiated wild-type mice, which produced high amount of IL-4, into normal syngeneic mice suppressed antigen-specific delayed type hypersensitivity and anti-tumor immune responses against transplanted highly immunogenic UV-induced skin tumors. Subsequent study also revealed that CD1d-deficient mice are resistant to UV-induced skin carcinogenesis (Matsumura et al., 2005). Although, the observed resistant characteristics of CD1d-deficient mice to UV-induced skin carcinogenesis may not be solely due to the lack of NKT cells, these results indicate that UV irradiation induced immunosuppressive NKT cells that may promote tumor development. Recently, it has been shown that epidermal Langerhans cells (LCs) are responsible for the induction of immunosuppressive NKT cell by UV radiation (Fukunaga et al., 2010). UV radiation activates migration of LCs to the skin draining lymph nodes. Adoptive transfer of LCs from the lymph node of UV-irradiated mice into wild-type mice, but not CD1d-deficient mice, resulted in antigen-specific immunosuppression. This study highlights the recent notion that LCs may not play a major role in cutaneous immune responses, but rather regulate immunity in infection and CHS, and play an important role in UV-induced immunosuppression. It has been well documented that the immunosuppressive mechanisms of action of NKT cells remains less clear, but appears to be dependent on IL-4, since immune suppression in mice transferred with LCs from UV-irradiated mice were completely blocked by neutralization of IL-4. However, how NKT cells in UV-irradiated host suppress anti-tumor immune responses remain largely unknown.

$CD25^+$ regulatory T cells. It was not until 1985 that Sakaguchi et al. resurrected the suppressor T cells, now renamed regulatory T cells, following almost two decades of abandonment in the field of immunology (Sakaguchi et al., 2007). First characterization of this T cell subset revealed that they constitutively expressed CD25 and suppressed autoimmunity. The current explosive developments in the field of regulatory T cells have shown that $CD25^+CD4^+$ regulatory T cells express the cell surface molecules such as CTLA-4, neurophilin-1, and folate receptor, and Foxp3 transcription factor. The findings at the cellular and molecular levels altogether provide firm evidence for their crucial roles in the establishment and maintenance of immunologic self-tolerance and immune homeostasis (Sakaguchi et al., 2007). Furthermore, it is increasingly clear that $CD25^+CD4^+Foxp3^+$ regulatory T cells play an important role in the suppression of anti-tumor immune responses (Nishikawa et al., 2008; Nishikawa et al., 2003; Nishikawa et al., 2005; Nishikawa et al., 2005). Importantly, we have shown that $CD25^+CD4^+Foxp3^+$ regulatory T cells significantly accelerate tumor development in a chemical carcinogen-induced primary tumor development model (Nishikawa et al., 2005). Recent studies revealed that $CD25^+CD4^+Foxp3^+$ regulatory T cells were also involved in the UV-induced immunosuppression. Loser et al. have demonstrated that receptor activator of NF-κB (RANK) and its ligand, RANKL, were involved in UV-induced immunosuppression via activation and/or expansion of $CD25^+CD4^+Foxp3^+$ regulatory T cells (Loser et al., 2006). They showed that UV irradiation induced the expression of RANKL on basal keratinocytes. Injection of specific RANKL antagonist, RANK-Fc, followed by UV irradiation and hapten immunization resulted in the abrogation of UV-induced hapten-specific immune suppression. Finally, it was found that RANK–RANKL signaling between RANK-expressing LCs and RANKL-overexpressing keratinocytes driven by K14 promoter transgenic mice resulted in the increased capacity of LCs to stimulate the proliferation of $CD25^+CD4^+Foxp3^+$ regulatory T cells. LCs stimulated by RANKL exhibit elevated expression of DEC205 and CD86 as well as increased IL-10 secretion, all of which have been shown to be associated with the DC-induced expansion of regulatory T cells (Loser et al., 2006; Mahnke et al., 2003; Maurer et al., 2003). In the study of Ghoreishi et al., transcutaneous immunization through UV-irradiated skin induced an increase in $CD25^+CD4^+Foxp3^+$ regulatory T cells that suppressed CTL responses against tumors (Ghoreishi & Dutz, 2006). In this study, IL-10 was not required for the induction and suppressive function of $CD25^+CD4^+Foxp3^+$ regulatory T cells. Such T cells were induced in IL-10-deficient mice and these regulatory T cells conferred suppression of immune responses upon transfer into IL-10-sufficient, but not IL-10-deficient mice. Therefore, it is suggested that UV-irradiation induces $CD25^+CD4^+Foxp3^+$ regulatory T cells independently of IL-10 expression, but these UV-induced regulatory T cells require IL-10 derived from other type of cells, in order to mediate anti-tumor immune responses and support tumor development in UV-irradiated hosts.

IL-10 producing regulatory T cells. Schwarz and colleagues have conducted a series of studies to characterize UV-induced regulatory T cells using a CHS model. In their studies, UV-induced regulatory T cells that confer suppression of CHS belong to the $CD4^+CD25^+$ subtype (Schwarz et al., 2004); co-express CTLA-4, GITR, and neuropilin-1 (Maeda et al., 2008; Schwarz et al., 2000); and bind the lectin dectin-2 (Aragane et al., 2003). While most of these phenotypic features are similar to $CD25^+CD4^+Foxp3^+$ regulatory T cells, these UV-induced regulatory T cells produced large amounts of IL-10 that mediates immunosuppression. Additionally, these UV-induced regulatory T cells exerted bystander suppression via the release of IL-10. These characteristics collectively indicate that this regulatory T cell subset belongs to Tr1 originally described by Groux et al. (Groux et al., 1997; Roncarolo et al., 2006; Vieira et al., 2004). The same group has also demonstrated that IL-10 negatively regulates CTL responses in UV-irradiated mice, which was associated with enhanced tumor growth (Loser et al., 2007). $CD4^+CD25^+$ T cells from UV-irradiated wild-type mice, but not those from UV-irradiated IL-10 deficient mice, could transfer the suppression of anti-tumor immune responses (Loser et al., 2007). Therefore, it is highly likely that UV-induced regulatory T cells reported by Schwarz et al. may also promote tumor development through production of IL-10. It appears that LCs with DNA-damage play an important role in the induction of this type of UV-induced regulatory T cells, since reduction of LCs containing CPDs in the regional lymph nodes by IL-12 prevented the development of UV-induced regulatory T cells. The effect of IL-12 on the prevention of UV-induced regulatory T cell development was not seen in mice deficient for DNA-repair enzymes.

4. UV radiation may induce tumor antigen-specific immune suppression thus contributing to the progression of emerging tumors

In most studies dealing with UV-induced immunosuppression and its impact on anti-tumor immunity, hosts are exposed to UV radiation before immunization, and only a few studies have examined the effect of UV irradiation on established immune responses (Nghiem et al., 2001; Nghiem et al., 2002; Ullrich et al., 2007). Based on the potent immunosuppressive effects of UV irradiation on a variety of immune responses, there is a high likelihood that it affects the efficacy of immune protection afforded by prior vaccination but may also provide tools to develop new therapies for allergic diseases and transplantation. Furthermore, it is also possible that exposure to UV radiation in hosts whose immunity is successfully controlling benign or premalignant tumors may induce tumor-specific immunosuppression and contribute to the development of clinically apparent tumors. In a series of studies, we have demonstrated that mice exposed to UV radiation one week after immunization exhibited reduced Th1- and Th2-driven Ab responses, suppressed airway inflammation in sensitized mice, and prolonged allograft survival in an Ag-specific manner (Hori et al., 2008; Wang et al., 2010; Wang et al., 2008). Additionally, we showed that UV irradiation following immunization led to the generation of $CD4^+$ regulatory T cells producing IL-10 and IFN-γ, and Ag-dependent secretion of IL-10 was responsible for the immunosuppression. These phenotypic and functional features were reminiscent of Tr1. However, $CD4^+$ T cells from UV-irradiated mice contained $Foxp3^+$ T cells lacking IL-10 expression (Wang et al., 2008). Recently, we generated a panel of T cell clones from UV-irradiated mice and examined their functional and phenotypic characteristics to better characterize the immunosuppressive cells. All of the T cell clones derived from UV-irradiated mice produced both IL-10 and IFN-γ, but not IL-4, and this strongly argues that a general shift of immunity from a Th1- to Th2-type immune response is not responsible for the UV-induced immune suppression (Beissert et al., 1996; Shreedhar et al., 1998). Notably, the T cell clones derived from UV-irradiated mice lacked expression of Foxp3 mRNA, but they uniformly expressed c-Maf mRNA. c-Maf was originally described as a Th2-specific transcription factor, but subsequent studies revealed that c-Maf transactivates IL-10 gene transcription independently of Th2 differentiation (Cao et al., 2005; Xu et al., 2009). More recent studies indicate that c-Maf transactivates IL-21, which acts as an autocrine growth factor for the expansion and/or maintenance of Tr1 cells (Apetoh et al., 2010; Pot et al., 2009). Although Th2 cells express c-Maf, it has also been shown that the expression levels of c-Maf mRNA are ~500-fold higher in Tr1 cells compared to Th2 cells (Pot et al., 2009). Therefore, c-Maf now can be regarded as a critical transcription factor for Tr1 cells. In addition, T cell clones from UV-irradiated mice exerted Ag-specific and bystander suppression of T cell activation in an IL-10-dependent but a contact-independent fashion. Taken together, these results indicate that UV-induced regulatory T cell subsets involve Tr1. We also found that IL-10 was required for the development of this regulatory T cell subset. $CD4^+$ T cells from UV-irradiated mice treated with anti-IL-10 no longer have immunosuppressive properties, clearly indicating that IL-10 is necessary for UV-induced regulatory T cells. Consistent with others, IL-10 is detectable in serum of mice exposed to UV radiation at dose of 15 or 30 kJ/m^2 (Beissert et al., 1996; Rivas & Ullrich, 1994; Shreedhar et al., 1998). In addition, treating UV-irradiated mice with anti-IL-10 has been reported to block the induction of systemic immune suppression (Rivas & Ullrich, 1992), which substantiates our results that neutralization of IL-10 suppresses the generation and function of regulatory T cells induced by UV-irradiation. Therefore, IL-10 that was possibly secreted by keratinocytes upon UV-irradiation (Rivas & Ullrich, 1992) appeared to play an obligatory role in the generation of Tr1-like regulatory T cells that mediated suppression of variety of immune responses. Although the precise mechanism by which UV induces Tr1-like regulatory T cells in vivo remains elusive, our preliminary experiments indicated that the effect of IL-10 induced by UV-irradiation on the generation of Tr1-like regulatory T cells was not a direct effect on T cells, because repetitive stimulation of $CD4^+$ T cells by anti-CD3 together with IL-10 in the presence, but not absence, of APC resulted in the generation of IL-10 producing Tr1-like regulatory T cells in vitro. These results confirm previous studies showing that IL-10 modulates APC and/or induces differentiation of $CD11c^{low}CD45RB^{high}$ DCs required to induce the generation of Tr1 in vitro and in vivo (Wakkach et al., 2001; Wakkach et al., 2003). However, it remains elusive whether UV induces such phenotypic changes or generation of such DCs. Importantly, using a murine tumor model in which ovalbumin (OVA) served as a surrogate tumor Ag, we demonstrated that exposure to UV radiation in OVA-immunized mice significantly accelerated the acceptance of the tumor as compared to those exposed to UV radiation alone, which is mediated antigen-specific regulatory T cells mentioned above. We also showed that these regulatory T cells suppress the induction and/or activation of cytotoxic T cells. All these results indicate that UV-irradiation after immunization induces Tr1 cells specific to the immunizing Ag and dominantly suppresses a variety of immune responses that control tumor progression. Accumulating evidence indicates that precancerous and malignant cells can induce specific immune response that leads to the elimination of malignant and/or transformed cell before they developed detectable tumors. Furthermore, recent multivariate analysis of a multi-country ecological study and population based, case-control study have shown a significant positive association between exposure to UV radiation and increase in the risks of non-Hodgkin's lymphoma and colon cancer, in addition to skin melanoma (Waltz & Chodick, 2008; Zhang et al., 2007). Even in the case with melanomas, some melanomas arise at such as palms, soles, and mucosal surfaces, which do not have obvious exposure to UV (Garibyan & Fisher, 2010). Therefore, it appears plausible that exposure to UV radiation in hosts whose immunity successfully controlling benign or premalignant tumors induces tumor-specific immunosuppression and contributes to tumor progression. In this regard, UV-induced immune suppression may also play an important role in the progression of various tumors, including some in which UV radiation does not play a direct causative role.

5. Molecules that trigger UV-induced immunosuppression

Immunologic reactions are evoked by an intricate network of signaling and cell activation. Therefore, UV-induced immunosuppression may also have evolved under the influence of altered molecules expressed in cells damaged by UV radiation. As is the case with a major role of DNA-damage played in the initiation of carcinogenesis, accumulating evidence indicates that UV-induced DNA-damage is an important trigger for UV-induced immunosuppression. The topical application of exogenous DNA repair enzymes to UV-irradiated skin has been shown to reduce UV-induced DNA-damage and resulted in the abrogation of UV-induced immunosuppression (Applegate et al., 1989; Kripke et al., 1992). Consistent with this finding, it has been shown that DNA-damage induced by the treatment of mice with HindIII-containing liposomes causes double-strand breaks and induces immunosuppression (Nishigori et al., 1998). Likewise, deficiency in DNA repair in XPA (xeroderma pigmentosum group A)-gene knockout mice exhibits enhanced susceptibility to UV-induced immunosuppression (Miyauchi-Hashimoto et al., 1996). IL-12 was the first cytokine being demonstrated to exert the capacity to prevent UV-induced immunosuppression (Muller et al., 1995; Schmitt et al., 1995; Schwarz et al., 1996). Because of its well-recognized immunostimulatory activities (Trinchieri, 2003), it was no wonder that exogenous administration of IL-12 recovered the immunosuppressive effects of UV radiation. However, recent studies unravel an unexpected capacity of IL-12 to reduce DNA-damage via induction or activation of the nucleotide excision repair (NER), the major endogenous DNA repair system (Schwarz et al., 2002). It has been demonstrated that IL-12 is unable to prevent UV-induced immunosuppression in mice deficient for NER (Schwarz et al., 2005). Using mouse models, the additional factors that influence the NER and reverse UV-induced immunosuppression have been demonstrated, including IL-18 (Schwarz et al., 2006), IL-23 (Majewski et al.), α-melanocyte-stimulating hormone (Bohm et al., 2005), infrared radiation (Jantschitsch et al., 2009), vitamin D (Tremezaygues et al., 2009), and even UV-A (Garssen et al., 2001) possibly through the induction of IL-12 (Shen et al., 1999); however, their relevance in human subjects remains to be determined. Although UV radiation induces different types of DNA lesions such as CPDs and 6-4PPs along with its isomeric secondary product, Dewar valence isomer, it was later found that repair of 6-4PPs had no effect on UV-induced immunosuppression (Jans et al., 2006). Using mice expressing the *P. tridacylus* CPD photolylase enzyme under the control of the basal keratinocyte-specific promoter keratin-14, which allows rapid, light-dependent removal of CPDs from basal keratinocytes only, it was demonstrated that removal of CPDs solely from basal epidermal cells in transgenic mice resulted in a major reduction in UV-induced carcinogenesis, but did not reverse UV-induced immunosuppression, whereas the removal from the entire skin reversed UV-induced immunosuppression (Jans et al., 2006). UV-induced DNA-damage in different cell types independently mediates carcinogenic or immunosuppressive properties of UV radiation. Collectively, these studies convincingly demonstrate that DNA-damage, especially in the form of CPDs, is a major molecular trigger in UV-induced immunosuppression.

In addition to CPDs, UV radiation induces the formation of cis-urocanic acid (cis-UCA) from its isomer trans-UCA. Trans-UCA is abundant in the skin because of the lack of the necessary enzymes in epidermal cells to catabolize UCA generated in the metabolic pathway of the essential amino acid histidine. Injection of cis-UCA (Beissert et al., 1997; De Fabo & Noonan, 1983; Norval et al., 1995) induces immunosuppression, whereas its removal by epidermal stripping, neutralization by antibodies, or blocking the binding to its receptor ($5\text{-}HT_{2A}$) with selective serotonin receptor antagonists, restores immune suppression induced by UV radiation (De Fabo & Noonan, 1983; Moodycliffe et al., 1996; Walterscheid et al., 2006). It also has been shown that neutralization of cis-UCA in vivo suppressed UV-induced carcinogenesis (Beissert et al., 2001). Despite all these documented abilities of cis-UCA to influence immune suppression and carcinogenesis, recent studies demonstrated that cis-UCA induces apoptosis in several human tumor cells including melanomas (Laihia et al., 2010; Laihia et al., 2009; Peuhu et al., 2010), and cis-UCA has been recognized as a potential anti-cancer agent.

Nevertheless, CPDs and cis-UCA, abundant molecules in UV-irradiated skin, are responsible for UV-induced immunosuppression. These molecules have been shown to induce cytokines such as IL-10, PGE2, and TGF-β (Curiel-Lewandrowski et al., 2003; Grewe et al., 2000; Kaneko et al., 2008; Kaneko et al., 2009; Nishigori et al., 1996), all of which may be involved in the development and/or activation of cells with regulatory activities (Allan et al., 2008). However, what still remains elusive is how these molecules induce various types of regulatory T cells that mediate antigen-specific and systemic immunosuppression.

6. Conclusion

Over the decades, it has become clear that UV irradiation has the potential to suppress a variety of immune reactions including anti-tumor immune responses through the generation of antigen-specific regulatory T cells. The concepts of 'regulatory T cells' and 'immune control of tumor' have experienced a very eventful past having been dogmatically disregarded and abandoned but being now highly appreciated and well recognized by the majority of immunologists. Major credit can be given to the researchers in the field of photoimmunology who persistently pursued and accumulated evidence supporting both concepts. However, it seems that the importance or physiological relevance of UV-induced skin cancers, wherein the existence of cancer immunity and regulatory T cells are so obvious, has never been established as a prominent model in the field of tumor immunology and immunology in general. As may be seen in this chapter, it is now quite clear that UV radiation plays an indisputable role in skin carcinogenesis, as a tumor initiator and progressor, and also in the development of cancer wherein UV radiation does not play a causative role.

Recent studies have begun to unravel the differential effects of UV radiation on the innate and the adaptive immune system (Schwarz, 2010). Although UV irradiation clearly suppresses adaptive immunity, it may activate innate immunity. It has been shown that only 30–50% of UVR doses that induced detectable sunburn are required for the suppression of immunity in humans, and therefore normal daily outdoor activities are likely to cause some degree of immunosuppression. Understanding that the skin is an organ that seems quite prone to autoimmunity, it is plausible that a certain degree of immunosuppression by daily solar exposure may be protective against autoimmunity, and that activation of innate immunity may compensate for the increased risks of microbial infection by suppression of adaptive immunity, which may function as a part of the protection mechanism acquired during evolution. This may argue against total sun protection for the sake of skin cancer prevention. Additionally, patients with allergic diseases that also receive benefit from UV-phototherapy may be through the induction of regulatory T cells (Wang, 2010). Thus, despite the fact that excessive and chronic UV radiation exposure remains one of the major environmental threats for human health, a better understanding of carcinogenic and immunosuppressive properties of UV radiation, and its underlying mechanisms is needed for the prevention and cure of skin cancer, but also for formulating therapeutic use of UV and future sun protection strategy.

7. Acknowledgements

The authors are very grateful to Dr. Kagemasa Kuribayashi for his insightful advice and encouragement that permit us to pursue the projects related to this review. The authors also thank Dr. Hiroshi Shiku for his continuous support. This work was supported in part by grants from Grant-in-Aid for Scientific Research (C) by the Ministry of Education, Culture, Sports, Science and Technology of Japan; and Long-range Research Initiative (LRI) by Japan Chemical Industry Association (JCIA, Tokyo, Japan) to T.K.

8. References

Aberg, F.; Pukkala, E.; Höckerstedt, K.; Sankila, R. & Isoniemi, H. (2008). Risk of malignant neoplasms after liver transplantation: a population-based study. *Liver Transpl,* Vol.14, No.10, (October 2008), pp. 1428-36, ISSN1527-6473

Allan, S.E.; Broady, R.; Gregori, S.; Himmel, M.E.; Locke, N.; Roncarolo, M.G.; Bacchetta, R. & Levings, M.K. (2008). CD4+ T-regulatory cells: toward therapy for human diseases. *Immunol Rev,* Vol.223, (June 2008), pp. 391-421, ISSN 1600-065X

Apetoh, L.; Quintana, F.J.; Pot, C.; Joller, N.; Xiao, S.; Kumar, D.; Burns, E.J.; Sherr, D.H.; Weiner, H.L. & Kuchroo, V.K. (2010). The aryl hydrocarbon receptor interacts with c-Maf to promote the differentiation of type 1 regulatory T cells induced by IL-27. *Nat Immunol,* Vol.11, No.9, (Sepember 2010), pp. 854-61, ISSN 1529-2916

Applegate, L.A.; Ley, R.D.; Alcalay, J. & Kripke, M.L. (1989). Identification of the molecular target for the suppression of contact hypersensitivity by ultraviolet radiation. *J Exp Med,* Vol.170, No.4, (October 1989), pp. 1117-31, ISSN 0022-1007

Aragane, Y.; Maeda, A.; Schwarz, A.; Tezuka, T.; Ariizumi, K. & Schwarz, T. (2003). Involvement of dectin-2 in ultraviolet radiation-induced tolerance. *J Immunol,* Vol.171, (September 2003), pp. 3801-7, ISSN 0022-1767

Bartel, D.P. (2004). MicroRNAs: genomics, biogenesis, mechanism, and function. *Cell,* Vol.116, No.2, (January 2004), pp. 281-97, ISSN 0092-8674

Beissert, S.; Hosoi, J.; Kuhn, R.; Rajewsky, K.; Muller, W. & Granstein, R.D. (1996). Impaired immunosuppressive response to ultraviolet radiation in interleukin-10-deficient mice. *J Invest Dermatol,* Vol.107, (October 1996), pp. 553-7, ISSN 0022-202X

Beissert, S.; Mohammad, T.; Torri, H.; Lonati, A.; Yan, Z.; Morrison, H. & Granstein, R.D. (1997). Regulation of tumor antigen presentation by urocanic acid. *J Immunol,* Vol.159, No.1, (July 1997), pp. 92-6, ISSN 0022-1767

Beissert, S.; Ruhlemann, D.; Mohammad, T.; Grabbe, S.; El-Ghorr, A.; Norval, M.; Morrison, H.; Granstein, R.D. & Schwarz, T. (2001). IL-12 prevents the inhibitory effects of cis-urocanic acid on tumor antigen presentation by Langerhans cells: implications for photocarcinogenesis. *J Immunol,* Vol.167, No.11, (December 2001), pp. 6232-8, ISSN 0022-1767

Beissert, S.; Schwarz, A. & Schwarz, T. (2006). Regulatory T cells. *J Invest Dermatol*, Vol.126, No.1, (January 2006), pp. 15-24, ISSN 0022-202X

Besaratinia, A. & Pfeifer, G.P. (2008). Sunlight ultraviolet irradiation and BRAF V600 mutagenesis in human melanoma. *Hum Mutat*, Vol.29, No.8, (Aug 2008), pp. 983-91, ISSN 1098-1004

Bohm, M.; Wolff, I.; Scholzen, T.E.; Robinson, S.J.; Healy, E.; Luger, T.A.; Schwarz, T. & Schwarz, A. (2005). alpha-Melanocyte-stimulating hormone protects from ultraviolet radiation-induced apoptosis and DNA damage. *J Biol Chem*, Vol.280, No.7, (February 2005), pp. 5795-802, ISSN 0021-9258

Boshoff, C. & Weiss, R. (2002). AIDS-related malignancies. Nat Rev Cancer, Vol.2, No.5, (May 2002), pp. 373-82, ISSN 1474-175X

Brash, D.E.; Rudolph, J.A.; Simon, J.A.; Lin, A.; McKenna, G.J.; Baden, H.P.; Halperin, A.J. & Ponten, J. (1991). A role for sunlight in skin cancer: UV-induced p53 mutations in squamous cell carcinoma. *Proc Natl Acad Sci U S A*, Vol.88, No.22, (November 1991), pp. 10124-8, ISSN 0027-8424

Brigl, M. & Brenner, M.B. (2004). CD1: antigen presentation and T cell function. Annu Rev Immunol, Vol.22, 2004), pp. 817-90, ISSN 0732-0582

Cao, S.; Liu, J.; Song, L. & Ma, X. (2005). The protooncogene c-Maf is an essential transcription factor for IL-10 gene expression in macrophages. *J Immunol*, Vol.174, No.6, (March 2005), pp. 3484-92, ISSN 0022-1767

Catto, J.W.; Alcaraz, A.; Bjartell, A.S.; De Vere White, R.; Evans, C.P.; Fussel, S.; Hamdy, F.C.; Kallioniemi, O.; Mengual, L.; Schlomm, T. & Visakorpi, T. (2011). MicroRNA in Prostate, Bladder, and Kidney Cancer: A Systematic Review. *Eur Urol*, Vol.59, No.5, (May 2011), pp. 671-81, ISSN 1873-7560

Chan, J.; Robinson, E.S.; Yeh, I.T. & McCarrey, J.R. (2002). Absence of ras gene mutations in UV-induced malignant melanomas correlates with a dermal origin of melanocytes in Monodelphis domestica. *Cancer Lett*, Vol.184, No.1, (October 2002), pp. 73-80, ISSN 0304-3835

Chaturvedi, A.K.; Pfeiffer, R.M.; Chang, L.; Goedert, J.J.; Biggar, R.J. & Engels, E.A. (2007). Elevated risk of lung cancer among people with AIDS. AIDS, Vol.21, No.2, (January 2007), pp. 207-13, ISSN 0269-9370

Clingen, P.H.; Arlett, C.F.; Roza, L.; Mori, T.; Nikaido, O. & Green, M.H. (1995). Induction of cyclobutane pyrimidine dimers, pyrimidine(6-4)pyrimidone photoproducts, and Dewar valence isomers by natural sunlight in normal human mononuclear cells. *Cancer Res*, Vol.55, No.11, (June 1995), pp. 2245-8, ISSN 0008-5472

Curiel-Lewandrowski, C.; Venna, S.S.; Eller, M.S.; Cruikshank, W.; Dougherty, I.; Cruz, P.D., Jr. & Gilchrest, B.A. (2003). Inhibition of the elicitation phase of contact hypersensitivity by thymidine dinucleotides is in part mediated by increased expression of interleukin-10 in human keratinocytes. Exp Dermatol, Vol.12, No.2, (Apr 2003), pp. 145-52, 0906-6705

D'Errico, M.; Calcagnile, A.; Canzona, F.; Didona, B.; Posteraro, P.; Cavalieri, R.; Corona, R.; Vorechovsky, I.; Nardo, T.; Stefanini, M. & Dogliotti, E. (2000). UV mutation signature in tumor suppressor genes involved in skin carcinogenesis in xeroderma pigmentosum patients. *Oncogene*, Vol.19, No.3, (Januart 2000), pp. 463-7, ISSN 0950-9232

Daya-Grosjean, L. & Sarasin, A. (2000). UV-specific mutations of the human patched gene in basal cell carcinomas from normal individuals and xeroderma pigmentosum patients. *Mutat Res*, Vol.450, No.1-2, (May 2000), pp. 193-9, ISSN 0027-5107

De Fabo, E.C. & Noonan, F.P. (1983). Mechanism of immune suppression by ultraviolet irradiation in vivo. I. Evidence for the existence of a unique photoreceptor in skin and its role in photoimmunology. J Exp Med, Vol.158, No.1, (July 1983), pp. 84-98, ISSN 0022-1007

de Gruiji, F.R. & van der Leun, J.C. (1982). Systemic influence of pre-irradiation of a limited skin area on UV-tumorigenesis. Photochem Photobiol, Vol.35, No.3, (March 1982), pp. 379-83, ISSN 0031-8655

de Gruijl, F.R. & Rebel, H. (2008). Early events in UV carcinogenesis--DNA damage, target cells and mutant p53 foci. *Photochem Photobiol*, Vol.84, No.2, (Mach 2008), pp. 382-7, ISSN 0031-8655

de Gruijl, F.R. & Van Der Leun, J.C. (1983). Follow up on systemic influence of partial pre-irradiation on UV-tumorigenesis. *Photochem Photobiol*, Vol.38, No.3, (September 1983), pp. 381-3, ISSN 0031-8655

de Gruijl, F.R.; van Kranen, H.J. & Mullenders, L.H. (2001). UV-induced DNA damage, repair, mutations and oncogenic pathways in skin cancer. *J Photochem Photobiol B*, Vol.63, No.1-3, (October 2001), pp. 19-27, ISSN 1011-1344

DeFabo, E.C. & Kripke, M.L. (1979). Dose-response characteristics of immunologic unresponsiveness to UV-induced tumors produced by UV irradiation of mice. *Photochem Photobiol*, Vol.30, No.3, (September 1979), pp. 385-90, ISSN 0031-8655

Diffey, B.L. (2002). Sources and measurement of ultraviolet radiation. *Methods*, Vol.28, No.1, (September 2002), pp. 4-13, ISSN 1046-2023

Dighe, A.S.; Richards, E.; Old, L.J. & Schreiber, R.D. (1994). Enhanced in vivo growth and resistance to rejection of tumor cells expressing dominant negative IFN γ receptors. *Immunity*, Vol.1, No.6, (September 1994), pp. 447-56, ISSN 1074-7613

Douki, T.; Perdiz, D.; Grof, P.; Kuluncsics, Z.; Moustacchi, E.; Cadet, J. & Sage, E. (1999). Oxidation of guanine in cellular DNA by solar UV radiation: biological role. *Photochem Photobiol*, Vol.70, No.2, (August 1999), pp. 184-90, ISSN 0031-8655

Douki, T.; Reynaud-Angelin, A.; Cadet, J. & Sage, E. (2003). Bipyrimidine photoproducts rather than oxidative lesions are the main type of DNA damage involved in the genotoxic effect of solar UVA radiation. *Biochemistry*, Vol.42, No.30, (August 2003), pp. 9221-6, ISSN 0006-2960

Dziunycz, P.; Iotzova-Weiss, G.; Eloranta, J.J.; Lauchli, S.; Hafner, J.; French, L.E. & Hofbauer, G.F. (2010). Squamous cell carcinoma of the skin shows a distinct microRNA profile modulated by UV radiation. J Invest Dermatol, Vol.130, No.11, (November 2010), pp. 2686-9, ISSN 1523-1747

Elmets, C.A.; Bergstresser, P.R.; Tigelaar, R.E.; Wood, P.J. & Streilein, J.W. (1983). Analysis of the mechanism of unresponsiveness produced by haptens painted on skin exposed to low dose ultraviolet radiation. J Exp Med, Vol.158, No.3, (September 1983), pp. 781-94, ISSN 0022-1007

Ely, J.O. & Ross, M.H. (1949). Absorption of ultraviolet light by living cells. *Nature*, Vol.163, No.4154, (June 1949), pp. 906, ISSN 0028-0836

Fisher, M.S. & Kripke, M.L. (1977). Systemic alteration induced in mice by ultraviolet light irradiation and its relationship to ultraviolet carcinogenesis. *Proc Natl Acad Sci USA*, Vol.74, No.4, (April 1977), pp. 1688-92, ISSN 0027-8424

Frisch, M.; Biggar, R.J.; Engels, E.A.; Goedert, J.J. & Group, A.-C.M.R.S. (2001). Association of cancer with AIDS-related immunosuppression in adults. *JAMA*, Vol.285, No.13, (April 2001), pp. 1736-45, ISSN 0098-7484

Fukunaga, A.; Khaskhely, N.M.; Ma, Y.; Sreevidya, C.S.; Taguchi, K.; Nishigori, C. & Ullrich, S.E. (2010). Langerhans cells serve as immunoregulatory cells by activating NKT cells. *J Immunol*, Vol.185, No.8, (October 2010), pp. 4633-40, ISSN 1550-6606

Gaddameedhi, S.; Kemp, M.G.; Reardon, J.T.; Shields, J.M.; Smith-Roe, S.L.; Kaufmann, W.K. & Sancar, A. (2010). Similar nucleotide excision repair capacity in melanocytes and melanoma cells. Cancer Res, Vol.70, No.12, (June 2010), pp. 4922-30, ISSN 1538-7445

Garibyan, L. & Fisher, D.E. (2010). How sunlight causes melanoma. *Curr Oncol Rep*, Vol.12, No.5, (Sepember 2010), pp. 319-26, ISSN 1534-6269

Garssen, J.; de Gruijl, F.; Mol, D.; de Klerk, A.; Roholl, P. & Van Loveren, H. (2001). UVA exposure affects UVB and cis-urocanic acid-induced systemic suppression of immune responses in Listeria monocytogenes-infected Balb/c mice. *Photochem Photobiol*, Vol.73, No.4, (April 2001), pp. 432-8, ISSN 0031-8655

Ghoreishi, M. & Dutz, J.P. (2006). Tolerance induction by transcutaneous immunization through ultraviolet-irradiated skin is transferable through $CD4^+CD25^+$ T regulatory cells and is dependent on host-derived IL-10. *J Immunol*, Vol.176, No.4, (February 2006), pp. 2635-44, ISSN 0022-1767

Ghosh, R.; Amstad, P. & Cerutti, P. (1993). UVB-induced DNA breaks interfere with transcriptional induction of c-fos. *Mol Cell Biol*, Vol.13, No.11, (Nov 1993), pp. 6992-9, ISSN 0270-7306

Grewe, M.; Stege, H.; Vink, A.; Klammer, M.; Ruzicka, T.; Roza, L. & Krutmann, J. (2000). Inhibition of intercellular adhesio nmolecule-1 (ICAM-1) expression in ultraviolet B-irradiated human antigen-presenting cells is restored after repair of cyclobutane pyrimidine dimers. *Exp Dermatol*, Vol.9, No.6, (December 2000), pp. 423-30, ISSN 0906-6705

Groux, H.; O'Garra, A.; Bigler, M.; Rouleau, M.; Antonenko, S.; de Vries, J.E. & Roncarolo, M.G. (1997). A $CD4^+$ T-cell subset inhibits antigen-specific T-cell responses and prevents colitis. *Nature*, Vol.389, (September 1997), pp. 737-42, ISSN 0028-0836

Guo, L.; Huang, Z.X.; Chen, X.W.; Deng, Q.K.; Yan, W.; Zhou, M.J.; Ou, C.S. & Ding, Z.H. (2009). Differential expression profiles of microRNAs in NIH3T3 cells in response to UVB irradiation. *Photochem Photobiol*, Vol.85, No.3, (May 2009), pp. 765-73, ISSN 0031-8655

Hanahan, D. & Weinberg, R.A. (2000). The hallmarks of cancer. Cell, Vol.100, No.1, (Jan 7 2000), pp. 57-70, ISSN 0092-8674

Hanahan, D. & Weinberg, R.A. (2011). Hallmarks of cancer: the next generation. *Cell*, Vol.144, No.5, (March 2011), pp. 646-74, ISSN 1097-4172

Harper, J.W. & Elledge, S.J. (2007). The DNA damage response: ten years after. Mol Cell, Vol.28, No.5, (December 2007), pp. 739-45, ISSN 1097-2765

Harrison, J.C. & Haber, J.E. (2006). Surviving the breakup: the DNA damage checkpoint. *Annu Rev Genet*, Vol.40, (June 2006), pp. 209-35, ISSN 0066-4197

Hoeijmakers, J.H. (2001). Genome maintenance mechanisms for preventing cancer. Nature, Vol.411, No.6835, (May 17 2001), pp. 366-74, ISSN 0028-0836

Holly, E.A.; Aston, D.A.; Cress, R.D.; Ahn, D.K. & Kristiansen, J.J. (1995). Cutaneous melanoma in women. I. Exposure to sunlight, ability to tan, and other risk factors related to ultraviolet light. Am J Epidemiol, Vol.141, No.10, (May 1995), pp. 923-33, ISSN 0002-9262

Hori, T.; Kuribayashi, K.; Uemoto, S.; Saito, K.; Wang, L.; Torii, M.; Shibutani, S.; Taniguchi, K.; Yagi, S.; Iida, T.; Yamamoto, C. & Kato, T. (2008). Alloantigen-specific prolongation of allograft survival in recipient mice treated by alloantigen immunization following ultraviolet-B irradiation. Transpl Immunol, Vol.19, No.1, (April 2008), pp. 45-54, ISSN 0966-3274

Hostetler, L.W.; Romerdahl, C.A. & Kripke, M.L. (1989). Specificity of antigens on UV radiation-induced antigenic tumor cell variants measured in vitro and in vivo. *Cancer Res*, Vol.49, No.5, (March 1989), pp. 1207-13, ISSN 0008-5472

Hussein, M.R.; Haemel, A.K. & Wood, G.S. (2003). Apoptosis and melanoma: molecular mechanisms. J Pathol, Vol.199, No.3, (March 2003), pp. 275-88, ISSN 0022-3417

IARC. (1992). IARC monographs on the evaluation of carcinogenic risks to humans. Solar and ultraviolet radiation. *IARC Monogr Eval Carcinog Risks Hum*, Vol.55, (1992), pp. 1-316, ISSN 1017-1606

Jacinto, F.V. & Esteller, M. (2007). Mutator pathways unleashed by epigenetic silencing in human cancer. *Mutagenesis*, Vol.22, No.4, (July 2007), pp. 247-53, ISSN 0267-8357

Jackson, S.P. & Bartek, J. (2009). The DNA-damage response in human biology and disease. *Nature*, Vol.461, No.7267, (October 2009), pp. 1071-8, ISSN 1476-4687

Jans, J.; Garinis, G.A.; Schul, W.; van Oudenaren, A.; Moorhouse, M.; Smid, M.; Sert, Y.G.; van der Velde, A.; Rijksen, Y.; de Gruijl, F.R.; van der Spek, P.J.; Yasui, A.; Hoeijmakers, J.H.; Leenen, P.J. & van der Horst, G.T. (2006). Differential role of basal keratinocytes in UV-induced immunosuppression and skin cancer. *Mol Cell Biol*, Vol.26, No.22, (November 2006), pp. 8515-26, ISSN 0270-7306

Jans, J.; Schul, W.; Sert, Y.G.; Rijksen, Y.; Rebel, H.; Eker, A.P.; Nakajima, S.; van Steeg, H.; de Gruijl, F.R.; Yasui, A.; Hoeijmakers, J.H. & van der Horst, G.T. (2005). Powerful skin cancer protection by a CPD-photolyase transgene. Curr Biol, Vol.15, No.2, (January 2005), pp. 105-15, ISSN 0960-9822

Jantschitsch, C.; Majewski, S.; Maeda, A.; Schwarz, T. & Schwarz, A. (2009). Infrared radiation confers resistance to UV-induced apoptosis via reduction of DNA damage and upregulation of antiapoptotic proteins. *J Invest Dermatol*, Vol.129, No.5, (May 2009), pp. 1271-9, ISSN 1523-1747

Jiveskog, S.; Ragnarsson-Olding, B.; Platz, A. & Ringborg, U. (1998). N-ras mutations are common in melanomas from sun-exposed skin of humans but rare in mucosal membranes or unexposed skin. *J Invest Dermatol*, Vol.111, No.5, (November 1998), pp. 757-61, ISSN 0022-202X

Kaneko, K.; Smetana-Just, U.; Matsui, M.; Young, A.R.; John, S.; Norval, M. & Walker, S.L. (2008). cis-Urocanic acid initiates gene transcription in primary human keratinocytes. *J Immunol*, Vol.181, No.1, (July 2008), pp. 217-24, ISSN 0022-1767

Kaneko, K.; Travers, J.B.; Matsui, M.S.; Young, A.R.; Norval, M. & Walker, S.L. (2009). cis-Urocanic acid stimulates primary human keratinocytes independently of serotonin or platelet-activating factor receptors. *J Invest Dermatol*, Vol.129, No.11, (November 2009), pp. 2567-73, ISSN 1523-1747

Kanellou, P.; Zaravinos, A.; Zioga, M.; Stratigos, A.; Baritaki, S.; Soufla, G.; Zoras, O. & Spandidos, D.A. (2008). Genomic instability, mutations and expression analysis of the tumour suppressor genes p14(ARF), p15(INK4b), p16(INK4a) and p53 in actinic keratosis. Cancer Lett, Vol.264, No.1, (June 2008), pp. 145-61, ISSN 0304-3835

Kaplan, D.H.; Shankaran, V.; Dighe, A.S.; Stockert, E.; Aguet, M.; Old, L.J. & Schreiber, R.D. (1998). Demonstration of an interferon gamma-dependent tumor surveillance system in immunocompetent mice. *Proc Natl Acad Sci U S A*, Vol.95, No.13, (June 1998), pp. 7556-61, ISSN 0027-842

Katiyar, S.K. (2007). UV-induced immune suppression and photocarcinogenesis: chemoprevention by dietary botanical agents. *Cancer Lett*, Vol.255, No.1, (Sepember 2007), pp. 1-11, ISSN 0304-3835

Kielbassa, C.; Roza, L. & Epe, B. (1997). Wavelength dependence of oxidative DNA damage induced by UV and visible light. *Carcinogenesis*, Vol.18, No.4, (April 1997), pp. 811-6, ISSN 0143-3334

Kreimer-Erlacher, H.; Seidl, H.; Back, B.; Kerl, H. & Wolf, P. (2001). High mutation frequency at Ha-ras exons 1-4 in squamous cell carcinomas from PUVA-treated psoriasis patients. *Photochem Photobiol*, Vol.74, No.2, (August 2001), pp. 323-30, ISSN 0031-8655

Kripke, M.L. (1974). Antigenicity of murine skin tumors induced by ultraviolet light. *J Natl Cancer Inst*, Vol.53, No.5, (November 1974), pp. 1333-6, ISSN 0027-8874

Kripke, M.L.; Cox, P.A.; Alas, L.G. & Yarosh, D.B. (1992). Pyrimidine dimers in DNA initiate systemic immunosuppression in UV-irradiated mice. *Proc Natl Acad Sci U S A*, Vol.89, No.16, (August 1992), pp. 7516-20, ISSN 0027-8424

Kripke, M.L. & Fisher, M.S. (1976). Immunologic parameters of ultraviolet carcinogenesis. *J Natl Cancer Inst*, Vol.57, No.1, (July 1976), pp. 211-5, ISSN 0027-8874

Kripke, M.L.; Lofgreen, J.S.; Beard, J.; Jessup, J.M. & Fisher, M.S. (1977). In vivo immune responses of mice during carcinogenesis by ultraviolet irradiation. *J Natl Cancer Inst*, Vol.59, No.4, (October 1977), pp. 1227-30, ISSN 0027-8874

Kripke, M.L.; Thorn, R.M.; Lill, P.H.; Civin, C.I.; Pazmino, N.H. & Fisher, M.S. (1979). Further characterization of immunological unresponsiveness induced in mice by ultraviolet radiation. Growth and induction of nonultraviolet-induced tumors in ultraviolet-irradiated mice. Transplantation, Vol.28, No.3, (Sepember 1979), pp. 212-7, ISSN 0041-1337

Laihia, J.K.; Kallio, J.P.; Taimen, P.; Kujari, H.; Kahari, V.M. & Leino, L. (2010). Protodynamic intracellular acidification by cis-urocanic acid promotes apoptosis of melanoma cells in vitro and in vivo. *J Invest Dermatol*, Vol.130, No.10, (October 2010), pp. 2431-9, ISSN 1523-1747

Laihia, J.K.; Pylkkanen, L.; Laato, M.; Bostrom, P.J. & Leino, L. (2009). Protodynamic therapy for bladder cancer: in vitro results of a novel treatment concept. *BJU Int*, Vol.104, No.9, (November 2009), pp. 1233-8, ISSN 1464-410X

Lippke, J.A.; Gordon, L.K.; Brash, D.E. & Haseltine, W.A. (1981). Distribution of UV light-induced damage in a defined sequence of human DNA: detection of alkaline-sensitive lesions at pyrimidine nucleoside-cytidine sequences. *Proc Natl Acad Sci U S A*, Vol.78, No.6, (June 1981), pp. 3388-92, ISSN 0027-8424

Livneh, Z. (2006). Keeping mammalian mutation load in check: regulation of the activity of error-prone DNA polymerases by p53 and p21. *Cell Cycle*, Vol.5, No.17, (September 2006), pp. 1918-22, ISSN 1551-4005

Loeffelbein, D.J.; Szilinski, K. & Hölzle, F. (2009). Immunosuppressive regimen influences incidence of skin cancer in renal and pancreatic transplant recipients. *Transplantation*, Vol.88, No.12, (December 2009), pp. 1398-9, ISSN 1534-6080

Loser, K.; Apelt, J.; Voskort, M.; Mohaupt, M.; Balkow, S.; Schwarz, T.; Grabbe, S. & Beissert, S. (2007). IL-10 controls ultraviolet-induced carcinogenesis in mice. *J Immunol*, Vol.179, No.1, (July 2007), pp. 365-71, ISSN 0022-1767

Loser, K.; Mehling, A.; Loeser, S.; Apelt, J.; Kuhn, A.; Grabbe, S.; Schwarz, T.; Penninger, J.M. & Beissert, S. (2006). Epidermal RANKL controls regulatory T-cell numbers via activation of dendritic cells. *Nat Med*, Vol.12, No.12, (December 2006), pp. 1372-9, ISSN 1078-8956

Maeda, A.; Beissert, S.; Schwarz, T. & Schwarz, A. (2008). Phenotypic and functional characterization of ultraviolet radiation-induced regulatory T cells. *J Immunol*, Vol.180, No.5, (March 2008), pp. 3065-71, ISSN 0022-1767

Mahnke, K.; Qian, Y.; Knop, J. & Enk, A.H. (2003). Induction of $CD4^+/CD25^+$ regulatory T cells by targeting of antigens to immature dendritic cells. *Blood*, Vol.101, No.12, (Junuary 2003), pp. 4862-9, ISSN 0006-4971

Majewski, S.; Jantschitsch, C.; Maeda, A.; Schwarz, T. & Schwarz, A. (2010). IL-23 antagonizes UVR-induced immunosuppression through two mechanisms: reduction of UVR-induced DNA damage and inhibition of UVR-induced regulatory T cells. *J Invest Dermatol*, Vol.130, No.2, (February 2010), pp. 554-62, ISSN 1523-1747

Markovitsi, D.; Gustavsson, T. & Banyasz, A. (2010). Absorption of UV radiation by DNA: spatial and temporal features. Mutat Res, Vol.704, No.1-3, (April 2010), pp. 21-8, ISSN 0027-5107

Matsumura, Y.; Moodycliffe, A.M.; Nghiem, D.X.; Ullrich, S.E. & Ananthaswamy, H.N. (2005). Inverse relationship between increased apoptosis and decreased skin cancer in UV-irradiated $CD1d^{-/-}$ mice. *Photochem Photobiol*, Vol.81, No.1, (January 2005), pp. 46-51, ISSN 0031-8655

Maurer, M.; Seidel-Guyenot, W.; Metz, M.; Knop, J. & Steinbrink, K. (2003). Critical role of IL-10 in the induction of low zone tolerance to contact allergens. *J Clin Invest*, Vol.112, No.3, (August 2003), pp. 432-9, ISSN 0021-9738

Mitchell, D.L.; Jen, J. & Cleaver, J.E. (1992). Sequence specificity of cyclobutane pyrimidine dimers in DNA treated with solar (ultraviolet B) radiation. *Nucleic Acids Res*, Vol.20, No.2, (January 1992), pp. 225-9, ISSN 0305-1048

Miyauchi-Hashimoto, H.; Tanaka, K. & Horio, T. (1996). Enhanced inflammation and immunosuppression by ultraviolet radiation in xeroderma pigmentosum group A (XPA) model mice. *J Invest Dermatol*, Vol.107, No.3, (September 1996), pp. 343-8, ISSN 0022-202X

Moloney, F.J.; Comber, H.; O'Lorcain, P.; O'Kelly, P.; Conlon, P.J. & Murphy, G.M. (2006). A population-based study of skin cancer incidence and prevalence in renal transplant recipients. *Br J Dermatol*, Vol.154, No.3, (March 2006), pp. 498-504, ISSN 0007-0963

Moodycliffe, A.M.; Bucana, C.D.; Kripke, M.L.; Norval, M. & Ullrich, S.E. (1996). Differential effects of a monoclonal antibody to cis-urocanic acid on the suppression of delayed and contact hypersensitivity following ultraviolet irradiation. *J Immunol*, Vol.157, No.7, (October 1996), pp. 2891-9, ISSN 0022-1767

Moodycliffe, A.M.; Nghiem, D.; Clydesdale, G. & Ullrich, S.E. (2000). Immune suppression and skin cancer development: regulation by NKT cells. *Nat Immunol*, Vol.1, No.6, (December 2000), pp. 521-5, ISSN 1529-2908

Mouret, S.; Baudouin, C.; Charveron, M.; Favier, A.; Cadet, J. & Douki, T. (2006). Cyclobutane pyrimidine dimers are predominant DNA lesions in whole human skin exposed to UVA radiation. *Proc Natl Acad Sci U S A*, Vol.103, No.37, (September 2006), pp. 13765-70, ISSN 0027-8424

Muller, G.; Saloga, J.; Germann, T.; Schuler, G.; Knop, J. & Enk, A.H. (1995). IL-12 as mediator and adjuvant for the induction of contact sensitivity in vivo. *J Immunol*, Vol.155, No.10, (November 1995), pp. 4661-8, ISSN 0022-1767

Nghiem, D.X.; Kazimi, N.; Clydesdale, G.; Ananthaswamy, H.N.; Kripke, M.L. & Ullrich, S.E. (2001). Ultraviolet A radiation suppresses an established immune response: Implications for sunscreen design. *J Invest Dermatol*, Vol.117, (November 2001), pp. 1193-9, ISSN 0022-1767

Nghiem, D.X.; Kazimi, N.; Mitchell, D.L.; Vink, A.A.; Ananthaswamy, H.N.; Kripke, M.L. & Ullrich, S.E. (2002). Mechanisms underlying the suppression of established immune responses by ultraviolet radiation. *J Invest Dermatol*, Vol.119, (September 2002), pp. 600-8, ISSN 0022-202X

Nishigori, C.; Yarosh, D.; O'Connor, A.; Shreedhar, V.K.; Ullrich, S.E.; Cox, P. & Kripke, M.L. (1998). HindIII liposomes suppress delayed-type hypersensitivity responses in vivo and induce epidermal IL-10 in vitro. *J Immunol*, Vol.161, No.6, (September 1998), pp. 2684-91, ISSN 0022-1767

Nishigori, C.; Yarosh, D.B.; Ullrich, S.E.; Vink, A.A.; Bucana, C.D.; Roza, L. & Kripke, M.L. (1996). Evidence that DNA damage triggers interleukin 10 cytokine production in UV-irradiated murine keratinocytes. *Proc Natl Acad Sci U S A*, Vol.93, No.19, (September 1996), pp. 10354-9, ISSN 0027-8424

Nishikawa, H.; Kato, T.; Hirayama, M.; Orito, Y.; Sato, E.; Harada, N.; Gnjatic, S.; Old, L.J. & Shiku, H. (2008). Regulatory T cell-resistant CD8+ T cells induced by glucocorticoid-induced tumor necrosis factor receptor signaling. *Cancer Res*, Vol.68, No.14, (Jul 15 2008), pp. 5948-54, ISSN 1538-7445

Nishikawa, H.; Kato, T.; Tanida, K.; Hiasa, A.; Tawara, I.; Ikeda, H.; Ikarashi, Y.; Wakasugi, H.; Kronenberg, M.; Nakayama, T.; Taniguchi, M.; Kuribayashi, K.; Old, L.J. & Shiku, H. (2003). $CD4^+$ $CD25^+$ T cells responding to serologically defined autoantigens suppress antitumor immune responses. *Proc Natl Acad Sci U S A*, Vol.100, No.19, (September 2003), pp. 10902-6, ISSN 0027-8424

Nishikawa, H.; Kato, T.; Tawara, I.; Saito, K.; Ikeda, H.; Kuribayashi, K.; Allen, P.M.; Schreiber, R.D.; Sakaguchi, S.; Old, L.J. & Shiku, H. (2005). Definition of target antigens for naturally occurring $CD4^+$ $CD25^+$ regulatory T cells. *J Exp Med*, Vol.201, No.5, (March 2005), pp. 681-6, ISSN 0022-1007

Nishikawa, H.; Kato, T.; Tawara, I.; Takemitsu, T.; Saito, K.; Wang, L.; Ikarashi, Y.; Wakasugi, H.; Nakayama, T.; Taniguchi, M.; Kuribayashi, K.; Old, L.J. & Shiku, H. (2005). Accelerated chemically induced tumor development mediated by $CD4^+CD25^+$ regulatory T cells in wild-type hosts. *Proc Natl Acad Sci U S A*, Vol.102, No.26, (June 2005), pp. 9253-7, ISSN 0027-8424

Noonan, F.P.; De Fabo, E.C. & Kripke, M.L. (1981). Suppression of contact hypersensitivity by ultraviolet radiation: an experimental model. *Springer Semin Immunopathol*, Vol.4, No.3, (1981), pp. 293-304, ISSN 0344-4325

Norval, M.; Gibbs, N.K. & Gilmour, J. (1995). The role of urocanic acid in UV-induced immunosuppression: recent advances (1992-1994). *Photochem Photobiol*, Vol.62, No.2, (August 1995), pp. 209-17, ISSN 0031-8655

Perdiz, D.; Grof, P.; Mezzina, M.; Nikaido, O.; Moustacchi, E. & Sage, E. (2000). Distribution and repair of bipyrimidine photoproducts in solar UV-irradiated mammalian cells. Possible role of Dewar photoproducts in solar mutagenesis. *J Biol Chem*, Vol.275, No.35, (September 2000), pp. 26732-42, ISSN 0021-9258

Peuhu, E.; Kaunisto, A.; Laihia, J.K.; Leino, L. & Eriksson, J.E. (2010). Molecular targets for the protodynamic action of cis-urocanic acid in human bladder carcinoma cells. BMC Cancer, Vol.10, (October 2010), pp. 521, ISSN 1471-2407

Ping, X.L.; Ratner, D.; Zhang, H.; Wu, X.L.; Zhang, M.J.; Chen, F.F.; Silvers, D.N.; Peacocke, M. & Tsou, H.C. (2001). PTCH mutations in squamous cell carcinoma of the skin. *J Invest Dermatol*, Vol.116, No.4, (April 2001), pp. 614-6, ISSN 0022-202X

Pot, C.; Jin, H.; Awasthi, A.; Liu, S.M.; Lai, C.Y.; Madan, R.; Sharpe, A.H.; Karp, C.L.; Miaw, S.C.; Ho, I.C. & Kuchroo, V.K. (2009). Cutting edge: IL-27 induces the transcription factor c-Maf, cytokine IL-21, and the costimulatory receptor ICOS that coordinately act together to promote differentiation of IL-10-producing Tr1 cells. *J Immunol*, Vol.183, No.2, (July 2009), pp. 797-801, ISSN 1550-6606

Pothof, J.; Verkaik, N.S.; Hoeijmakers, J.H. & van Gent, D.C. (2009). MicroRNA responses and stress granule formation modulate the DNA damage response. *Cell Cycle*, Vol.8, No.21, (November 2009), pp. 3462-8, ISSN 1551-4005

Rees, J. (1994). Genetic alterations in non-melanoma skin cancer. *J Invest Dermatol*, Vol.103, No.6, (December 1994), pp. 747-50, ISSN 0022-202X

Rigel, D.S. (2008). Cutaneous ultraviolet exposure and its relationship to the development of skin cancer. *J Am Acad Dermatol*, Vol.58, No.5 Suppl 2, (May 2008), pp. S129-32, ISSN 1097-6787

Rivas, J.M. & Ullrich, S.E. (1992). Systemic suppression of DTH by supernatants from UV-irradiated keratinocytes: an essential role for keratinocyte-derived IL-10. *J Immunol*, Vol.149, (December 1992), pp. 3865-71, ISSN 0022-1767

Rivas, J.M. & Ullrich, S.E. (1994). The role of IL-4, IL-10, and TNF-α in the immune suppression induced by ultraviolet radiation. *J Leukoc Biol*, Vol.56, (December 1994), pp. 769-75, ISSN 0741-5400

Roberts, L.K.; Lynch, D.H. & Daynes, R.A. (1982). Evidence for two functionally distinct cross-reactive tumor antigens associated with ultraviolet light and chemically induced tumors. *Transplantation*, Vol.33, No.4, (April 1982), pp. 352-60, ISSN 0041-1337

Rochette, P.J.; Therrien, J.P.; Drouin, R.; Perdiz, D.; Bastien, N.; Drobetsky, E.A. & Sage, E. (2003). UVA-induced cyclobutane pyrimidine dimers form predominantly at thymine-thymine dipyrimidines and correlate with the mutation spectrum in rodent cells. *Nucleic Acids Res*, Vol.31, No.11, (June 2003), pp. 2786-94, ISSN 1362-4962

Roncarolo, M.G.; Gregori, S.; Battaglia, M.; Bacchetta, R.; Fleischhauer, K. & Levings, M.K. (2006). Interleukin-10-secreting type 1 regulatory T cells in rodents and humans. *Immunol Rev*, Vol.212, (August 2006), pp. 28-50, ISSN 0105-2896

Runger, T.M. (2007). How different wavelengths of the ultraviolet spectrum contribute to skin carcinogenesis: the role of cellular damage responses. *J Invest Dermatol*, Vol.127, No.9, (Sepember 2007), pp. 2103-5, ISSN 1523-1747

Sakaguchi, S.; Wing, K. & Miyara, M. (2007). Regulatory T cells - a brief history and perspective. Eur J Immunol, Vol.37 Suppl 1, (November 2007), pp. S116-23, ISSN 0014-2980

Saridaki, Z.; Liloglou, T.; Zafiropoulos, A.; Koumantaki, E.; Zoras, O. & Spandidos, D.A. (2003). Mutational analysis of CDKN2A genes in patients with squamous cell carcinoma of the skin. *Br J Dermatol*, Vol.148, No.4, (April 2003), pp. 638-48, ISSN 0007-0963

Schmitt, D.A.; Owen-Schaub, L. & Ullrich, S.E. (1995). Effect of IL-12 on immune suppression and suppressor cell induction by ultraviolet radiation. *J Immunol*, Vol.154, No.10, (May 1995), pp. 5114-20, ISSN 0022-1767

Schwarz, A.; Beissert, S.; Grosse-Heithmeyer, K.; Gunzer, M.; Bluestone, J.A.; Grabbe, S. & Schwarz, T. (2000). Evidence for functional relevance of CTLA-4 in ultraviolet-radiation-induced tolerance. *J Immunol*, Vol.165, (August 2000), pp. 1824-31, ISSN 0022-1767

Schwarz, A.; Grabbe, S.; Aragane, Y.; Sandkuhl, K.; Riemann, H.; Luger, T.A.; Kubin, M.; Trinchieri, G. & Schwarz, T. (1996). Interleukin-12 prevents ultraviolet B-induced local immunosuppression and overcomes UVB-induced tolerance. *J Invest Dermatol*, Vol.106, No.6, (Jun e1996), pp. 1187-91, ISSN 0022-202X

Schwarz, A.; Maeda, A.; Kernebeck, K.; van Steeg, H.; Beissert, S. & Schwarz, T. (2005). Prevention of UV radiation-induced immunosuppression by IL-12 is dependent on DNA repair. J Exp Med, Vol.201, No.2, (January 2005), pp. 173-9, ISSN 0022-1007

Schwarz, A.; Maeda, A.; Stander, S.; van Steeg, H. & Schwarz, T. (2006). IL-18 reduces ultraviolet radiation-induced DNA damage and thereby affects photoimmunosuppression. *J Immunol*, Vol.176, No.5, (March 2006), pp. 2896-901, ISSN 0022-1767

Schwarz, A.; Maeda, A.; Wild, M.K.; Kernebeck, K.; Gross, N.; Aragane, Y.; Beissert, S.; Vestweber, D. & Schwarz, T. (2004). Ultraviolet radiation-induced regulatory T cells not only inhibit the induction but can suppress the effector phase of contact hypersensitivity. *J Immunol*, Vol.172, (January 2004), pp. 1036-43, ISSN 0022-1767

Schwarz, A.; Stander, S.; Berneburg, M.; Bohm, M.; Kulms, D.; van Steeg, H.; Grosse-Heitmeyer, K.; Krutmann, J. & Schwarz, T. (2002). Interleukin-12 suppresses ultraviolet radiation-induced apoptosis by inducing DNA repair. *Nat Cell Biol*, Vol.4, No.1, (January 2002), pp. 26-31, ISSN 1465-7392

Schwarz, T. (2010). The dark and the sunny sides of UVR-induced immunosuppression: photoimmunology revisited. *J Invest Dermatol*, Vol.130, No.1, (January 2010), pp. 49-54, ISSN 1523-1747

Selcuklu, S.D.; Donoghue, M.T. & Spillane, C. (2009). miR-21 as a key regulator of oncogenic processes. *Biochem Soc Trans*, Vol.37, No.Pt 4, (August 2009), pp. 918-25, ISSN 1470-8752

Shankaran, V.; Ikeda, H.; Bruce, A.T.; White, J.M.; Swanson, P.E.; Old, L.J. & Schreiber, R.D. (2001). IFNγ and lymphocytes prevent primary tumour development and shape tumour immunogenicity. *Nature*, Vol.410, No.6832, (April 2001), pp. 1107-11, ISSN 0028-0836

Shen, J.; Bao, S. & Reeve, V.E. (1999). Modulation of IL-10, IL-12, and IFN-γ in the epidermis of hairless mice by UVA (320-400 nm) and UVB (280-320 nm) radiation. *J Invest Dermatol*, Vol.113, No.6, (December 1999), pp. 1059-64, ISSN 0022-202X

Shreedhar, V.; Giese, T.; Sung, V.W. & Ullrich, S.E. (1998). A cytokine cascade including prostaglandin E2, IL-4, and IL-10 is responsible for UV-induced systemic immune suppression. *J Immunol*, Vol.160, (April 1998), pp. 3783-9, ISSN 0022-1767

Smyth, M.J.; Crowe, N.Y. & Godfrey, D.I. (2001). NK cells and NKT cells collaborate in host protection from methylcholanthrene-induced fibrosarcoma. *Int Immunol*, Vol.13, No.4, (April 2001), pp. 459-63, ISSN 0953-8178

Soufir, N.; Moles, J.P.; Vilmer, C.; Moch, C.; Verola, O.; Rivet, J.; Tesniere, A.; Dubertret, L. & Basset-Seguin, N. (1999). P16 UV mutations in human skin epithelial tumors. Oncogene, Vol.18, No.39, (Sepember 1999), pp. 5477-81, ISSN 0950-9232

Sparrow, L.E.; Eldon, M.J.; English, D.R. & Heenan, P.J. (1998). p16 and p21WAF1 protein expression in melanocytic tumors by immunohistochemistry. *Am J Dermatopathol*, Vol.20, No.3, (June 1998), pp. 255-61, ISSN 0193-1091

Spellman, C.W. & Daynes, R.A. (1977). Modification of immunological potential by ultraviolet radiation. II. Generation of suppressor cells in short-term UV-irradiated mice. *Transplantation*, Vol.24, No.2, (August 1977), pp. 120-6, ISSN 0041-1337

Spellman, C.W. & Daynes, R.A. (1984). Cross-reactive transplantation antigens between UV-irradiated skin and UV-induced tumors. *Photodermatol*, Vol.1, No.4, (August 1984), pp. 164-9, ISSN 0108-9684

Spellman, C.W.; Woodward, J.G. & Daynes, R.A. (1977). Modification of immunological potential by ultraviolet radiation. I. Immune status of short-term UV-irradiated mice. *Transplantation*, Vol.24, No.2, (August 1977), pp. 112-9, ISSN 0041-1337

Spencer, J.M.; Kahn, S.M.; Jiang, W.; DeLeo, V.A. & Weinstein, I.B. (1995). Activated ras genes occur in human actinic keratoses, premalignant precursors to squamous cell carcinomas. *Arch Dermatol*, Vol.131, No.7, (July 1995), pp. 796-800, ISSN 0003-987X

Sreevidya, C.S.; Fukunaga, A.; Khaskhely, N.M.; Masaki, T.; Ono, R.; Nishigori, C. & Ullrich, S.E. (2010). Agents that reverse UV-Induced immune suppression and photocarcinogenesis affect DNA repair. *J Invest Dermatol*, Vol.130, No.5, (May 2010), pp. 1428-37, ISSN 1523-1747

Street, S.E.; Cretney, E. & Smyth, M.J. (2001). Perforin and interferon-gamma activities independently control tumor initiation, growth, and metastasis. *Blood*, Vol.97, No.1, (January 2001), pp. 192-7, ISSN 0006-4971

Street, S.E.A.; Trapani, J.A.; MacGregor, D. & Smyth, M.J. (2002). Suppression of lymphoma and epithelial malignancies effected by interferon gamma. *J Exp Med*, Vol.196, No.1, (July 2002), pp. 129-34, ISSN 0022-1007

Toda, M.; Wang, L.; Ogura, S.; Torii, M.; Kurachi, M.; Kakimi, K.; Nishikawa, H.; Matsushima, K.; Shiku, H.; Kuribayashi, K. & Kato, T. (2011). UV irradiation of immunized mice induces type 1 regulatory T cells that suppress tumor antigen specific cytotoxic T lymphocyte responses. *Int J Cancer*, (201), in press

Toews, G.B.; Bergstresser, P.R. & Streilein, J.W. (1980). Epidermal Langerhans cell density determines whether contact hypersensitivity or unresponsiveness follows skin painting with DNFB. *J Immunol*, Vol.124, No.1, (January 1980), pp. 445-53, ISSN 0022-1767

Tremezaygues, L.; Seifert, M.; Tilgen, W. & Reichrath, J. (2009). 1,25-dihydroxyvitamin D(3) protects human keratinocytes against UV-B-induced damage: In vitro analysis of cell viability/proliferation, DNA-damage and -repair. *Dermatoendocrinol*, Vol.1, No.4, (July 2009), pp. 239-45, ISSN 1938-198

Trinchieri, G. (2003). Interleukin-12 and the regulation of innate resistance and adaptive immunity. *Nat Rev Immunol*, Vol.3, No.2, (February 2003), pp. 133-46, ISSN 1474-1733

Tyrrell, R.M. (1994). The molecular and cellular pathology of solar ultraviolet radiation. *Mol Aspects Med*, Vol.15, No.1, (January 1994), pp. 1-77, ISSN 0098-2997

Ullrich, S.E. & Kripke, M.L. (1984). Mechanisms in the suppression of tumor rejection produced in mice by repeated UV irradiation. *J Immunol*, Vol.133, No.5, (November 1984), pp. 2786-90, ISSN 0022-1767

Ullrich, S.E.; Nghiem, D.X. & Khaskina, P. (2007). Suppression of an established immune response by UVA--a critical role for mast cells. *Photochem Photobiol*, Vol.83, No.5, (September 2007), pp. 1095-100, ISSN 0031-8655

Urbach, F. (1991). Potential health effects of climatic change: effects of increased ultraviolet radiation on man. *Environ Health Perspect*, Vol.96, (December 1991), pp. 175-6, ISSN 0091-6765

Vajdic, C.M.; McDonald, S.P.; McCredie, M.R.E.; van Leeuwen, M.T.; Stewart, J.H.; Law, M.; Chapman, J.R.; Webster, A.C.; Kaldor, J.M. & Grulich, A.E. (2006). Cancer incidence before and after kidney transplantation. *JAMA*, Vol.296, No.23, (December 2006), pp. 2823-31, ISSN 1538-3598

van der Schroeff, J.G.; Evers, L.M.; Boot, A.J. & Bos, J.L. (1990). Ras oncogene mutations in basal cell carcinomas and squamous cell carcinomas of human skin. *J Invest Dermatol*, Vol.94, No.4, (April 1990), pp. 423-5, ISSN 0022-202X

Vesely, M.D.; Kershaw, M.H.; Schreiber, R.D. & Smyth, M.J. (2011). Natural innate and adaptive immunity to cancer. *Annu Rev Immunol*, Vol.29, (April 2011), pp. 235-71, ISSN 1545-3278

Vieira, P.L.; Christensen, J.R.; Minaee, S.; J., O.N.E.; Barrat, F.J.; Boonstra, A.; Barthlott, T.; Stockinger, B.; Wraith, D.C. & O'Garra, A. (2004). IL-10 secreting regulatory T cells do not express Foxp3 but have comparable regulatory function to naturally occurring CD4+CD25+ regulatory T cells. *J Immunol*, Vol.172, (May 2004), pp. 5986-93, ISSN 0022-1767

Wakkach, A.; Cottrez, F. & Groux, H. (2001). Differentiation of regulatory T cells 1 is induced by CD2 costimulation. *J Immunol*, Vol.167, (September 2001), pp. 3107-13, ISSN 0022-1767

Wakkach, A.; Founier, N.; Brun, V.; Breittmayer, J.-P.; Cottrez, F. & Groux, H. (2003). Characterization of dendritic cells that induce tolerance and T regulatory 1 cell differentiation in vivo. *Immunity*, Vol.18, (May 2003), pp. 605-17, ISSN 1074-7613

Walterscheid, J.P.; Nghiem, D.X.; Kazimi, N.; Nutt, L.K.; McConkey, D.J.; Norval, M. & Ullrich, S.E. (2006). Cis-urocanic acid, a sunlight-induced immunosuppressive factor, activates immune suppression via the 5-HT2A receptor. *Proc Natl Acad Sci U S A*, Vol.103, No.46, (November 2006), pp. 17420-5, ISSN 0027-8424

Waltz, P. & Chodick, G. (2008). Assessment of ecological regression in the study of colon, breast, ovary, non-Hodgkin's lymphoma, or prostate cancer and residential UV. Eur J Cancer Prev, Vol.17, No.3, (June 2008), pp. 279-86, ISSN 1473-5709

Wang, L.; Saito, K.; Toda, M.; Hori, T.; Torii, M.; Ma, N.; Katayama, N.; Shiku, H.; Kuribayashi, K. & Kato, T. (2010). UV irradiation after immunization induces type 1 regulatory T cells that suppress Th2-type immune responses via secretion of IL-10. *Immunobiology*, Vol.215, (May 2010), pp. 124-32, ISSN 1878-3279

Wang, L.; Toda, M.; Saito, K.; Hori, T.; Horii, T.; Shiku, H.; Kuribayashi, K. & Kato, T. (2008). Post-immune UV-irradiation induces Tr1-like regulatory T cells that suppress humoral immune responses. *Int Immunol*, Vol.20, (January 2008), pp. 57-70, ISSN 1460-2377

Wogan, G.N.; Hecht, S.S.; Felton, J.S.; Conney, A.H. & Loeb, L.A. (2004). Environmental and chemical carcinogenesis. *Semin Cancer Biol*, Vol.14, No.6, (December 2004), pp. 473-86, ISSN 1044-579X

Wood, R.D.; Mitchell, M. & Lindahl, T. (2005). Human DNA repair genes, 2005. *Mutat Res*, Vol.577, No.1-2, (September 2005), pp. 275-83, ISSN 0027-5107

Xu, J.; Yang, Y.; Qiu, G.; Lal, G.; Wu, Z.; Levy, D.E.; Ochando, J.C.; Bromberg, J.S. & Ding, Y. (2009). c-Maf regulates IL-10 expression during Th17 polarization. *J Immunol*, Vol.182, No.10, (May 2009), pp. 6226-36, ISSN 1550-6606

Yarosh, D.; Alas, L.G.; Yee, V.; Oberyszyn, A.; Kibitel, J.T.; Mitchell, D.; Rosenstein, R.; Spinowitz, A. & Citron, M. (1992). Pyrimidine dimer removal enhanced by DNA repair liposomes reduces the incidence of UV skin cancer in mice. *Cancer Res*, Vol.52, No.15, (August 1992), pp. 4227-31, ISSN 0008-5472

Yarosh, D.; Klein, J.; O'Connor, A.; Hawk, J.; Rafal, E. & Wolf, P. (2001). Effect of topically applied T4 endonuclease V in liposomes on skin cancer in xeroderma pigmentosum: a randomised study. Xeroderma Pigmentosum Study Group. *Lancet*, Vol.357, No.9260, (March 2001), pp. 926-9, ISSN 0140-6736

Zhang, H.; Ping, X.L.; Lee, P.K.; Wu, X.L.; Yao, Y.J.; Zhang, M.J.; Silvers, D.N.; Ratner, D.; Malhotra, R.; Peacocke, M. & Tsou, H.C. (2001). Role of PTCH and p53 genes in early-onset basal cell carcinoma. *Am J Pathol*, Vol.158, No.2, (February 2001), pp. 381-5, ISSN 0002-9440

Zhang, X.; Rosenstein, B.S.; Wang, Y.; Lebwohl, M.; Mitchell, D.M. & Wei, H. (1997). Induction of 8-oxo-7,8-dihydro-2'-deoxyguanosine by ultraviolet radiation in calf thymus DNA and HeLa cells. *Photochem Photobiol*, Vol.65, No.1, (January 1997), pp. 119-24, ISSN 0031-8655

Zhang, Y.; Holford, T.R.; Leaderer, B.; Boyle, P.; Zhu, Y.; Wang, R.; Zou, K.; Zhang, B.; Wise, J.P., Sr.; Qin, Q.; Kilfoy, B.; Han, J. & Zheng, T. (2007). Ultraviolet radiation exposure and risk of non-Hodgkin's lymphoma. *Am J Epidemiol*, Vol.165, No.11, (June 2007), pp. 1255-64, ISSN 0002-9262

Ziegler, A.; Jonason, A.S.; Leffell, D.J.; Simon, J.A.; Sharma, H.W.; Kimmelman, J.; Remington, L.; Jacks, T. & Brash, D.E. (1994). Sunburn and p53 in the onset of skin cancer. *Nature*, Vol.372, No.6508, (December 1994), pp. 773-6, ISSN 0028-0836

Ziegler, A.; Leffell, D.J.; Kunala, S.; Sharma, H.W.; Gailani, M.; Simon, J.A.; Halperin, A.J.; Baden, H.P.; Shapiro, P.E.; Bale, A.E. & et al. (1993). Mutation hotspots due to sunlight in the p53 gene of nonmelanoma skin cancers. *Proc Natl Acad Sci U S A*, Vol.90, No.9, (May 1993), pp. 4216-20, ISSN 0027-8424

3

Genetic Predisposition to Cutaneous Squamous Cell Carcinoma

Yi-Zhen Ng[1,2], Jasbani H.S Dayal[1] and Andrew P. South[1]
[1]*Division of Cancer Research, Medical Research Institute, Level 7 Clinical Research Centre, Ninewells Hospital and Medical School, University of Dundee, Dundee,*
[2]*Epithelial Biology Group, A*STAR Institute of Medical Biology,*
[1]*UK*
[2]*Singapore*

1. Introduction

Ultraviolet (UV) radiation is the most ubiquitous mutagen known and as a direct result the skin is by far the most common site for cancer in Caucasian populations. In United Kingdom, non-melanoma skin cancer (NMSC) is the most frequent occurring cancer registration with over 98,854 cases in 2008, although estimates place it higher due to under-reporting (CRUK, 2011a). Approximately three-quarters of NMSC are benign basal cell carcinomas (BCCs), while the remaining quarter consists predominantly of cutaneous squamous cell carcinomas (cSCC). NMSC accounts for 1 in 4 skin cancer deaths, the majority of which is attributed to the more malignant cSCC (Office for National Statistics). The overall prognosis is generally excellent for NMSC with only 491 deaths reported in UK in 2008 (mortality rate of 0.5 per 100,000 population) (CRUK, 2011b). However, those patients presenting with regional metastasis have poor outcome; 5-year survival in this group is 25-50% (Epstein, 1984; Veness *et al.*, 2007).

A number of high-risk groups exist such as organ transplant recipients (OTR), patients with recessive dystrophic epidermolysis bullosa (RDEB) and xeroderma pigmentosum (XP), where individuals are predisposed to developing cSCC with considerable morbidity and mortality (Kraemer *et al.*, 1994; Euvrard *et al.*, 2003; Fine *et al.*, 2009). The incidence of cSCC can be up to 250 times higher in OTRs compared to the general population (Hartevelt *et al.*, 1990). Up to 70% of XP patients can develop malignant skin neoplasms (Kraemer *et al.*, 1994). OTRs with metastatic skin cancer (mostly cSCC in regional lymph node basins) have a poor prognosis with 3-year disease specific survival of 56% (Martinez *et al.*, 2003). Comparatively, RDEB patients have a worse prognosis with more than 80% deaths from metastatic disease within 5 years of diagnosis of their first cSCC (Fine *et al.*, 2009).

While great strides have been made in understanding the molecular pathogenesis of BCC, where mutations in *PTCH1* or *SMO* result in aberrant patched/hedgehog intracellular signaling (Johnson *et al.*, 1996; Xie *et al.*, 1998; Epstein, 2008), the mechanisms and pathways implicated in cSCC are yet to be fully elucidated. This chapter will discuss what can be learnt from studying inherited diseases that predispose patients to developing cSCC.

1.1 Known molecular mechanisms in cSCC tumourigenesis

Cancer is a genetic disease that arises as a result of an accumulation of structural and/or functional defects in the DNA double helix. The current paradigm for understanding tumourigenesis is crystallized by Hanahan and Weinberg in their 2000 and 2011 reviews where fundamental events termed "hallmarks of cancer" are required in the multi-step development of human tumours (Hanahan and Weinberg, 2000, 2011). Originally, six hallmarks of cancer were postulated: (i) sustaining proliferative signaling, (ii) evading growth suppressors, (iii) activating invasion and metastasis, (iv) enabling replicative immortality, (v) inducing angiogenesis and (vi) resisting cell death (Hanahan and Weinberg, 2000). A further two "emerging hallmarks" were later added: deregulation of cellular energetics and evasion of immune destruction. At the same time, two "enabling characteristics" which enable the acquisition of the hallmarks of cancer were also described. These are genomic instability and tumour-promoting immune response (Hanahan and Weinberg, 2011). In particular, genomic instability is "enabling" in the sense that it can lead to aberrant expression of key genes that can have an effect on important cellular mechanisms such as apoptosis, DNA repair, and proliferation.

Exposure to UV, particularly UV-B, can result in genetic abnormalities, notably mutations in the tumour suppressor *TP53* gene, "the guardian of the genome" (Brash et al., 1991; Lane, 1992). Aberrant mutations in this gene have also been observed early on in solar keratoses (Taguchi *et al.*, 1994), Bowen's disease (Campbell *et al.*, 1993) and in ~58% of invasive cSCC (Brash *et al.*, 1991). *TP53* mutations are a widespread phenomenon in human tumours and have a unique UV signature (C→T dipyrimidine substitution) in skin tumours (Brash *et al.*, 1991). In line with this, germline *TP53* mutations in Li-Fraumeni patients can result in an early onset of cancer which includes, but is not limited to, cSCC. Li-Fraumeni, as a cSCC predisposing syndrome will be discussed later in greater detail in this review.

Another gene that has been associated with cSCC is the *RAS* oncogene. *RAS* was first implicated in the initiation of cSCC when *H-ras* mutations were found in the benign papillomas of mice treated with the 7,12-dimethylbenz[a]anthracene (Balmain *et al.*, 1984). In laboratories, expression of oncogenic *RAS* in human keratinocytes was able to recapitulate tumours in mice (Boukamp *et al.*, 1990; Dajee *et al.*, 2003). However the data based on *RAS* mutations in human cSCC is ambiguous. Various independent studies conducted thus far have revealed heterogeneity in their expression and correlation to cSCC development. In North African XP patients, *RAS* genes were found to be at least twice as mutated (50%) compared to control tumours (22%) (Daya-Grosjean *et al.*, 1993). In contrast, a separate study found only 1 mutation in 26 cSCCs from XP patients (Sato *et al.*, 1994). Our lab have demonstrated lack of *RAS* mutations in 10 cSCCs (Pourreyron *et al.*, 2007) while whole exome sequencing have recently identified activating *HRAS* mutation in only one from 8 cSCC (Durinck *et al.*, 2011). This whole exome sequencing study also identified a high proportion of truncating mutations in *NOTCH1* and *NOTCH2* genes, an observation also reported in head and neck SCC (Agrawal *et al.*, 2011; Stransky *et al.*, 2011), suggesting that NOTCH may act as a tumour suppressor in a high proportion of SCC. The identification of an increased risk of developing well differentiated cSCC in patients receiving kinase inhibitors, particularly melanoma patients receiving B-RAF inhibitors (Arnault *et al.*, 2009; Flaherty *et al.*, 2009), has rekindled interest in this area, especially since the identification that inhibition of RAF, which is downstream of RAS, can lead to RAS hyperactivation (Heidorn *et al.*, 2010; Poulikakos *et al.*, 2010). Whether there is a difference between inhibitor (chemically) induced cSCC, and UV induced cSCC remains to be investigated.

Further genes such as cell cycle inhibitor *CDKN2A* (Brown *et al.*, 2004), *MYC* (Pelisson *et al.*, 1996) and *PIK3CA* (Waterman *et al.*, 2007) have also been implicated in cSCC development (Green and Khavari, 2004). Although these correlations provide clues to the pathways involved in cSCC pathogenesis, definitive causal relationships remain elusive.

Here we focus on cSCC and review the genetic and molecular basis behind inherited disorders which are associated with a predisposition to cSCC. In particular, we will examine what is currently known about the pathogenesis in the patient group where cSCC has the biggest impact on mortality - RDEB.

2. Cancer predisposition

Abnormalities in tumour suppressor genes (TSG) and/or oncogenes (OG) that control important cellular mechanisms which are crucial for normal cell functioning can either be acquired during an individual's lifetime or inherited and predispose individuals to cancer. Clinically, an individual is suspected of an inherited predisposition to cancer if (i) other family members have been diagnosed with cancer, (ii) cancer is detected at a young age, (iii) multifocal or bilateral primary tumours are formed or (iv) two or more primary tumours are detected. This inherited predisposition to cancer or familial cancer syndrome (FCS) accounts for 5-10% of all reported cancers and is characterised by mutations, deletions and amplifications of specific TSG's and/or OG's within affected families.

Linkage analysis and positional cloning has enabled the identification of key high penetrance genes responsible for cancer predisposition such as the *BRCA1* (Hall *et al.*, 1990; Narod *et al.*, 1991; Miki *et al.*, 1994) and *BRCA2* (Wooster *et al.*, 1995) genes in breast cancer and *CDKN2A* in melanoma (Goldstein *et al.*, 2001). However, a mutation in such high penetrance genes is only detected in ~25% of familial cancers, thereby suggesting the prevalence of more complex and diverse molecular and genetic interactions in cancer predisposition. Genome wide association studies (GWAS) of affected families have also allowed the identification of other low penetrance genes, suggesting the involvement of multiple gene clusters in cancer susceptibility. This may also enable a better understanding of the genetic mechanisms underlying sporadic cancers (Hemel and Domchek, 2010).

2.1 Familial cancer syndromes and cSCC predisposition

A number of FCS are associated with an increased risk of developing cSCC: Blooms syndrome, Cowden syndrome, Fanconi anemia, Li-Fraumeni syndrome (LFS), Rothmund-Thomson syndrome (RTS), Werner's syndrome and xeroderma pigmentosum. A significant number of individuals within affected families have been shown to carry mutations in specific DNA repair genes that subsequently increase the risk of developing skin cancer, such as *BLM* (Blooms syndrome), *PTEN* (Cowden syndrome), *FANCA-N* (Fanconi's Anemia), *TP53* (LFS), *RECQL4* (RTS), *WRN* (Werner's syndrome), and *XPA-G* (XP).

Blooms syndrome

Blooms syndrome is a rare autosomal recessive disorder characterised by genomic instability. The *BLM* gene that resides on chromosome 15q26.1 is a member of the DNA helicase family and is commonly mutated in individuals diagnosed with Blooms syndrome. A loss of function of this gene results in error prone DNA repair and replication (Ellis *et al.*,

1995; German *et al.*, 2007). Due to increased chromatin exchange and extensive chromosomal instability observed in these individuals, this disease is also referred to as the chromosome breakage syndrome.

The phenotypic characteristics of individuals with Blooms syndrome include severe growth retardation, small stature, infertility, diabetes and chronic pulmonary disease. Skin specific abnormalities appear after first exposure to sunlight and manifest as an erythematous telangiectatic rash. Due to photosensitivity, skin cancer, in particular, cSCC develops in ~14% of individuals and is diagnosed at a mean age of 31.8 years (German, 1997). However, the most common cause of death in Blooms syndrome patients is due to other malignancies such as leukemia and lymphoma.

Cowden syndrome

Cowden syndrome is inherited in an autosomal dominant pattern and is characterised by the development of multiple hamartomas. This disease involves the loss of function of the phosphatase and tensin homolog (PTEN) in about 80-85% of affected individuals (Li *et al.*, 1997; Liaw *et al.*, 1997; Nelen *et al.*, 1996). *PTEN* is a tumour suppressor gene that negatively regulates the protein kinase B (AKT) signaling pathway, which in turn inhibits the phosphorylation and regulation of key genes known to assist carcinogenesis by increasing cell proliferation and anti-apoptotic activity (Segrelles *et al.*, 2002).

Reduced *PTEN* levels in mice have been previously shown to aid malignant transformation of skin lesions in cSCC (Ming and He, 2009; Suzuki *et al.*, 1998). *PTEN* null mice with mutations specifically induced in keratinocytes exhibit hyperkeratosis and epidermal hyperplasia along with the development of cSCC and papillomas. Additionally, these mutant mice have ruffled and shaggy hair with cuticles separated from their hair shafts (Suzuki *et al.*, 2003). A more recent study has also suggested a role of UV-B radiation in the suppression of PTEN via the ERK/AKT signaling pathway in mouse skin (Ming *et al.*, 2009).

The estimated risk of developing Cowden syndrome is 1 in 200,000 with the majority of cases presenting thyroid, breast and endometrium tumours (Starink *et al.*, 1986). Although >90% of affected individuals present abnormalities of the skin including, acral keratoses and trichilemmomas, most of these lesions are not neoplastic and do not contribute towards skin cancer related deaths (Blumenthal and Dennis, 2008).

Fanconi anemia

Fanconi anemia is a rare genetic disease that can either be inherited in an autosomal recessive or X-linked recessive manner. Thirteen genes involved in the inheritance of this disease have so far been identified but the mechanism underlying their interaction is not fully understood (Bagby, 2003; Bagby and Alter, 2006). Some of these genes are associated with breast cancer susceptibility such as the *FANCD1*, which was identified as the *BRCA2* gene (Howlett *et al.*, 2002) and *FANCJ*, also known as *BRIP1* (Seal *et al.*, 2006).

This disease is characterised by an increase in the number of chromosome breaks and bone marrow failure in affected individuals. A number of heterogeneous physical birth defects such as, short stature, dangling thumbs, microcephaly and dislocated hips are also observed. Clinically, this disease can be identified by the use of DNA cross-linkers such as mitomycin-C that increase the rate of chromosome breaks in cultured Fanconi anemia primary cells (Poon *et al.*, 1974).

The risk of developing cancer in individuals diagnosed with Fanconi anemia is estimated at 76% by 45 years of age (Alter, 2003). The majority of people diagnosed are predisposed to leukemia, in particular, acute myeloid leukemia (~95%), hepatocellular carcinoma and Wilm's tumours (Alter and Olson, 2009). Only a fraction of individuals are diagnosed with NMSC and no studies have reported any significant number of aggressive or metastatic cSCCs.

Li-Fraumeni syndrome

Families with Li-Fraumeni cancer syndrome are predisposed to NMSC that include cSCC (Benjamin and Ananthaswamy, 2007; Srivastava *et al.*, 1992). Up to 60% of LFS individuals have mutations in the *TP53* tumour suppressor gene (Malkin, 1994). The *TP53* gene is a transcription transactivator that resides on chromosome 17p13.1 and is reported to be mutated in ~60% cSCC patients (Brash *et al.*, 1991). This gene is activated in response to DNA damage that can result from exposure to UV radiations. In particular, *TP53* has been shown to protect skin cells from damage caused by exposure to UV-B radiation (Smith and Fornace, 1997). Hence, cells with mutant *TP53* gene are unable to maintain the integrity of their DNA, which can lead to the development of precancerous skin lesions known as actinic keratosis. Although a small number of individuals with LFS are predisposed to cSCC, there are no reports associating LFS with cSCC related mortality. LFS families instead have a higher susceptibility of developing life threatening brain tumours, soft tissue sarcoma and breast cancer (Olivier *et al.*, 2003).

Rothmund-Thomson syndrome

Rothmund-Thomson syndrome is an inherited autosomal recessive disorder that is predominantly associated with poikiloderma of the face, neck and extremities. It has been previously reported that 5-10% of RTS individuals are predisposed to skin cancer, with cSCC being the most common type. Approximately, two thirds of RTS patients have mutations in the *RECQL4* gene (Kitao *et al.*, 1999), which is a member of the RecQ DNA helicase family and resides on chromosome 8q24.3. A normal function of this gene is required to suppress random DNA recombination and assist in DNA repair and proper chromosome segregation. A mutation in the *RECQL4* gene is associated with abnormalities of chromosome 8 including both numerical (trisomy 8) and structural (duplication of part of chromosome 8q) aberrations. Karyotypic analysis have confirmed a gain of chromosome 8q in a significant number of cSCC patients (Jin *et al.*, 1999), thereby suggesting an underlying link between genes residing on chromosome 8 (*RECQL4, cMYC*) and cSCC predisposition in a subset of RTS patients. Although a significant number of RTS patients are associated with cSCC with multiple cSCCs diagnosed at an early age (Haneke and Gutschmidt, 1979; Borg *et al.*, 1998), the exact underlying mechanism and the incidence of metastasis has not been extensively studied.

Werner's syndrome

Werner's syndrome or progeria adultorum (premature aging of adults) is mainly associated with thin, tight skin, short stature, bilateral cataracts, graying and thinning of hair and sclerodermatous skin changes. Like Blooms syndrome, Werner's syndrome is inherited in an autosomal recessive manner and is also associated with chromosomal instability and increased cancer susceptibility. More than 90% of Werner's syndrome patients carry a mutation in the *WRN* gene residing on chromosome 8p12, which is involved in important cellular mechanisms such as DNA repair, replication and recombination (Huang *et al.*, 2006). The average life expectancy of individuals diagnosed with Werner's syndrome is 45-50 years with an early onset of carcinogenesis in a significant number of patients (40%) and a high incidence of thyroid and skin cancer (Yamamoto *et al.*, 2003). Individuals diagnosed with this syndrome are 10 times more likely to develop epithelial cancers and sarcomas. The majority of skin cancers (~20%) diagnosed are acral lentiginous melanomas (up to 14%) and relatively aggressive cSCC's (5%) that metastasise to the lymph nodes and internal organs (Machino *et al.*, 1984). It has been previously reported that malignant tumours occur at an average age of 41 years in the Japanese population diagnosed with Werner's syndrome. There is further evidence to suggest higher cancer related mortality (6.1%) than the Japanese general population (0.3%) as a result of metastasis (Yamamoto *et al.*, 2003).

Xeroderma Pigmentosum

Xeroderma Pigmentosum is an inherited autosomal recessive neurocutaneous disorder that is caused as a result of mutations in genes involved in the nucleotide excision repair (NER) mechanism. XP patients have heterogeneous mutations in these genes and are grouped accordingly into seven groups (*XP-A* to *XP-G*) (Kraemer, 1993; Kraemer *et al.*, 2007). This disease is phenotypically characterised by dry, pigmented skin with premature ageing and photosensitivity. In addition to skin abnormalities, neurological defects including microcephaly and spasticity are also observed. It has been previously reported that up to 70% of XP patients develop malignant skin neoplasms, in which ~50% are NMSC (Kraemer *et al.*, 1994). The incidence of metastasis in XP related cSCC is reported to be 4%, which is comparable to the general population (2-4%) (Kraemer *et al.*, 1987). Other neoplasms associated with XP include brain and lung cancer but the relative incidence of developing these tumours is lower compared to skin cancer.

2.2 Inherited skin disorders and cSCC predisposition

Hereditary skin disorders that result in photosensitivity, ulceration or blistering of the skin can also be complicated by cSCC predisposition. These include, albinism, Bazex syndrome, Darier disease, epidermolysis bullosa (EB), epidermodysplasia verruciformis (EV), Ferguson-Smith diesease, Huriez syndrome, Keratitis-Ichthyosis-Deafness (KID) and XX sex reversal with palmar plantar keratoderma, and will be discussed below. Although all of the aforementioned skin disorders contribute to the development of cSCC, the recessive dystrophic subtype of EB is associated with by far the highest cSCC related mortality and will be discussed in detail in section 3 (Reed *et al.*, 1975; Fine *et al.*, 2009).

Albinism

Albinism is a heterogeneous group of disorders with an autosomal recessive inheritance pattern and is associated with aberrant melanin production. Albinism can be broadly grouped into (i) oculocutaneous albinism (OCA) and (ii) ocular albinism (OA). Individuals diagnosed with OCA have low levels of melanin in the skin, eyes and hair and are characterised by pale light skin that is photosensitive and prone to developing skin cancer (Perry and Silverberg, 2001). OA on the contrary is mainly associated with abnormal pigmentation of the optic system with no differences observed in the skin of the affected individuals

Three OCA subcategories exist as per the genetic classification of the disease, OCA1 (*tyrosinase* gene, 11q14-21), OCA2 (*P protein* gene, 15q11-13) and OCA3 (*tyrosinase* related gene, 9p23) (Summers, 2009). Mutations in the *tyrosinase* gene causes type 1 OCA. The enzyme tyrosinase is involved in the conversion of tyrosine into melanin (by converting dopaquinone to either eumelanin or pheomelanin) that protects skin cells against the deleterious effects of UV radiations (Oetting and King, 1993). Type 2 OCA results from mutations in the gene encoding the P protein (pink-eyed dilution protein homolog or melanocyte-specific transporter protein) that is responsible for the transport of tyrosine prior to melanin production by melanocytes (Saitoh *et al.*, 2000). The third type of OCA is caused due to the mutations in tyrosine related proteins 1 and 2 that are involved in the production of eumelanin. In a study involving 111 South African (black population) albinos, the incidence of NMSC was reported to be as high as 23%. Additionally, BCC was found to be less common than cSCC in these individuals (Kromberg *et al.*, 1987; Kromberg *et al.*, 1989).

Bazex syndrome

Acrokeratosis paraneoplastica or Bazex syndrome is a rare inherited skin disorder (Bazex and Griffiths, 1980). This disease presents in the form of psoriasiform-erythematous plaques in the hands, feet, nose and earlobes. The most common feature of Bazex is the occurrence of an internal malignancy along with one of the cutaneous psoriasiform lesions (Pecora *et al.*, 1983; Sharma *et al.*, 2006). The most frequently occurring malignancy in Bazex syndrome is SCC of the aero-digestive tract. In some cases cervical lymph node metastasis is also reported where the primary tumours have not been identified (Viteri *et al.*, 2005). Bazex syndrome is not primarily linked with cSCC and the number of cases reported in literature are low (Hara *et al.*, 1995) with no indication of cSCC associated mortality and/or metastasis (Sarkar *et al.*, 1998)

Darier disease

Darier-White disease or keratosis follicularis is an autosomal dominant inherited skin disorder characterized by the occurrence of wart-like, yellowish and mildly greasy blemishes that emit a strong odor. In some cases abnormalities of the nail and mucous membrane have been observed such as having an irregular nail texture and blemishes on gums, tongue and throat. Epilepsy and learning disabilities have also been reported in some affected individuals. The prevalence of Darier disease is estimated at 1 in 30,000 in Scotland alone. Lower number of cases are reported from other countries such as Denmark (1 in 100,000) and Wales (1 in 36,000) but the worldwide prevalence of this disease is unknown (Sehgal and Srivastava, 2005).

Mutation in the *ATP2A2* gene located on chromosome 12q23-24.1 is responsible for this disease (Sakuntabhai *et al.*, 1999a; Sakuntabhai *et al.*, 1999b). However, the severity of the disease has been shown to vary between individuals carrying the same mutation due to environmental factors such as exposure to UV radiation and hot climatic conditions. A mutation in the *ATP2A2* gene reduces the level of its' protein product the SERCA2 enzyme (an intracellular Ca^{2+} pump), which in turn reduces calcium levels in the endoplasmic reticulum, rendering it dysfunctional (Byrne, 2006). The complete molecular mechanism underlying the *ATP2A2* gene mutation causing blemishes solely localized to the skin is not fully understood. However, it has been postulated that skin cells are the only cell type without a backup system for calcium transport, therefore the disease manifests in the skin even if SERCA2 is expressed in other organs. Further preliminary studies have also shown that synthesis and trafficking of desmosomal proteins can be altered as a result of low calcium levels (Dhitavat *et al.*, 2004). Moreover, abnormal expression levels of keratin 10 and 14 have also been associated with altered calcium regulation in Darier disease (Leinonen *et al.*, 2009).

The most serious complication of Darier disease is the onset of bacterial and viral infections that can lead to fatal outcomes. Anecdotal case studies have reported cSCC in Darier disease

(Orihuela *et al.*, 1995; Downs *et al.*, 1997; Vazquez *et al.*, 2002) but none have reported metastasis related mortality and the life expectancy of these individuals is comparable to the normal population.

Epidermolysis Bullosa

Inherited EB is a group of rare skin fragility disorders characterized by chronic blistering of the skin and mucosae following minor mechanical trauma. Based on a large American study, EB incidence was reported to be 19.6 per million live births between 1986 and 1990 along with a prevalence of 8.22 per million within the population studied (Fine *et al.*, 1999)

In the revised 2008 classification, EB is divided into four main groups based on the ultrastructural level of blister formation in the basement membrane zone (BMZ) (Fine *et al.*, 2008). The four groups are EB simplex (EBS), junctional EB (JEB), dystrophic EB (DEB) and Kindler syndrome (KS), and have either intraepidermal, intra-lamina lucida, sub-lamina densa or a mixed level of dermal-epidermal cleavage, respectively. Kindler syndrome (KS), RDEB and JEB are associated with a predisposition to developing cSCC (Fine *et al.*, 2009; Yazdanfar and Hashemi, 2009; Yuen and Jonkman, 2011) of which JEB and KS will be discussed here and RDEB later in Section 3.

Kindler syndrome

Kindler syndrome (KS) is associated with photosensitivity, extensive skin blistering, and progressive poikiloderma. It is a rare autosomal recessive disorder caused as a result of mutation in the *FERMT1* gene that resides on chromosome 20p12.3 (Siegel *et al.*, 2003). This gene encodes a protein (kindlin-1) that is involved in linking the actin cytoskeleton with the extra cellular matrix (ECM) and regulating the secretion of various basement membrane factors by the basal keratinocytes. KS unlike other skin related disorders results from defects in the actin-ECM interaction instead of the keratin-ECM interaction (Ashton *et al.*, 2004; Arita *et al.*, 2007).

Up to 10% of individuals suffering from KS develop NMSC, mostly cSCC, with the youngest patient reported being a 16 year old boy (Arita *et al.*, 2007; Lai-Cheong *et al.*, 2009; Yazdanfar and Hashemi, 2009). Owing to a low incidence of KS (only about 100 cases reported worldwide) a detailed analysis of metastasis and cSCC related death has not been possible. However, anecdotal case studies have reported the prevalence of aggressive cSCC that metastasise to the axillary lymph nodes. These cSCC tumours have been shown to recur following radiation therapy, thereby necessitating amputation of the affected limbs (Emanuel *et al.*, 2006).

Junctional Epidermolysis Bullosa

JEB is inherited in an autosomal recessive manner and is characterized by skin cleavage in the lamina lucida of the BMZ. JEB can be further classified into two main subtypes - the lethal JEB- Herlitz (JEB-H) and JEB-other. In JEB-H, there is a lack of laminin-332 expression (laminin-5) due to premature termination codon mutations in the gene of any of the three polypeptide components (*LAMA3, LAMB3* and *LAMC2*) of laminin 332 (Christiano and Uitto, 1996; Kivirikko *et al.*, 1996). Extensive blistering occurs soon after birth. Due to the severe blistering and fragile internal mucosae, most infants die early. JEB-other (includes localized and generalized non-Herlitz JEB and JEB with pyloric atresia), may involve type XVII collagen or $\alpha6\beta4$ integrin gene in addition to laminin-332 (McGrath e*t al.*, 1995; Kivirikko *et al.*, 1995; Vidal *et al.*, 1995). Patients usually survive to adulthood in generalized non-Herlitz JEB as severity of the disease decrease with age.

Although, an association between JEB and cSCC was not found in the large study conducted by Fine and colleagues (Fine *et al.*, 2009), a recent retrospective study of 28 non-Herlitz JEB patients revealed an increased incidence of aggressive cSCC, albeit at a lower frequency than in sg-RDEB patients with a lifetime risk of 25% (Yuen and Jonkman, 2011). The first cSCC occurred at an average age of 50. Multiple cSCCs were common and tended to be in the lower extremities (Yuen and Jonkman, 2011).

Epidermodysplasia Verruciformis

Human papillomavirus (HPV) infection has long been implicated in the development of cSCC in the rare genodermatosis epidermodysplasia verruciformis (EV) (Orth *et al.*, 1978). Mutations in *EVER1* and *EVER2* genes result in susceptibility to beta- human papillomavirus (β-HPV) infection and a high risk of skin cancer - about 50% of the patients eventually develop cSCC (Ramoz *et al.*, 2002). Onset of lesions usually appears within the first decade, with cSCCs appearing at an average age of 20 at sun-exposed areas (de Oliveira *et al.*, 2003; Gul *et al.*, 2007). Although the tumours are generally localized, aggressive metastatic cSCCs resulting in mortality have been reported (Kaspar *et al.*, 1991; de Oliveira *et al.*, 2003; Gul *et al.*, 2007).

Due to the high incidence of cSCC in transplant patients it has long been postulated that a viral etiology exists. However, a role of HPV has long been debated (Harwood and Proby, 2002) and the available data are not clear. Transgenic mice expressing the complete early regions of HPV8 develop skin papillomas and varying degrees of epidermal dysplasia, with 6% of the transgenic mice eventually developing malignant tumours (Marcuzzi *et al.*, 2009). In humans although associations were found between HPVs and cSCC in the general population (Masini *et al.*, 2003), the ubiquitous presence of the various HPV types in normal skin makes it difficult to draw any definitive conclusions (Astori *et al.*, 1998). Recently, Arron and colleagues were able to show conclusively by harnessing transcriptome sequencing technology that β-HPV is not active in cSCC, thereby demonstrating no role for HPV in maintaining cSCC tumours (Arron *et al.*, 2011). However this data does not exclude a role for HPV in tumour initiation.

Ferguson-Smith disease

Multiple self-healing squamous epithelioma or Ferguson-Smith disease is associated with the occurrence of multiple invasive skin tumours that spontaneously heal leaving pitted scars and is mainly reported in individuals originating from western Scotland (Ferguson-Smith *et al.*, 1971). Recently, this autosomal dominant inherited skin disease was linked to mutations in the *TGFBR1* gene on chromosome 9q22.33 (Goudie *et al.*, 2011). This gene encodes a protein that aids in the transduction of TGF-beta signaling from the cell to the cytoplasm, thereby, assisting in the regulation of important cellular mechanisms including cell division, differentiation and adhesion. As the name suggests, this disorder involves the development of multiple self-healing cSCCs that emerge and regress with no cases of metastasis or mortality having been reported. Whether *TGFBR1* mutations are common in the large proportion of benign and sometimes spontaneously regressing cSCC is unknown.

Huriez syndrome

Huriez syndrome is characterised by palmoplantar keratoderma, congenital scleroatrophy and hypoplasia of the nails. This syndrome is inherited in an autosomal dominant manner and linkage analysis has enabled the mapping of possible Huriez syndrome susceptibility genes on chromosome 4q23 (Lee *et al.*, 2000). Huriez disease is often associated with aggressive and metastatic cSCC (Hamm *et al.*, 1996). cSCC develops in ~15% of individuals diagnosed with this disease (Sekar SC, 2008) , especially in the scleroatrophic areas in the affected individuals. The clinical manifestations of cSCC in Huriez syndrome are very similar to Marjolin's ulcer where malignant lesions appear in ulcers, scarred and/or burnt tissue. Further parallels exist between Marjolin's ulcer and RDEB, and will be discussed further in section 3.

Keratitis-Ichthyosis-deafness

KID was first coined in 1981 (Skinner *et al.*, 1981) owing to the three distinct phenotypic characteristics including vascularising keratitis, localized or generalised skin ichthyosis and severe hearing disability. Since its first description in 1915, approximately 100 cases have been reported so far in literature. KID is a rare genetic disorder that is inherited in an autosomal dominant pattern. Mutations in the *GJB2* gene encoding the gap junction protein Connexin 26 are reported in affected individuals (Terrinoni *et al.*, 2010). Gap junctions are membrane channels connecting adjacent cells, which are involved in the reciprocal transport of small molecules and ions including Ca^{2+} between neighboring cells. These junctions play an important role in cell proliferation, growth and differentiation.
A significant percentage of KID syndrome patients have been diagnosed with follicular tumours and cSCC (Madariaga *et al.*, 1986; Conrado *et al.*, 2007). The largest study (n=14) to date has shown that about 29% of affected individuals develop cSCC and SCC of the oral mucosa at an early age with the mean age of 25 years (Mazereeuw-Hautier *et al.*, 2007). Although, some studies have documented the occurrence of cSCC in KID syndrome, most of these are less aggressive forms with no reports of metastasis or cSCC related deaths.

XX sex reversal and Palmar Plantar Keratoderma

XX sex reversal and Palmar Plantar Keratoderma (PPK) reported in a Sicilian family also predisposes to cSCC (Micali *et al.*, 2005). Since, none of the females in the affected family were diagnosed with PPK or sex reversal, the study spanning three generations has suggested that loss of function of a single gene is responsible for PPK, sex reversal and subsequent cSCC predisposition (Radi *et al.*, 2005). Linkage analysis has led to the identification of a locus on chromosome 1q34-35 and further sequencing studies have enabled the isolation of a homozygous mutation in the *RSPO1* gene (Parma *et al.*, 2006), which is shown to enhance Wnt signaling. Although, the males carrying the 46XX genotype along with PPK are reported to develop cSCC that metastasizes to other internal organs, the cSCC related incidence has not been fully reported due to the low number of cases documented in literature.

3. Recessive Dystrophic Epidermolysis Bullosa

DEB is caused exclusively by mutations in the *COL7A1* gene which encodes type VII collagen (Ryynänen *et al.*, 1991; Hovnanian *et al.*, 1992; Christiano *et al.*, 1994). Type VII collagen is the main constituent of anchoring fibrils, which secure the basement membrane to its underlying dermis (Burgeson, 1993). Both keratinocytes and fibroblasts are able to synthesise type VII collagen (Marinkovich *et al.*, 1993; Vindevoghel *et al.*, 1997; Woodley *et al.*, 2003). Ultra-structurally, DEB is characterized by skin cleavage at the sub-lamina densa with absent or reduced anchoring fibrils, leading to skin blistering (Tidman and Eady, 1985; McGrath *et al.*, 1993; Uitto *et al.*, 1994; Uitto *et al.*, 1999). As the skin cleavage occurs below the basement membrane, blisters form in the dermis and tend to heal with scar formation

(Bruckner-Tuderman, 2001). Other typical clinical manifestations of DEB are nail dystrophy and milia formation.

This genetic disorder can be inherited either as an autosomal dominant (DDEB) or recessive (RDEB) trait. Blistering severity in DEB patients varies considerably. In general, RDEB differs clinically from DDEB in that it is significantly more debilitating - mild friction is sufficient to induce blisters in RDEB, whereas considerable force like sharp knocks and glancing blows are required in DDEB (Eady *et al.*, 2004). In addition, blistering can extend to the oral cavity, gastro-intestinal tract and eyes in RDEB patients, leading to soft tissue scarring, microstomia, ankyloglossia and dental caries (Fine *et al.*, 2008; Fine and Mellerio, 2009). Importantly and unlike RDEB, no evidence for an increased incidence of cSCC was reported in a large study of 442 DDEB patients (Fine *et al.*, 2009) although case reports do exist in the literature (Song and Dicksheet, 1985; McGrath *et al.*, 1992b; Christiano *et al.*, 1999).

RDEB is further sub-divided on the basis of clinical features into: RDEB severe generalized, RDEB generalized other and RDEB inversa (Fine, 1999; Fine *et al.*, 2009). RDEB severe generalized (sg-RDEB, previously known as RDEB Hallopeau-Siemens) is, as the name suggests, the most severe mutilating subtype of RDEB. There is severe blistering and extensive atrophic scarring and the patients are usually anaemic. As a result, physical development is stunted, with delayed puberty and osteoporosis. RDEB generalized other (RDEB-O, previously known as mitis RDEB) is the second major form of RDEB. While it shares many cutaneous and extracutaneous similarities with sg-RDEB, RDEB-O generally has milder clinical manifestations, with blistering and scarring that is more comparable to that in DDEB. In the third classification - RDEB inversa (RDEB-I), blisters are present at birth but later become localized to acral areas as well as skin folds such as lateral neck, groin and axillary vaults.

The most severe form of RDEB, sg-RDEB is primarily associated with nonsense mutations, insertions, deletions or out-of-frame splicing mutations in both alleles of *COL7A1*, which produce frameshift and/or premature termination codons (PTC). PTC mutations lead to mRNA instability, resulting in dramatic reduction or a complete absence of anchoring fibrils in the skin, thereby causing a more severe disease phenotype (Christiano *et al.*, 1997; Uitto and Richard, 2004; Varki *et al.*, 2007). In RDEB-O, missense mutation or in-frame deletion in one or both *COL7A1* alleles leads to the altered conformation of polypeptides. This altered conformation prevents the proper assembly of the polypeptides into anchoring fibrils. Therefore, only some anchoring fibrils are observed under electron microscope or detected using immunohistochemistry methods (Uitto and Richard, 2004; Varki *et al.*, 2007). These mutant anchoring fibrils are not able to fulfill their role in dermal-epidermal adhesion, which is consistent with the phenotype of moderate blistering observed in this DEB sub-type (Woodley *et al.*, 2008).

3.1 RDEB patients develop malignant cSCC

Case reports of multiple, metastatic and life-threatening skin cancer in RDEB patients arising on damaged tissue date as far back as 1975 (Reed *et al.*, 1975). A recent study examined the risk for skin cancer over a 20-year period in the 3280 EB patients in the US EB registry, the largest cohort to date, convincingly demonstrated that RDEB patients, comprising 421 individuals, are at high risk of developing aggressive and life-threatening cSCC (Fine *et al.*, 2009). The cumulative risk of developing cSCC in patients with severe-generalized RDEB (sg-RDEB) stands at more than 90% by the age of 50 (Fine *et al.*, 2009). While there have been a few cases of malignant melanoma in RDEB (Chorny *et al.*, 1993; Fine *et al.*, 2009) the overwhelming majority of the tumours that occur in RDEB patients are cSCC. A correlation exists between severity of blistering and development of cSCC. The cumulative risk of developing cSCC is highest in sg-RDEB (where skin blistering is most severe and extensive) followed by RDEB-O (which has milder clinical manifestations) and finally RDEB-I (where blistering becomes localized to acral areas and skin folds with age). This is further supported by the observation that the most common site for cSCCs in RDEB is persistent skin wounds followed by long-term cutaneous scars rather than sun-exposed areas. However, no detailed analysis has been carried out to examine the *COL7A1* mutation spectrum in a large cohort of RDEB patients who eventually develop cSCC. Such clinical, genetic and immunohistological data could shed further light on the relationships between the loss of type VII collagen, formation of anchoring fibrils, severity of blistering and the risk of developing cSCC.

Perplexingly, although most cSCCs in RDEB patients are histo-pathologically moderately differentiated (McGrath *et al.*, 1992b), these cSCCs are biologically aggressive and have the propensity to recur or metastasize to distant sites, eventually causing the death of the patient. In fact, most RDEB patients will develop multiple cSCCs (median number per RDEB patient = 3-3.5) and die from metastatic disease despite surgical excision (Fine *et al.*, 2009). The cancer survival rates for RDEB patients are dismal: more than 80% die from metastatic cSCC in 5 years after initial tumour presentation. These statistics stand in stark contrast to those of the general US population where the lifetime risk of developing cSCC is only 7-11% and the overall mortality rate for NMSC considerably lower at 0.69 per 100,000 per year (Miller and Weinstock, 1994; Lewis and Weinstock, 2007).

The large numbers of cSCC in RDEB patients are only matched and exceeded by XP patients. However, clinical observations point to clear differences in pathogenesis of cSCC in XP and RDEB. Unlike RDEB, metastasis in XP patients is rare. Additionally, XP have a high rate of internal malignancies such as a 20-fold increase in incidence of brain tumours, not observed in RDEB (Daya-Grosjean and Sarasin, 2005).

Clinical similarities exist between the cSCCs in both JEB and RDEB patients - multiple cSCCs are common and there is a preponderance of cSCCs in areas of chronic blistering, erosion and scarring in both groups (Fine *et al.*, 2009; Yuen and Jonkman, 2011). These observations point to the possible involvement of a disrupted basement membrane and wounded permissive microenvironment in cSCC carcinogenesis; however, the data are not clear in JEB. Also other blistering and inflammatory skin diseases exist which are not cancer prone. What is clear is that *COL7A1* plays an important role in cSCC but the conspicuous absence of cancer in other mucousal tissues such as oral and GI tracts, which can also blister, in RDEB patients and are reported to express *COL7A1*, is perplexing. Furthermore, although a significant number of studies have been undertaken that seek to explain the high incidence and aggressive nature of cSCC in RDEB patients no single experiment or investigation has provided conclusive answers to these questions and often the data can be conflicting and controversial.

3.2 Expression of type VII collagen in cancers

Since the development of reliable monoclonal antibodies (Sakai *et al.*, 1986; Leigh *et al.*, 1988) numerous studies to examine the expression of type VII collagen in a wide range of malignant tissues have been conducted. The resulting data have yielded diverging results, which are summarized in Table 1 and discussed herein. It is apparent that type VII collagen can be differentially expressed in different tumour types. Protein expression is observed in brain tumours (Paulus *et al.*, 1995), female genital tract SCC (Wetzels *et al.*, 1991), oral SCC (Kainulainen *et al.*, 1997) and head and neck SCC (Wetzels *et al.*, 1991; Wetzels *et al.*, 1992b).

Up-regulation of the protein and/or mRNA is seen in esophageal SCC (Baba *et al.*, 2006; Kita *et al.*, 2009), colorectal carcinoma (Visser *et al.*, 1993; Skovbjerg *et al.*, 2009) and thyroid carcinoma (Lohi *et al.*, 1998). In the case of esophageal SCC, increased expression of *COL7A1* mRNA and its corresponding protein is correlated to a poorer five- year survival rate (Baba *et al.*, 2006; Kita *et al.*, 2009), while evidence in colorectal cancer suggests that the up-regulation of *COL7A1* mRNA and protein is an early event that occurs in both adenomas and carcinoma (Visser *et al.*, 1993; Skovbjerg *et al.*, 2009).

Reference	Tissue	Type VII Expression and Localization
(Paulus *et al.*, 1995)	Brain tumours (choroid plexus papilloma, pineoblastoma, pituitary adenoma)	Presence of type VII collagen expression
(Wetzels *et al.*, 1991)	Lung SCC Head and Neck SCC Female genital tract SCC	Expression seen in carcinomas with squamous differentiation
(Kainulainen *et al.*, 1997)	Oral SCC	Linear staining pattern around tumour and cytoplasmic staining in large number of tumours. Some fibroblast-like stromal cells also stained positive.
(Wetzels *et al.*, 1992b)	Head and Neck SCC	Expression in basement membranes of all 42 tumours, independent of the tumour grade. Expression observed in cytoplasm of 36% of tumour cells. In more than half of the cases, a stronger staining in the tumour centre was seen, which weakens towards the tumour periphery.
(Lohi *et al.*, 1998)	Normal thyroid follicular epithelium, thyroid carcinoma	Absent from normal thyroid follicular epithelium Expression of protein in most thyroid carcinomas
(Visser *et al.*, 1993)	Normal mucosa of colon, adenoma and adenocarcinoma	No expression in normal mucosa, but expression is detected in basement membrane of dysplastic epithelium. A stronger expression in well and moderately differentiated carcinoma
(Skovbjerg *et al.*, 2009)	Colorectal cancer	The *COL7A1* mRNA levels were statistically significantly higher in adenoma and colorectal cancer tissue as compared to healthy tissues, indicating that this is an early event in carcinogenesis
(Baba *et al.*, 2006)	Esophageal SCC	Expression of type VII collagen was closely related to poor prognosis. Cytoplasmic expression of type VII collagen was detected in 35% of the samples.

(Kita *et al.*, 2009)	Esophageal SCC	The expression levels COL7A1 mRNA is higher in malignant tissues than normal tissues and is significantly correlated with depth of tumor invasion and lymphatic invasion. Patients with high levels of *COL7A1* mRNA (n=4) have a worse five-year survival rate than otherwise (n=22).
(Dumas *et al.*, 1999)	BCC and cSCC	Expression tends to decrease on the leading edge of invasive tumor mass in BCC and SCC. Reduction of type VII collagen expression is greater in SCC than BCC, when compared to normal skin
(Yasaka *et al.*, 1994)	BCC	Reduced staining in the basement membrane of some nests of BCCs along with intra-tumoral staining in all tumours
(Jones *et al.*, 1989)	BCC	Localized to the basement membrane zone of tumor cells and some stromal staining observed at the tumour stromal interface
(Bechetoille *et al.*, 2000)	Melanoma cell lines growing on de-epidermised dermis	Local invasion of human metastatic melanoma cells through the basement membrane of a de-epidermised dermis is correlated with discontinuities of type VII collagen
(Kirkham *et al.*, 1989)	Melanoma	Discontinuities of type VII collagen in the basement membrane observed in melanomas thicker than 0.9mm
(Tani *et al.*, 1996)	Normal gastric epithelium Gastric carcinoma	Punctate expression in basement membrane of normal surface epithelium. Basement membrane of most tumors were devoid of type VII collagen expression, although some occasional staining is observed at sites containing laminin-332
(Nagle *et al.*, 1994)	Prostate carcinoma	Loss of type VII collagen expression
(Bonkhoff, 1998)	Prostate carcinoma	Early stromal invasion is associated with the loss of both hemidesmosomal proteins and type VII collagen but invasive tumor cells then go on to produce basement membrane-like matrices
(Wetzels *et al.*, 1992a)	Lung Carcinoma	Expression seen in lung SCCs, with a corresponding reduction in expression with decreasing differentiation. Type VII collagen was not identified in adenocarcinomas, small cell carcinomas or carcinoids.

Table 1. Type VII collagen expression in malignant tissues

Conversely, down-regulation of the protein and/or mRNA is observed in cSCC (Dumas *et al.*, 1999), melanoma tumours (Kirkham *et al.*, 1989) and cell lines (Bechetoille *et al.*, 2000), lung SCCs (Wetzels *et al.*, 1992a), BCCs (Jones *et al.*, 1989; Yasaka *et al.*, 1994; Dumas *et al.*, 1999), gastric carcinoma (Tani *et al.*, 1996) and prostate carcinoma (Nagle *et al.*, 1994; Bonkhoff, 1998). In prostate carcinogenesis, evidence points to the loss of type VII collagen as an early event which leads to dysplasia, (Bonkhoff, 1998). In addition, anticancer drugs shown to be effective against prostate cancer down-regulate *COL7A1* expression *in vitro* (Hurst et al., 2008). While the lack of type VII collagen in these cancers seems to correlate with dysplasia, the lack of an increased risk of lung, BCC, gastric and prostate cancers in RDEB patients would suggest that the loss of type VII collagen is more likely to be a consequence of tumourigenesis rather than a key driver in the aforementioned cancers.
Interestingly, a weaker staining is observed at the tumour periphery, along with decreased type VII collagen reported in both cutaneous (Dumas *et al.*, 1999) and head and neck SCC (Wetzels *et al.*, 1992b). Local invasion of human metastatic melanoma cells through the basement membrane of a de-epidermised dermis is correlated with discontinuities of type VII collagen staining along basement membrane (Bechetoille *et al.*, 2000). This experiment parallels earlier observations that discontinuities of type VII collagen staining appear when malignant melanomas progress past a thickness of 0.9mm (Kirkham *et al.*, 1989).
Cytoplasmic type VII collagen immuno-staining has also been demonstrated in cSCC (Dumas *et al.*, 1999), oral SCC (Kainulainen *et al.*, 1997), and head and neck SCC (Wetzels *et al.*, 1992b). Similar intracellular expression of type VII collagen has been reported in RDEB SCC (Kanitakis *et al.*, 1997) and transiently in wounded normal and RDEB skin (McGrath *et al.*, 1992a), suggesting cytoplasmic type VII collagen may be involved in tumour development and/or wound healing. Cellular signaling via type VII collagen has recently been identified (reviewed by Rodeck and Uitto and discussed in the following section (Rodeck and Uitto, 2007)) and may have considerable impact on the processes of tumorigenesis and wound healing. But overall it is difficult to distill the immunohistochemical and mRNA expression data into any sweeping conclusive statement as to whether aberrant expression of type VII collagen contributes to human cancer and in what way.

3.3 Search for mechanisms involved in RDEB SCC tumourigenesis

The mechanism behind the aggressive nature of RDEB SCC has thus far remained elusive. One possibility recently explored was that the chronically wounded environment in RDEB patients may enable HPV infection and contribute toward cSCC tumourigenesis. Research within our lab has found that the aggressive nature of RDEB SCC cannot be accounted for by the overall prevalence of alpha- or beta-HPV infection through demonstrating comparative data for non-RDEB SCC (Purdie *et al.*, 2010). As discussed in the introduction, various independent studies conducted thus far have revealed heterogeneity in the incidence of *RAS* mutations in human cSCC and we have been unable to detect *RAS* mutations in six RDEB SCC patients and four non-RDEB SCC patient samples (Pourreyron *et al.*, 2007). Similar to non-RDEB SCC data a proportion of RDEB tumours harbour *TP53* mutation and *CDKN2A* methylation/ aberrant expression (Arbiser *et al.*, 2004; Watt *et al.*, 2011). In the following section we discuss the various ideas and studies investigating aspects of RDEB and RDEB SCC pathology.

Tumours – wounds that do not heal

Given the constantly wounded environment in RDEB, parallels can be drawn between RDEB SCC and Marjolin's ulcers. Marjolin's ulcer refers to a malignant lesion that arises in areas of chronic inflammation such as burns and ulcers. A retrospective study of 412 case reports between 1923 and 2004 on Marjolin's ulcers found cSCC to be the most frequent cancer at 71%, followed by BCC at 21 % and melanoma at 6% (Kowal-Vern and Criswell, 2005). The cSCCs tended to be aggressive - local recurrence, regional lymph node metastases and distant metastases were found in 16%, 22% and 14% of the cases respectively and the mortality rate was 21%. In Marjolin's ulcer, the mean latency period is 31 years while almost 50% of sg-RDEB patients develop their first cSCC at the age of 30 (Fine *et al.*, 2009). Both Marjolin's Ulcers and RDEB SCCs are much more aggressive than UV-induced cSCC from the general population. Certainly this clinical parallel exists and is yet to be fully explored.

Tissue stress and "activated" keratinocytes

Goldberg and colleagues postulated that repetitive tissue stress could be the underlying driving force for tumour promotion in RDEB where there is an altered interaction of keratinocytes with their chronically stressed microenvironment (Goldberg *et al.*, 1988). In support of this theory, Smoller *et al.* found a "growth-activated" state characterized by upregulation of filaggrin, involucrin and specific cytokeratins in biopsies taken from RDEB healed wounds (n=6) and in all actinic keratoses (n=10) (Smoller *et al.*, 1990a; Smoller *et al.*, 1990b). In contrast, healed wounds of the simplex form of epidermolysis bullosa (Barkan *et al.*, 2010), which usually heal without scarring and are not predisposed to cSCC, did not exhibit this "activated" state (n=4). These observations lead the investigators to speculate that this growth activation could be a reason for cSCC development.

Contribution of type VII collagen to RDEB SCC tumourigenesis

Given the inverse relationship between severity of DEB and type VII collagen expression (McGrath *et al.*, 1993), it has long been hypothesized that the absence of type VII collagen in RDEB patients is a major contributing factor to the aggressive nature of SCC. However, given the absence of significant cSCC incidence in DDEB patients (Fine et al., 2009) and no reports of unaffected RDEB family members developing cSCC, little evidence exists for *COL7A1* being a classical tumour suppressor gene. A number of studies have investigated *COL7A1* and type VII collagen manipulation in different experimental systems.

Chen and colleagues observed that re-expression of full-length type VII collagen into RDEB keratinocytes and RDEB fibroblasts using lentivirus resulted in reduced cell migration and increased cell adhesion (Chen *et al.*, 2002). Subsequently, intravenous injection of RDEB fibroblasts re-expressing type VII collagen into athymic mice led to improved wound healing compared to non-gene corrected RDEB fibroblasts (Woodley *et al.*, 2007). Following this and at odds with the data in RDEB patient cells, it was shown that type VII collagen increased migration in normal keratinocytes and fibroblasts, identifying that a 684 amino acid residue within the triple helical domain of type VII collagen conferred this increase (Chen *et al.*, 2008). These data suggest that the ability of type VII collagen to influence migration and adhesion is dependent on the cellular context and possibly the status of endogenous *COL7A1*.

Martins and colleagues knocked-down expression of type VII collagen in non-RDEB SCC keratinocytes *in vitro* and showed that loss of type VII collagen promoted migration and invasion, increased epithelial mesenchymal transition (EMT) and reduced terminal epithelial differentiation, characteristics usually associated with tumourigenesis (Martins *et al.*, 2009). This work agrees with the data demonstrating decreased migration in RDEB cells upon reintroduction of wild type *COL7A1* and may suggest similarities between RDEB non-tumour cells and non-RDEB tumour cells.

Ortiz-Urda and colleagues demonstrated that type VII collagen, specifically the NC1 domain, was required for RAS-driven tumourigenesis in a model where primary keratinocytes are transformed with oncogenic RAS-V12 and the NF-κB super-repressor IκBαM (Ortiz-Urda *et al.*, 2005). Injection of transformed RDEB cells without detectable type VII collagen did not grow quickly as tumours in mice, whereas those expressing NC1 fragment grew rapidly. The fibronectin-like sequences within the NC1 domain have multiple functions and facilitate binding to laminin beta3 domain V-III to not only activate phosphoinositol-3-kinase signaling, but also promote tumor cell invasion, prevent apoptosis and promote neoplasia (Waterman *et al.*, 2007). These results suggested that RDEB patients who still express the NC1 domain may be more susceptible to developing cSCC, while conversely, sg-RDEB patients without any detectable type VII collagen expression will be less likely to develop cSCC. However, it has been demonstrated that RDEB patients without any detectable type VII collagen can still develop cSCCs (Pourreyron *et al.*, 2007; Rodeck and Uitto, 2007).

The above studies highlight the importance of type VII collagen in tumourigenesis but also suggest that cellular context is important in how type VII collagen exerts its influence. It is clear that, regardless of the amount and type of mutated type VII collagen expressed, cSCC will develop in RDEB patients.

Immune surveillance in RDEB

As discussed earlier, avoidance of immune destruction is a recognized hallmark of cancer which can enable growth and dissemination (Hanahan and Weinberg, 2011). In the only study of its kind to date, natural killer cell activity was observed to be reduced in RDEB, DDEB, JEB and malabsorption patients but not in EBS and normal patients (Tyring *et al.*, 1989), which the authors suggest may be responsible for the development of cSCC in RDEB patients.

Basic fibroblast growth factor in RDEB

Elevated levels of urinary basic fibroblast growth factor (bFGF) were observed in more than 51% of 39 RDEB patients, 21% of 33 unaffected family members and 13% of 30 EBS patients also had elevated levels (Arbiser *et al.*, 1998). It is only in JEB that elevated bFGF levels were not observed in this study. Although the authors postulate that bFGF might promote tumourigenesis through its mitogenic or angiogenic effect, the presence of elevated levels in unaffected family members would suggest other confounding factors may determine bFGF levels. Furthermore, no direct correlation was found between the levels of bFGF to the presence of cSCC in RDEB patients.

Matrix metalloproteinase expression in RDEB

During wound healing, matrix metalloproteinase (MMPs) play a vital role in cell migration, tissue remodeling and inflammation (Gill and Parks, 2008). Given the constant wounded environment in RDEB, there have been reports of elevated levels of MMPs in the fragile skin (Bodemer *et al.*, 2003; Bruckner-Tuderman *et al.*, 1992; Sato *et al.*, 1995). *MMP1* gene, which encodes a type VII collagen degrading enzyme, has recently emerged as being a modifier gene involved in RDEB. A single nucleotide polymorphism in *MMP1* promoter increased expression of MMP1 protein (Titeux *et al.*, 2008). This increased expression of MMP1 resulted in a faster degradation of type VII collagen, and a worse disease severity in RDEB patients. How this modifier gene relates to the development of cSCC in RDEB patients is yet to be determined. While the presence of this modifier gene may provide an explanation for the phenotypic variation observed in some DEB patients with the same *COL7A1* mutations, it is unlikely to be the sole modifier. In support of this notion, recent observations by a separate group did not find a correlation between RDEB disease severity and MMP1 genotype (Kern *et al.*, 2009).

MMP protein expression has been investigated in RDEB cSCC: MMP-7 protein levels were detected in both RDEB SCC (25 of 25 samples) and UV induced cSCC (60 of 61 samples) but only detected in 1 of 27 normal skin samples (Kivisaari *et al.*, 2008). The intensity of MMP-7 immunostaining was correlated significantly and positively with the histological grade of RDEB SCC tumour, which was not observed in sporadic UV-induced cSCC. Specific knockdown of MMP-7 using RNAi in cSCC cell-lines inhibits shedding of heparin-binding epidermal growth factor-like growth factor (HB-EGF), resulting in attenuation of EGF signalling and reduced cell proliferation (Kivisaari *et al.*, 2010). Another cSCC specific marker, which has been suggested to be involved in RDEB tumourigenesis, is mucin-1. This marker is found in all RDEB SCCs (n=25), JEB SCC (n=5) and 52 of 55 UV induced cSCCs (Cooper *et al.*, 2004).

IGFB3 and RDEB SCC

Gene expression profiling was studied using microarray comparing RDEB SCC (n=3) and non-RDEB SCC tissue (n=3) with the corresponding peri-tumoural skin found decreased expression of death-associated kinase-3 and insulin-like growth factor-binding protein-3 (*IGFBP-3*) genes in RDEB SCC compared to non-RDEB SCC (Mallipeddi *et al.*, 2004). In particular, the reduced expression of IGFBP-3 was confirmed using semi-quantitative RT-PCR, real-time PCR and immunohistochemistry. The authors speculate that the diminished levels of IGFBP result in reduced tumour cell apoptosis by allowing cSCC to grow unchecked. However, further work has yet to demonstrate the biological implications of reduced levels of IGFBP in RDEB SCC development. It is also important to note that overall there were very few differences between RDEB and non-RDEB SCC expression profiles in this experiment (Mallipeddi *et al.*, 2004).

Are there differences between RDEB SCC and non-RDEB SCC?

The clinical data would suggest defined pathology unique to RDEB SCC yet numerous molecular and histological studies identify only similarities with UV induced cSCC in the general population (Tyring *et al.*, 1989; Arbiser *et al.*, 1998; Arbiser *et al.*, 2004; Cooper *et al.*, 2004; Mallipeddi *et al.*, 2004; Kivisaari *et al.*, 2008; Purdie *et al.*, 2010) and those which report differences are neither replicated nor significantly powered to make definitive conclusions (Mallipeddi *et al.*, 2004; Ortiz-Urda *et al.*, 2005). To date no single study has identified a distinct difference in the histology or expression of markers both at the mRNA or protein level when comparing cSCC from RDEB patients with cSCC in the general population. We have recently tried to address this question with a gene expression study utilising microarrays containing more than 47,000 probes to interrogate RNA isolated from primary cSCC keratinocytes isolated from RDEB and non-RDEB patients (Watt *et al.*, 2011). Disappointingly, yet consistent with previous studies, no significant differences between the tumour groups were identified: unsupervised clustering of this array data demonstrated lack of separation between RDEB and non-RDEB cSCC samples (Fig. 1). However, the dendrogram was able to clearly separate non-cSCC (NHK and EBK) from cSCC (SCC and RDEB SCC) keratinocytes, and further interrogation of this data has identified markers common to all cSCC which have potential for development as therapeutic targets in RDEB

SCC (Watt *et al.*, 2011). Overall, this data suggests that the aggressive nature of RDEB SCC may not be accounted for by differences in the tumour keratinocytes.

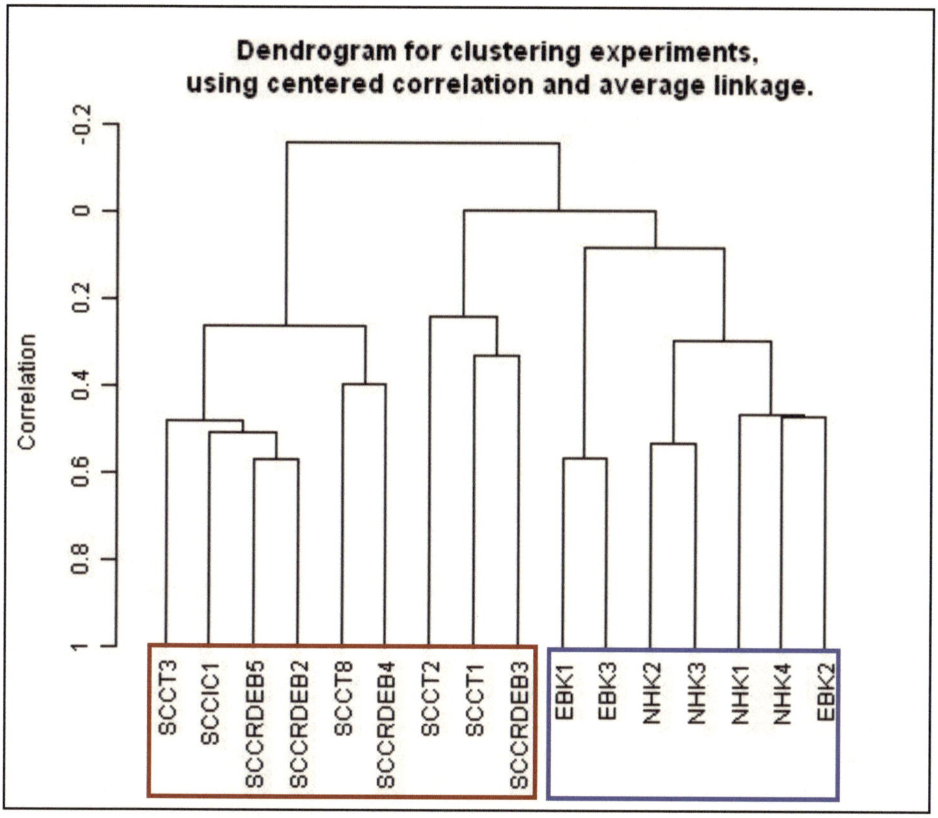

Fig. 1. Unsupervised clustering of *in vitro* keratinocyte gene expression data separates tumour from normal but is unable to distinguish RDEB cSCC from non-RDEB cSCC. Although cSCC keratinocyte samples (red box) cluster independently of non-cSCC keratinocyte samples (blue box), no clear separation of RDEB SCC and non-RDEB SCC keratinocytes is found. NHK = normal skin samples, EB = cells isolated from RDEB skin, SCC = UV-induced cSCC. SCCRDEB = cSCC from RDEB patient (adapted from Watt et al., 2011).

3.4 RDEB SCC and the tumour microenvironment

Increasing evidence now points to the dermal component as being a major factor in wound healing and cSCC invasion in non-RDEB individuals (Gaggioli *et al.*, 2007; Erez *et al.*, 2010). In particular, fibroblasts have been shown to play a role in cancer initiation and progression via stromal-epithelial interactions (Bhowmick *et al.*, 2004). They can provide oncogenic signals such as fibroblast growth factors, which act in a paracrine manner to the transformed tumour keratinocytes. These stromal cells are said to be "activated", becoming more proliferative and secreting more ECM proteins like type I collagen and fibronectin. Such fibroblasts are also known as cancer-associated fibroblasts (CAF) (Kalluri and Zeisberg, 2006).

The observation that little differences were observed between RDEB tumour and non-RDEB tumour keratinocytes, and in the light of recent recognition of the importance of the tumour microenvironment prompted us to investigate the other major type VII collagen secreting cell type of the surrounding stroma in RDEB skin and RDEB SCC - the dermal fibroblasts (Marinkovich *et al.*, 1993; Goto *et al.*, 2006).
To study this, we have undertaken gene expression profiling comparing cultured primary human dermal fibroblasts isolated from reduction surgery samples (normal), RDEB skin from patients yet to be diagnosed with cSCC, cSCC tumours arising in the general population and those from RDEB patients. Preliminary results are promising. Based on the microarray data, RDEB and cSCC fibroblasts share similar gene expression profile in culture and that the RDEB SCC fibroblasts are most dysregulated at the mRNA level out of all three disease states compared to normal fibroblasts (Ng *et al.*, 2010). These data suggests that the dermal microenvironment may be conducive to tumourigenesis and that transformation of RDEB to RDEB cSCC fibroblast may be crucial in accounting for the aggressive nature of cSCCs in RDEB patients.

3.5 Future directions in RDEB SCC

At present there is no cure for RDEB. However, several molecular therapies, which aim to correct EB, are currently undergoing clinical trials. One of the most promising therapies for RDEB patients is bone marrow transplantation. Following normal donor marrow-derived cells injection in murine *COL7A1*$^{(-/-)}$ models, successful re-expression of type VII collagen forming rudimentary anchoring fibrils and reduced blister formation was observed in the skin (Tolar *et al.*, 2009). These positive results prompted human clinical trials involving bone marrow transplant therapy in RDEB patients. The latest published clinical trial results are encouraging (Wagner *et al.*, 2010). Six out of seven children underwent successful transplantation after which they experienced improved wound healing and reduced blister formation between 30-130 days post transplantation, increased type VII collagen deposition and a sustained presence of donor cells in their skin. One patient died about 6 months post-transplantation as a consequence of graft rejection and infection. Hence, while this approach holds much promise, it is not without its inherent risks. Furthermore, immune-suppression in solid organ transplant patients has been linked to a high risk for developing skin cancer. Given that RDEB patients are already predisposed to develop cSCC, it remains to be seen if immunosuppression in the RDEB patients undergoing bone marrow transplantation will further accelerate cSCC development or whether improving the clinical condition will result in a reduction in cSCC incidence.

4. Conclusion

While most efforts and funding have been directed towards understanding the complex nature of skin cancer in the general population, sometimes it is through the study of the rare genetic disorders, such as xeroderma pigmentosum and RDEB, which offers insights into the biology of cSCC tumourigenesis by virtue of their known genetic mutation(s) leading to a specific phenotype. Through the study of XP, we know the importance of DNA repair in correcting UV damage in the skin. In the case of RDEB, the reasons for the development of numerous life-threatening cSCCs are still not fully elucidated, but evidence points towards a role for a permissive tumour microenvironment.

5. References

Agrawal N, Frederick MJ, Pickering CR, Bettegowda C, Chang K, Li RJ, *et al.* (2011) Exome sequencing of head and neck squamous cell carcinoma reveals inactivating mutations in NOTCH1. *Science* Epub 2011 Jul 28. doi: 10.1126/science.1206923.

Alter BP (2003) Cancer in Fanconi anemia, 1927-2001. *Cancer* 97:425-440.

Alter BP, Olson SB (2009) Wilms tumor, AML, and medulloblastoma in a child with cancer prone syndrome of total premature chromatid separation and Fanconi anemia. *Pediatr Blood Cancer* 54:488; author reply 489.

Arbiser JL, Fine JD, Murrell D, Paller A, Connors S, Keough K, *et al.* (1998) Basic fibroblast growth factor: a missing link between collagen VII, increased collagenase, and squamous cell carcinoma in recessive dystrophic epidermolysis bullosa. *Mol Med* 4:191-195.

Arbiser JL, Fan CY, Su X, Van Emburgh BO, Cerimele F, Miller MS, *et al.* (2004) Involvement of p53 and p16 tumor suppressor genes in recessive dystrophic epidermolysis bullosa-associated squamous cell carcinoma. *J Invest Dermatol* 123:788-790.

Arita K, Wessagowit V, Inamadar AC, Palit A, Fassihi H, Lai-Cheong JE, *et al.* (2007) Unusual molecular findings in Kindler syndrome. *Br J Dermatol* 157:1252-1256.

Arnault JP, Wechsler J, Escudier B, Spatz A, Tomasic G, Sibaud V, *et al.* (2009) Keratoacanthomas and squamous cell carcinomas in patients receiving sorafenib. *J Clin Oncol* 27:e59-61.

Arron ST, Ruby JG, Dybbro E, Ganem D, Derisi JL (2011) Transcriptome sequencing demonstrates that human papillomavirus is not active in cutaneous squamous cell carcinoma. *J Invest Dermatol* 131:1745-1753.

Ashton GH, McLean WH, South AP, Oyama N, Smith FJ, Al-Suwaid R, *et al.* (2004) Recurrent mutations in kindlin-1, a novel keratinocyte focal contact protein, in the autosomal recessive skin fragility and photosensitivity disorder, Kindler syndrome. *J Invest Dermatol* 122:78-83.

Astori G, Lavergne D, Benton C, Hockmayr B, Egawa K, Garbe C, *et al.* (1998) Human Papillomaviruses are Commonly Found in Normal Skin of Immunocompetent Hosts. *J Invest Dermatol* 110:752-755.

Baba Y, Iyama K, Honda S, Ishikawa S, Miyanari N, Baba H (2006) Cytoplasmic expression of type VII collagen is related to prognosis in patients with esophageal squamous cell carcinoma. *Oncology* 71:221-228.

Bagby GC, Jr. (2003) Genetic basis of Fanconi anemia. *Curr Opin Hematol* 10:68-76.

Bagby GC, Alter BP (2006) Fanconi anemia. *Semin Hematol* 43:147-156.

Balmain A, Ramsden M, Bowden GT, Smith J (1984) Activation of the mouse cellular Harvey-ras gene in chemically induced benign skin papillomas. *Nature* 307:658-660.

Barkan D, El Touny LH, Michalowski AM, Smith JA, Chu I, Davis AS, *et al.* (2010) Metastatic growth from dormant cells induced by a col-I-enriched fibrotic environment. *Cancer Res* 70:5706-5716.

Bazex A, Griffiths A (1980) Acrokeratosis paraneoplastica--a new cutaneous marker of malignancy. *Br J Dermatol* 103:301-306.

Bechetoille N, Haftek M, Staquet MJ, Cochran AJ, Schmitt D, Berthier-Vergnes O (2000) Penetration of human metastatic melanoma cells through an authentic dermal-epidermal junction is associated with dissolution of native collagen types IV and VII. *Melanoma Res* 10:427-434.

Benjamin CL, Ananthaswamy HN (2007) p53 and the pathogenesis of skin cancer. *Toxicol Appl Pharmacol* 224:241-248.

Bhowmick NA, Chytil A, Plieth D, Gorska AE, Dumont N, Shappell S, *et al.* (2004) TGF-beta signaling in fibroblasts modulates the oncogenic potential of adjacent epithelia. *Science* 303:848-851.

Blumenthal GM, Dennis PA (2008) PTEN hamartoma tumor syndromes. *Eur J Hum Genet* 16:1289-1300.

Bodemer C, Tchen SI, Ghomrasseni S, Seguier S, Gaultier F, Fraitag S, *et al.* (2003) Skin expression of metalloproteinases and tissue inhibitor of metalloproteinases in sibling patients with recessive dystrophic epidermolysis and intrafamilial phenotypic variation. *J Invest Dermatol* 121:273-279.

Bonkhoff H (1998) Analytical molecular pathology of epithelial-stromal interactions in the normal and neoplastic prostate. *Anal Quant Cytol Histol* 20:437-442.

Borg MF, Olver IN, Hill MP (1998) Rothmund-Thomson syndrome and tolerance of chemoradiotherapy. *Australas Radiol* 42:216-218.

Boukamp P, Stanbridge EJ, Foo DY, Cerutti PA, Fusenig NE (1990) c-Ha-ras oncogene expression in immortalized human keratinocytes (HaCaT) alters growth potential in vivo but lacks correlation with malignancy. *Cancer Res* 50:2840-2847.

Brash DE, Rudolph JA, Simon JA, Lin A, McKenna GJ, Baden HP, *et al.* (1991) A role for sunlight in skin cancer: UV-induced p53 mutations in squamous cell carcinoma. *Proc Natl Acad Sci U S A* 88:10124-10128.

Brown VL, Harwood CA, Crook T, Cronin JG, Kelsell DP, Proby CM (2004) p16INK4a and p14ARF tumor suppressor genes are commonly inactivated in cutaneous squamous cell carcinoma. *J Invest Dermatol* 122:1284-1292.

Bruckner-Tuderman L, Winberg JO, Anton-Lamprecht I, Schnyder UW, Gedde-Dahl T, Jr. (1992) Anchoring fibrils, collagen VII, and neutral metalloproteases in recessive dystrophic epidermolysis bullosa inversa. *J Invest Dermatol* 99:550-558.

Bruckner-Tuderman L (2001) Dermal-epidermal adhesion. In: *Cell adhesion and migration in skin disease* (Barker J, McGrath J, eds), Amsterdam: Harwood Academic Publishers, 133-163.

Burgeson RE (1993) Type VII collagen, anchoring fibrils, and epidermolysis bullosa. *J Invest Dermatol* 101:252-255.

Byrne CR (2006) The focal nature of Darier's disease lesions: calcium pumps, stress, and mutation? *J Invest Dermatol* 126:702-703.

Campbell C, Quinn AG, Ro YS, Angus B, Rees JL (1993) p53 mutations are common and early events that precede tumor invasion in squamous cell neoplasia of the skin. *J Invest Dermatol* 100:746-748.

Chen M, Kasahara N, Keene DR, Chan L, Hoeffler WK, Finlay D, *et al.* (2002) Restoration of type VII collagen expression and function in dystrophic epidermolysis bullosa. *Nat Genet* 32:670-675.

Chen M, Hou Y, Wang X, Martin S, Li W, Woodley D (2008) A 684 helical domain of type VII collagen promotes in vivo skin wound closure by enhancing fibroblast and keratinocyte migration [Abstract]. *J Invest Dermatol* 128:S48.

Chorny JA, Shroyer KR, Golitz LE (1993) Malignant melanoma and a squamous cell carcinoma in recessive dystrophic epidermolysis bullosa. *Arch Dermatol* 129:1212.

Christiano AM, Anhalt G, Gibbons S, Bauer EA, Uitto J (1994) Premature termination codons in the type VII collagen gene (COL7A1) underlie severe, mutilating recessive dystrophic epidermolysis bullosa. *Genomics* 21:160-168.

Christiano AM, Uitto J (1996) Molecular complexity of the cutaneous basement membrane zone. Revelations from the paradigms of epidermolysis bullosa. *Exp Dermatol* 5:1-11.

Christiano AM, Amano S, Eichenfield LF, Burgeson RE, Uitto J (1997) Premature termination codon mutations in the type VII collagen gene in recessive dystrophic epidermolysis bullosa result in nonsense-mediated mRNA decay and absence of functional protein. *J Invest Dermatol* 109:390-394.

Christiano AM, Crollick J, Pincus S, Uitto J (1999) Squamous cell carcinoma in a family with dominant dystrophic epidermolysis bullosa: a molecular genetic study. *Exp Dermatol* 8:146-152.

Conrado LA, Marques SA, Lastoria JC, Cuce LC, Marques ME, Dillon NL (2007) Keratitis-ichthyosis-deafness (KID) syndrome with squamous cell carcinoma. *Int J Dermatol* 46:403-406.

Cooper HL, Cook IS, Theaker JM, Mallipeddi R, McGrath J, Friedmann P, *et al.* (2004) Expression and glycosylation of MUC1 in epidermolysis bullosa-associated and sporadic cutaneous squamous cell carcinomas. *Br J Dermatol* 151:540-545.

CRUK (2011a) CancerStats report: Incidence 2008 UK [Online] Available from: http://info.cancerresearchuk.org/prod_consump/groups/cr_common/@nre/@sta/documents/generalcontent/cr_072111.pdf (Accessed June 2011).

CRUK (2011b) Latest UK cancer incidence year and mortality year summary - age standardised rates [Online] Available from: http://info.cancerresearchuk.org/prod_consump/groups/cr_common/@nre/@sta/documents/generalcontent/cr_072108.pdf (Accessed June 2011).

Dajee M, Lazarov M, Zhang JY, Cai T, Green CL, Russell AJ, *et al.* (2003) NF-kappaB blockade and oncogenic Ras trigger invasive human epidermal neoplasia. *Nature* 421:639-643.

Daya-Grosjean L, Robert C, Drougard C, Suarez H, Sarasin A (1993) High mutation frequency in ras genes of skin tumors isolated from DNA repair deficient xeroderma pigmentosum patients. *Cancer Res* 53:1625-1629.

Daya-Grosjean L, Sarasin A (2005) The role of UV induced lesions in skin carcinogenesis: an overview of oncogene and tumor suppressor gene modifications in xeroderma pigmentosum skin tumors. *Mutat Res* 571:43-56.

de Oliveira WR, Festa Neto C, Rady PL, Tyring SK (2003) Clinical aspects of epidermodysplasia verruciformis. *J Eur Acad Dermatol Venereol* 17:394-398.

Dhitavat J, Fairclough RJ, Hovnanian A, Burge SM (2004) Calcium pumps and keratinocytes: lessons from Darier's disease and Hailey-Hailey disease. *Br J Dermatol* 150:821-828.

Downs AM, Ward KA, Peachey RD (1997) Subungual squamous cell carcinoma in Darier's disease. *Clin Exp Dermatol* 22:277-279.

Dumas V, Kanitakis J, Charvat S, Euvrard S, Faure M, Claudy A (1999) Expression of basement membrane antigens and matrix metalloproteinases 2 and 9 in cutaneous basal and squamous cell carcinomas. *Anticancer Res* 19:2929-2938.

Durinck S, Ho C, Wang NJ, Liao W, Jakkula LR, Collisson EA, *et al.* (2011) Temporal dissection of tumorigenesis in primary cancers. *Cancer Discovery* Epub 2011 June 29. doi: 10.1158/2159-8290.cd-11-0028

Eady RAJ, Fine J-D, Burge SM (2004) Genetic blistering diseases. In: *Rook's textbook of dermatology* (Burns T, Breathnach S, Cox N, Griffiths C, eds) 7th ed., Vol. 2, Oxford: Wiley-Blackwell.

Ellis NA, Groden J, Ye TZ, Straughen J, Lennon DJ, Ciocci S, *et al.* (1995) The Bloom's syndrome gene product is homologous to RecQ helicases. *Cell* 83:655-666.

Emanuel PO, Rudikoff D, Phelps RG (2006) Aggressive squamous cell carcinoma in Kindler syndrome. *Skinmed* 5:305-307.

Epstein E, Sr. (1984) Metastases of sun-induced SCC. *J Dermatol Surg Oncol* 10:418.

Epstein EH (2008) Basal cell carcinomas: attack of the hedgehog. *Nat Rev Cancer* 8:743-754.

Erez N, Truitt M, Olson P, Hanahan D (2010) Cancer-associated fibroblasts are activated in incipient neoplasia to orchestrate tumor-promoting inflammation in an NF-kappaB- dependent manner. *Cancer Cell* 17:135-147.

Euvrard S, Kanitakis J, Claudy A (2003) Skin cancers after organ transplantation. *N Engl J Med* 348:1681-1691.

Ferguson-Smith MA, Wallace DC, James ZH, Renwick JH (1971) Multiple self-healing squamous epithelioma. *Birth Defects Orig Artic Ser* 7:157-163.

Fine J-D (1999) The classification of inherited epidermolysis bullosa. In: *Epidermolysis bullosa: clinical, epidemiologic and laboratory advances and the findings of the national epidermolysis bullosa registry* (Fine J-D, Bauer E, McGuire J, Moshell A, eds), Baltimore: The Johns Hopkins University Press., 20-47.

Fine J-D, Johnson LB, Suchindran C, Moshell A, Jr TG-D (1999) The epidemology of inherited epidermolysis bullosa: Findings in U.S., Canadian and European Study Populations. In: *Epidermolysis bullosa: clinical, epidemiologic and laboratory advances and the findings of the national epidermolysis bullosa registry* (Fine J-D, Bauer E, McGuire J, Moshell A, eds), Baltimore: The Johns Hopkins University Press., 101-113.

Fine J-D, Eady RAJ, Bauer EA, Bauer JW, Bruckner-Tuderman L, Heagerty A, *et al.* (2008) The classification of inherited epidermolysis bullosa (EB): Report of the Third International Consensus Meeting on Diagnosis and Classification of EB. *J Am Acad Dermatol* 58:931-950.

Fine JD, Johnson LB, Weiner M, Li KP, Suchindran C (2009) Epidermolysis bullosa and the risk of life-threatening cancers: the National EB Registry experience, 1986-2006. *J Am Acad Dermatol* 60:203-211.

Fine JD, Mellerio JE (2009) Extracutaneous manifestations and complications of inherited epidermolysis bullosa: part I. Epithelial associated tissues. *J Am Acad Dermatol* 61:367-384.

Flaherty K, Puzanov I, Sosman J (2009) Phase I study of PLX4032: proof of concept for V600E BRAF mutation as a therapeutic target in human cancer [Abstract]. *J Clin Oncol* 27:155.

Gaggioli C, Hooper S, Hidalgo-Carcedo C, Grosse R, Marshall JF, Harrington K, *et al.* (2007) Fibroblast-led collective invasion of carcinoma cells with differing roles for RhoGTPases in leading and following cells. *Nat Cell Biol* 9:1392-1400.

German J (1997) Bloom's syndrome. XX. The first 100 cancers. *Cancer Genet Cytogenet* 93:100-106.

German J, Sanz MM, Ciocci S, Ye TZ, Ellis NA (2007) Syndrome-causing mutations of the BLM gene in persons in the Bloom's Syndrome Registry. *Hum Mutat* 28:743-753.

Gill SE, Parks WC (2008) Metalloproteinases and their inhibitors: regulators of wound healing. *Int J Biochem Cell Biol* 40:1334-1347.

Goldberg GI, Eisen AZ, Bauer EA (1988) Tissue stress and tumor promotion. Possible relevance to epidermolysis bullosa. *Arch Dermatol* 124:737-741.

Goldstein AM, Liu L, Shennan MG, Hogg D, Tucker MA, Struewing JP (2001) A common founder for the V126D CDKN2A mutation in seven North American melanoma-prone families. *Br J Cancer* 85:527-530.

Goto M, Sawamura D, Ito K, Abe M, Nishie W, Sakai K, *et al.* (2006) Fibroblasts show more potential as target cells than keratinocytes in COL7A1 gene therapy of dystrophic epidermolysis bullosa. *J Invest Dermatol* 126:766-772.

Goudie DR, D'Alessandro M, Merriman B, Lee H, Szeverenyi I, Avery S, *et al.* (2011) Multiple self-healing squamous epithelioma is caused by a disease-specific spectrum of mutations in TGFBR1. *Nat Genet* 43:365-369.

Green CL, Khavari PA (2004) Targets for molecular therapy of skin cancer. *Semin Cancer Biol* 14:63-69.

Gul U, Kilic A, Gonul M, Cakmak SK, Bayis SS (2007) Clinical aspects of epidermodysplasia verruciformis and review of the literature. *Int J Dermatol* 46:1069-1072.

Hall JM, Lee MK, Newman B, Morrow JE, Anderson LA, Huey B, *et al.* (1990) Linkage of early-onset familial breast cancer to chromosome 17q21. *Science* 250:1684-1689.

Hamm H, Traupe H, Brocker EB, Schubert H, Kolde G (1996) The scleroatrophic syndrome of Huriez: a cancer-prone genodermatosis. *Br J Dermatol* 134:512-518.

Hanahan D, Weinberg RA (2000) The hallmarks of cancer. *Cell* 100:57-70.

Hanahan D, Weinberg RA (2011) Hallmarks of cancer: the next generation. *Cell* 144:646-674.

Haneke E, Gutschmidt E (1979) Premature multiple Bowen's disease in poikiloderma congenitale with warty hyperkeratoses. *Dermatologica* 158:384-388.

Hara M, Hunayama M, Aiba S, Suetake T, Watanabe M, Tanaka M, *et al.* (1995) Acrokeratosis paraneoplastica (Bazex syndrome) associated with primary cutaneous squamous cell carcinoma of the lower leg, vitiligo and alopecia areata. *Br J Dermatol* 133:121-124.

Hartevelt MM, Bavinck JN, Kootte AM, Vermeer BJ, Vandenbroucke JP (1990) Incidence of skin cancer after renal transplantation in The Netherlands. *Transplantation* 49:506-509.

Harwood CA, Proby CM (2002) Human papillomaviruses and non-melanoma skin cancer. *Current Opinion in Infectious Diseases* 15:101-114.

Heidorn SJ, Milagre C, Whittaker S, Nourry A, Niculescu-Duvas I, Dhomen N, *et al.* (2010) Kinase-dead BRAF and oncogenic RAS cooperate to drive tumor progression through CRAF. *Cell* 140:209-221.

Hemel D, Domchek SM (2010) Breast cancer predisposition syndromes. *Hematol Oncol Clin North Am* 24:799-814.

Hovnanian A, Duquesnoy P, Blanchet-Bardon C, Knowlton RG, Amselem S, Lathrop M, *et al.* (1992) Genetic linkage of recessive dystrophic epidermolysis bullosa to the type VII collagen gene. *J Clin Invest* 90:1032-1036.

Howlett NG, Taniguchi T, Olson S, Cox B, Waisfisz Q, De Die-Smulders C, *et al.* (2002) Biallelic inactivation of BRCA2 in Fanconi anemia. *Science* 297:606-609.

Huang S, Lee L, Hanson NB, Lenaerts C, Hoehn H, Poot M, *et al.* (2006) The spectrum of WRN mutations in Werner syndrome patients. *Hum Mutat* 27:558-567.

Hurst R, Elliott RM, Goldson AJ, Fairweather-Tait SJ (2008) Se-methylselenocysteine alters collagen gene and protein expression in human prostate cells. *Cancer Letter* 269:117-126.

Jin Y, Martins C, Jin C, Salemark L, Jonsson N, Persson B, *et al.* (1999) Nonrandom karyotypic features in squamous cell carcinomas of the skin. *Genes Chromosomes Cancer* 26:295-303.

Johnson RL, Rothman AL, Xie J, Goodrich LV, Bare JW, Bonifas JM, *et al.* (1996) Human homolog of patched, a candidate gene for the basal cell nevus syndrome. *Science* 272:1668-1671.

Jones JC, Steinman HK, Goldsmith BA (1989) Hemidesmosomes, collagen VII, and intermediate filaments in basal cell carcinoma. *J Invest Dermatol* 93:662-671.

Kainulainen T, Grenman R, Oikarinen A, Greenspan DS, Salo T (1997) Distribution and synthesis of type VII collagen in oral squamous cell carcinoma. *J Oral Pathol Med* 26:414-418.

Kalluri R, Zeisberg M (2006) Fibroblasts in cancer. *Nat Rev Cancer* 6:392-401.

Kanitakis J, Barthelemy H, Faure M, Claudy A (1997) Intracellular expression of type VII collagen in squamous cell carcinoma complicating dystrophic epidermolysis bullosa. *Br J Dermatol* 137:310-313.

Kaspar TA, Wagner RF, Jr., Jablonska S, Niimura M, Tyring SK (1991) Prognosis and treatment of advanced squamous cell carcinoma secondary to epidermodysplasia verruciformis: a worldwide analysis of 11 patients. *J Dermatol Surg Oncol* 17:237-240.

Kern JS, Gruninger G, Imsak R, Muller ML, Schumann H, Kiritsi D, *et al.* (2009) Forty-two novel COL7A1 mutations and the role of a frequent single nucleotide polymorphism in the MMP1 promoter in modulation of disease severity in a large European dystrophic epidermolysis bullosa cohort. *Br J Dermatol* 161:1089-1097.

Kirkham N, Price ML, Gibson B, Leigh IM, Coburn P, Darley CR (1989) Type VII collagen antibody LH 7.2 identifies basement membrane characteristics of thin malignant melanomas. *J Pathol* 157:243-247.

Kita Y, Mimori K, Tanaka F, Matsumoto T, Haraguchi N, Ishikawa K, *et al.* (2009) Clinical significance of LAMB3 and COL7A1 mRNA in esophageal squamous cell carcinoma. *Eur J Surg Oncol* 35:52-58.

Kitao S, Shimamoto A, Goto M, Miller RW, Smithson WA, Lindor NM, *et al.* (1999) Mutations in RECQL4 cause a subset of cases of Rothmund-Thomson syndrome. *Nat Genet* 22:82-84.

Kivirikko S, McGrath JA, Baudoin C, Aberdam D, Ciatti S, Dunnill MG, McMillan JR, Eady RA, Ortonne JP, Meneguzzi G, *et al.* (1995) A homozygous nonsense mutation in the alpha 3 chain gene of laminin 5 (LAMA3) in lethal (Herlitz) junctional epidermolysis bullosa. *Hum Mol Genet.* 4: 959-962.

Kivirikko S, McGrath JA, Pulkkinen L, Uitto J, Christiano AM (1996) Mutational hotspots in the LAMB3 gene in the lethal (Herlitz) type of junctional epidermolysis bullosa. *Hum Mol Genet* 5:231-237.

Kivisaari AK, Kallajoki M, Mirtti T, McGrath JA, Bauer JW, Weber F, *et al.* (2008) Transformation-specific matrix metalloproteinases (MMP)-7 and MMP-13 are expressed by tumour cells in epidermolysis bullosa-associated squamous cell carcinomas. *Br J Dermatol* 158:778-785.

Kivisaari AK, Kallajoki M, Ala-aho R, McGrath JA, Bauer JW, Konigova R, *et al.* (2010) Matrix metalloproteinase-7 activates heparin-binding epidermal growth factor-like growth factor in cutaneous squamous cell carcinoma. *Br J Dermatol* 163:726-735.

Kowal-Vern A, Criswell BK (2005) Burn scar neoplasms: a literature review and statistical analysis. *Burns* 31:403-413.

Kraemer KH, Lee MM, Scotto J (1987) Xeroderma pigmentosum. Cutaneous, ocular, and neurologic abnormalities in 830 published cases. *Arch Dermatol* 123:241-250.

Kraemer KH (1993) Xeroderma pigmentosum. In: GeneReviews [Online] Available from: http://www.ncbi.nlm.nih.gov/entrez/query.fcgi?cmd=Retrieve&db=PubMed&dopt=Citation&list_uids=20301571 (Pagon RA BT, Dolan CR , Stephens K ed): University of Washington, Seattle (Accessed June 2011).

Kraemer KH, Lee MM, Andrews AD, Lambert WC (1994) The role of sunlight and DNA repair in melanoma and nonmelanoma skin cancer. The xeroderma pigmentosum paradigm. *Arch Dermatol* 130:1018-1021.

Kraemer KH, Patronas NJ, Schiffmann R, Brooks BP, Tamura D, DiGiovanna JJ (2007) Xeroderma pigmentosum, trichothiodystrophy and Cockayne syndrome: a complex genotype-phenotype relationship. *Neuroscience* 145:1388-1396.

Kromberg JG, Castle D, Zwane EM, Jenkins T (1989) Albinism and skin cancer in Southern Africa. *Clin Genet* 36:43-52.

Kromberg JG, Zwane E, Castle D, Jenkins T (1987) Albinism in South African blacks. *Lancet* 2:388-389.

Lai-Cheong JE, Tanaka A, Hawche G, Emanuel P, Maari C, Taskesen M, *et al.* (2009) Kindler syndrome: a focal adhesion genodermatosis. *Br J Dermatol* 160:233-242.

Lane DP (1992) Cancer. p53, guardian of the genome. *Nature* 358:15-16.

Lee YA, Stevens HP, Delaporte E, Wahn U, Reis A (2000) A gene for an autosomal dominant scleroatrophic syndrome predisposing to skin cancer (Huriez syndrome) maps to chromosome 4q23. *Am J Hum Genet* 66:326-330.

Leigh IM, Eady RA, Heagerty AH, Purkis PE, Whitehead PA, Burgeson RE (1988) Type VII collagen is a normal component of epidermal basement membrane, which shows altered expression in recessive dystrophic epidermolysis bullosa. *J Invest Dermatol* 90:639-642.

Leinonen PT, Hagg PM, Peltonen S, Jouhilahti EM, Melkko J, Korkiamaki T, *et al.* (2009) Reevaluation of the normal epidermal calcium gradient, and analysis of calcium levels and ATP receptors in Hailey-Hailey and Darier epidermis. *J Invest Dermatol* 129:1379-1387.

Lewis KG, Weinstock MA (2007) Trends in nonmelanoma skin cancer mortality rates in the United States, 1969 through 2000. *J Invest Dermatol* 127:2323-2327.

Li J, Yen C, Liaw D, Podsypanina K, Bose S, Wang SI, *et al.* (1997) PTEN, a putative protein tyrosine phosphatase gene mutated in human brain, breast, and prostate cancer. *Science* 275:1943-1947.

Liaw D, Marsh DJ, Li J, Dahia PL, Wang SI, Zheng Z, *et al.* (1997) Germline mutations of the PTEN gene in Cowden disease, an inherited breast and thyroid cancer syndrome. *Nat Genet* 16:64-67.

Lohi J, Leivo I, Owaribe K, Burgeson RE, Franssila K, Virtanen I (1998) Neoexpression of the epithelial adhesion complex antigens in thyroid tumours is associated with proliferation and squamous differentiation markers. *J Pathol* 184:191-196.

Machino H, Miki Y, Teramoto T, Shiraishi S, Sasaki MS (1984) Cytogenetic studies in a patient with porokeratosis of Mibelli, multiple cancers and a forme fruste of Werner's syndrome. *Br J Dermatol* 111:579-586.

Madariaga J, Fromowitz F, Phillips M, Hoover HC, Jr. (1986) Squamous cell carcinoma in congenital ichthyosis with deafness and keratitis. A case report and review of the literature. *Cancer* 57:2026-2029.

Malkin D (1994) p53 and the Li-Fraumeni syndrome. *Biochim Biophys Acta* 1198:197-213.

Mallipeddi R, Wessagowit V, South AP, Robson AM, Orchard GE, Eady RA, *et al.* (2004) Reduced expression of insulin-like growth factor-binding protein-3 (IGFBP-3) in Squamous cell carcinoma complicating recessive dystrophic epidermolysis bullosa. *J Invest Dermatol* 122:1302-1309.

Marcuzzi GP, Hufbauer M, Kasper HU, Weissenborn SJ, Smola S, Pfister H (2009) Spontaneous tumour development in human papillomavirus type 8 E6 transgenic mice and rapid induction by UV-light exposure and wounding. *J Gen Virol* 90:2855-2864.

Marinkovich MP, Keene DR, Rimberg CS, Burgeson RE (1993) Cellular origin of the dermal-epidermal basement membrane. *Developmental Dynamics* 197:255-267.

Martinez JC, Otley CC, Stasko T, Euvrard S, Brown C, Schanbacher CF, *et al.* (2003) Defining the clinical course of metastatic skin cancer in organ transplant recipients: a multicenter collaborative study. *Arch Dermatol* 139:301-306.

Martins V, Vyas J, Chen M, Purdie K, Mein C, South A, *et al.* (2009) Increased invasive behaviour in cutaneous squamous cell carcinoma with loss of basement-membrane type VII collagen. *J Cell Sci* 122:1788-1799.

Masini C, Fuchs PG, Gabrielli F, Stark S, Sera F, Ploner M, *et al.* (2003) Evidence for the association of human papillomavirus infection and cutaneous squamous cell carcinoma in immunocompetent individuals. *Arch Dermatol* 139:890-894.

Mazereeuw-Hautier J, Bitoun E, Chevrant-Breton J, Man SY, Bodemer C, Prins C, *et al.* (2007) Keratitis-ichthyosis-deafness syndrome: disease expression and spectrum of connexin 26 (GJB2) mutations in 14 patients. *Br J Dermatol* 156:1015-1019.

McGrath JA, Leigh IM, Eady RA (1992a) Intracellular expression of type VII collagen during wound healing in severe recessive dystrophic epidermolysis bullosa and normal human skin. *Br J Dermatol* 127:312-317.

McGrath JA, Schofield OM, Mayou BJ, McKee PH, Eady RA (1992b) Epidermolysis bullosa complicated by squamous cell carcinoma: report of 10 cases. *J Cutan Pathol* 19:116-123.

McGrath JA, Ishida-Yamamoto A, O'Grady A, Leigh IM, Eady RA (1993) Structural variations in anchoring fibrils in dystrophic epidermolysis bullosa: correlation with type VII collagen expression. *J Invest Dermatol* 100:366-372.

McGrath JA, Gatalica B, Christiano AM, Li K, Owaribe K, McMillan JR, Eady RA, Uitto J. (1995) Mutations in the 180-kD bullous pemphigoid antigen (BPAG2), a hemidesmosomal transmembrane collagen (COL17A1), in generalized atrophic benign epidermolysis bullosa. *Nat Genet.* 11: 83-86.

Micali G, Nasca MR, Innocenzi D, Frasin LA, Radi O, Parma P, *et al.* (2005) Association of palmoplantar keratoderma, cutaneous squamous cell carcinoma, dental anomalies, and hypogenitalism in four siblings with 46,XX karyotype: a new syndrome. *J Am Acad Dermatol* 53:S234-239.

Miki Y, Swensen J, Shattuck-Eidens D, Futreal PA, Harshman K, Tavtigian S, *et al.* (1994) A strong candidate for the breast and ovarian cancer susceptibility gene BRCA1. *Science* 266:66-71.

Miller DL, Weinstock MA (1994) Nonmelanoma skin cancer in the United States: incidence. *J Am Acad Dermatol* 30:774-778.

Ming M, Han W, Maddox J, Soltani K, Shea CR, Freeman DM, *et al.* (2009) UVB-induced ERK/AKT-dependent PTEN suppression promotes survival of epidermal keratinocytes. *Oncogene* 29:492-502.

Ming M, He YY (2009) PTEN: new insights into its regulation and function in skin cancer. *J Invest Dermatol* 129:2109-2112.

Nagle RB, Knox JD, Wolf C, Bowden GT, Cress AE (1994) Adhesion molecules, extracellular matrix, and proteases in prostate carcinoma. *J Cell Biochem Suppl* 19:232-237.

Narod SA, Feunteun J, Lynch HT, Watson P, Conway T, Lynch J, *et al.* (1991) Familial breast-ovarian cancer locus on chromosome 17q12-q23. *Lancet* 338:82-83.

Nelen MR, Padberg GW, Peeters EA, Lin AY, van den Helm B, Frants RR, *et al.* (1996) Localization of the gene for Cowden disease to chromosome 10q22-23. *Nat Genet* 13:114-116.

Ng Y, Pourreyron, Salas-Alanis J, Murrell D, McGrath J, Lane E, *et al.* (2010) Tumour microenvironment is implicated by dermal fibroblast expression profiling in the development of aggressive squamous cell carcinoma in patients with recessive dystrophic epidermolysis bullosa [Abstract]. *J Invest Dermatol* 130:S83.

Oetting WS, King RA (1993) Molecular basis of type I (tyrosinase-related) oculocutaneous albinism: mutations and polymorphisms of the human tyrosinase gene. *Hum Mutat* 2:1-6.

Office for National Statistics (2010) Mortality statistics: Deaths registered in 2009 - Review of the national statistician on deaths in england and wales, 2009. Available from: http://www.statistics.gov.uk/downloads/theme_health/dr2009/dr-09.pdf (Accessed May 2011).

Olivier M, Goldgar DE, Sodha N, Ohgaki H, Kleihues P, Hainaut P, *et al.* (2003) Li-Fraumeni and related syndromes: correlation between tumor type, family structure, and TP53 genotype. *Cancer Res* 63:6643-6650.

Orihuela E, Tyring SK, Pow-Sang M, Dozier S, Cirelli R, Arany I, *et al.* (1995) Development of human papillomavirus type 16 associated squamous cell carcinoma of the scrotum in a patient with Darier's disease treated with systemic isotretinoin. *J Urol* 153:1940-1943.

Orth G, Jablonska S, Favre M, Croissant O, Jarzabek-Chorzelska M, Rzesa G (1978) Characterization of two types of human papillomaviruses in lesions of epidermodysplasia verruciformis. *Proc Natl Acad Sci U S A* 75:1537-1541.

Ortiz-Urda S, Garcia J, Green CL, Chen L, Lin Q, Veitch DP, *et al.* (2005) Type VII collagen is required for Ras-driven human epidermal tumorigenesis. *Science* 307:1773-1776.

Parma P, Radi O, Vidal V, Chaboissier MC, Dellambra E, Valentini S, *et al.* (2006) R-spondin1 is essential in sex determination, skin differentiation and malignancy. *Nat Genet* 38:1304-1309.

Paulus W, Baur I, Liszka U, Drlicek M, Leigh I, Bruckner-Tuderman L (1995) Expression of type VII collagen, the major anchoring fibril component, in normal and neoplastic human nervous system. *Virchows Arch* 426:199-202.

Pecora AL, Landsman L, Imgrund SP, Lambert WC (1983) Acrokeratosis paraneoplastica (Bazex' syndrome). Report of a case and review of the literature. *Arch Dermatol* 119:820-826.

Pelisson I, Soler C, Chardonnet Y, Euvrard S, Schmitt D (1996) A possible role for human papillomaviruses and c-myc, c-Ha-ras, and p53 gene alterations in malignant cutaneous lesions from renal transplant recipients. *Cancer Detect Prev* 20:20-30.

Perry PK, Silverberg NB (2001) Cutaneous malignancy in albinism. *Cutis* 67:427-430.

Poon PK, O'Brien RL, Parker JW (1974) Defective DNA repair in Fanconi's anaemia. *Nature* 250:223-225.

Poulikakos PI, Zhang C, Bollag G, Shokat KM, Rosen N (2010) RAF inhibitors transactivate RAF dimers and ERK signalling in cells with wild-type BRAF. *Nature* 464:427-430.

Pourreyron C, Cox G, Mao X, Volz A, Baksh N (2007) Patients with recessive dystrophic epidermolysis bullosa develop squamous-cell carcinoma regardless of type VII collagen expression. *J Invest Dermatol* 127:2438-2444.

Purdie KJ, Pourreyron C, Fassihi H, Cepeda-Valdes R, Frew JW, Volz A, *et al.* (2010) No evidence that human papillomavirus is responsible for the aggressive nature of recessive dystrophic epidermolysis bullosa-associated squamous cell carcinoma. *J Invest Dermatol* 130:2853-2855.

Radi O, Parma P, Imbeaud S, Nasca MR, Uccellatore F, Maraschio P, *et al.* (2005) XX sex reversal, palmoplantar keratoderma, and predisposition to squamous cell carcinoma: genetic analysis in one family. *Am J Med Genet A* 138A:241-246.

Ramoz N, Rueda LA, Bouadjar B, Montoya LS, Orth G, Favre M (2002) Mutations in two adjacent novel genes are associated with epidermodysplasia verruciformis. *Nat Genet* 32:579-581.

Reed WB, Roenigk H, Dorner W, Welsh O, Martin FJO (1975) Epidermal neoplasms with epidermolysis bullosa dystrophica with the first report of carcinoma with the acquired type. *Arch Dermatol Res* 253:1-14.

Rodeck U, Uitto J (2007) Recessive dystrophic epidermolysis bullosa-associated squamous-cell carcinoma: an enigmatic entity with complex pathogenesis. *J Invest Dermatol* 127:2295-2296.

Ryynänen M, Knowlton RG, Parente MG, Chung LC, Chu ML, Uitto J (1991) Human type VII collagen: genetic linkage of the gene (COL7A1) on chromosome 3 to dominant dystrophic epidermolysis bullosa. *Am J Hum Genet* 49:797-803.

Saitoh S, Oiso N, Wada T, Narazaki O, Fukai K (2000) Oculocutaneous albinism type 2 with a P gene missense mutation in a patient with Angelman syndrome. *J Med Genet* 37:392-394.

Sakai LY, Keene DR, Morris NP, Burgeson RE (1986) Type VII collagen is a major structural component of anchoring fibrils. *J Cell Biol* 103:1577-1586.

Sakuntabhai A, Burge S, Monk S, Hovnanian A (1999a) Spectrum of novel ATP2A2 mutations in patients with Darier's disease. *Hum Mol Genet* 8:1611-1619.

Sakuntabhai A, Ruiz-Perez V, Carter S, Jacobsen N, Burge S, Monk S, *et al.* (1999b) Mutations in ATP2A2, encoding a Ca2+ pump, cause Darier disease. *Nat Genet* 21:271-277.

Sarkar B, Knecht R, Sarkar C, Weidauer H (1998) Bazex syndrome (acrokeratosis paraneoplastica). *Eur Arch Otorhinolaryngol* 255:205-210.

Sato M, Nishigori C, Lu Y, Zghal M, Yagi T, Takebe H (1994) Far less frequent mutations in ras genes than in the p53 gene in skin tumors of xeroderma pigmentosum patients. *Mol Carcinog* 11:98-105.

Sato T, Nomura K, Hashimoto I (1995) Expression of collagenase and stromelysin in skin fibroblasts from recessive dystrophic epidermolysis bullosa. *Arch Dermatol Res* 287:428-433.

Seal S, Thompson D, Renwick A, Elliott A, Kelly P, Barfoot R, *et al.* (2006) Truncating mutations in the Fanconi anemia J gene BRIP1 are low-penetrance breast cancer susceptibility alleles. *Nat Genet* 38:1239-1241.

Segrelles C, Ruiz S, Perez P, Murga C, Santos M, Budunova IV, *et al.* (2002) Functional roles of Akt signaling in mouse skin tumorigenesis. *Oncogene* 21:53-64.

Sehgal VN, Srivastava G (2005) Darier's (Darier-White) disease/keratosis follicularis. *Int J Dermatol* 44:184-192.

Sekar SC SC (2008) Huriez syndrome. *Indian J Dermatol Venereol Leprol* 74:409-410.

Sharma V, Sharma NL, Ranjan N, Tegta GR, Sarin S (2006) Acrokeratosis paraneoplastica (Bazex syndrome): case report and review of literature. *Dermatol Online J* 12:11.

Siegel DH, Ashton GH, Penagos HG, Lee JV, Feiler HS, Wilhelmsen KC, *et al.* (2003) Loss of kindlin-1, a human homolog of the Caenorhabditis elegans actin-extracellular-matrix linker protein UNC-112, causes Kindler syndrome. *Am J Hum Genet* 73:174-187.

Skinner BA, Greist MC, Norins AL (1981) The keratitis, ichthyosis, and deafness (KID) syndrome. *Arch Dermatol* 117:285-289.

Skovbjerg H, Anthonsen D, Lothe IM, Tveit KM, Kure EH, Vogel LK (2009) Collagen mRNA levels changes during colorectal cancer carcinogenesis. *BMC Cancer* 9:136.

Smith ML, Fornace AJ, Jr. (1997) p53-mediated protective responses to UV irradiation. *Proc Natl Acad Sci U S A* 94:12255-12257.

Smoller BA, McNutt NS, Carter DM, Gottlieb AB, Hsu A, Krueger J (1990a) Recessive dystrophic epidermolysis bullosa skin displays a chronic growth-activated immunophenotype. Implications for carcinogenesis. *Arch Dermatol* 126:78-83.

Smoller BR, Krueger J, McNutt NS, Hsu A (1990b) "Activated" keratinocyte phenotype is unifying feature in conditions which predispose to squamous cell carcinoma of the skin. *Mod Pathol* 3:171-175.

Song IC, Dicksheet S (1985) Management of squamous cell carcinoma in a patient with dominant-type epidermolysis bullosa dystrophica: a surgical challenge. *Plast Reconstr Surg* 75:732-736.

Srivastava S, Tong YA, Devadas K, Zou ZQ, Sykes VW, Chen Y, *et al.* (1992) Detection of both mutant and wild-type p53 protein in normal skin fibroblasts and demonstration of a shared 'second hit' on p53 in diverse tumors from a cancer-prone family with Li-Fraumeni syndrome. *Oncogene* 7:987-991.

Starink TM, van der Veen JP, Arwert F, de Waal LP, de Lange GG, Gille JJ, *et al.* (1986) The Cowden syndrome: a clinical and genetic study in 21 patients. *Clin Genet* 29:222-233.

Stransky N, Egloff AM, Tward AD, Kostic AD, Cibulskis K, Sivachenko A, *et al.* (2011) The mutational landscape of head and neck squamous cell carcinoma. *Science* Epub 2011 July 28. doi: 10.1126/science.1208130.

Summers CG (2009) Albinism: classification, clinical characteristics, and recent findings. *Optom Vis Sci* 86:659-662.

Suzuki A, de la Pompa JL, Stambolic V, Elia AJ, Sasaki T, del Barco Barrantes I, *et al.* (1998) High cancer susceptibility and embryonic lethality associated with mutation of the PTEN tumor suppressor gene in mice. *Curr Biol* 8:1169-1178.

Suzuki A, Itami S, Ohishi M, Hamada K, Inoue T, Komazawa N, *et al.* (2003) Keratinocyte-specific Pten deficiency results in epidermal hyperplasia, accelerated hair follicle morphogenesis and tumor formation. *Cancer Res* 63:674-681.

Taguchi M, Watanabe S, Yashima K, Murakami Y, Sekiya T, Ikeda S (1994) Aberrations of the tumor suppressor p53 gene and p53 protein in solar keratosis in human skin. *J Invest Dermatol* 103:500-503.

Tani T, Karttunen T, Kiviluoto T, Kivilaakso E, Burgeson RE, Sipponen P, *et al.* (1996) Alpha 6 beta 4 integrin and newly deposited laminin-1 and laminin-5 form the adhesion mechanism of gastric carcinoma. Continuous expression of laminins but not that of collagen VII is preserved in invasive parts of the carcinomas: implications for acquisition of the invading phenotype. *Am J Pathol* 149:781-793.

Terrinoni A, Codispoti A, Serra V, Bruno E, Didona B, Paradisi M, *et al.* (2010) Connexin 26 (GJB2) mutations as a cause of the KID syndrome with hearing loss. *Biochem Biophys Res Commun* 395:25-30.

Tidman MJ, Eady RA (1985) Evaluation of anchoring fibrils and other components of the dermal-epidermal junction in dystrophic epidermolysis bullosa by a quantitative ultrastructural technique. *J Invest Dermatol* 84:374-377.

Titeux M, Pendaries V, Tonasso L, Decha A, Bodemer C, Hovnanian A (2008) A frequent functional SNP in the MMP1 promoter is associated with higher disease severity in recessive dystrophic epidermolysis bullosa. *Hum Mutat* 29:267-276.

Tolar J, Ishida-Yamamoto A, Riddle M, McElmurry RT, Osborn M, Xia L, *et al.* (2009) Amelioration of epidermolysis bullosa by transfer of wild-type bone marrow cells. *Blood* 113:1167-1174.

Tyring SK, Chopra V, Johnson L, Fine JD (1989) Natural killer cell activity is reduced in patients with severe forms of inherited epidermolysis bullosa. *Arch Dermatol* 125:797-800.

Uitto J, Pulkkinen L, Christiano AM (1994) Molecular basis of the dystrophic and junctional forms of epidermolysis bullosa: mutations in the type VII collagen and kalinin (laminin 5) genes. *J Invest Dermatol* 103:39S-46S.

Uitto J, Pulkkinen L, Christiano AM (1999) The molecular basis of dystrophic forms of epidermolysis bullosa. In: *Epidermolysis bullosa: clinical, epidemiologic and laboratory advances and the findings of the national epidermolysis bullosa registry* (Fine J-D, Bauer E, McGuire J, Moshell A, eds), Baltimore: The Johns Hopkins University Press., 326-350.

Uitto J, Richard G (2004) Progress in epidermolysis bullosa: genetic classification and clinical implications. *Am J Med Genet C Semin Med Genet* 131C:61-74.

Varki R, Sadowski S, Uitto J, Pfendner E (2007) Epidermolysis bullosa. II. Type VII collagen mutations and phenotype-genotype correlations in the dystrophic subtypes. *J Med Genet* 44:181-192.

Vazquez J, Morales C, Gonzalez LO, Lamelas ML, Ribas A (2002) Vulval squamous cell carcinoma arising in localized Darier's disease. *Eur J Obstet Gynecol Reprod Biol* 102:206-208.

Veness MJ, Porceddu S, Palme CE, Morgan GJ (2007) Cutaneous head and neck squamous cell carcinoma metastatic to parotid and cervical lymph nodes. *Head Neck* 29:621-631.

Vidal, F., Aberdam, D., Miquel, C., Christiano, A. M., Pulkkinen, L., Uitto, J., Ortonne, J.-P., Meneguzzi, G. (1995) Integrin beta-4 mutations associated with junctional epidermolysis bullosa with pyloric atresia. *Nat Genet.* 10: 229-234.

Vindevoghel L, Chung KY, Davis A, Kouba D, Kivirikko S, Alder H, *et al.* (1997) A GT-rich sequence binding the transcription factor Sp1 is crucial for high expression of the human type VII collagen gene (COL7A1) in fibroblasts and keratinocytes. *J Biol Chem* 272:10196-10204.

Visser R, Arends JW, Leigh IM, Bosman FT (1993) Patterns and composition of basement membranes in colon adenomas and adenocarcinomas. *J Pathol* 170:285-290.

Viteri A, Munoz A, Barcelo R (2005) Acrokeratosis paraneoplastica (Bazex syndrome) preceeding the diagnosis of metastatic squamous cell carcinoma of the esophagus. *J Am Acad Dermatol* 52:711-712.

Wagner JE, Ishida-Yamamoto A, McGrath JA, Hordinsky M, Keene DR, Woodley DT, *et al.* (2010) Bone marrow transplantation for recessive dystrophic epidermolysis bullosa. *N Engl J Med* 363:629-639.

Waterman EA, Sakai N, Nguyen NT, Horst BAJ, Veitch DP, Dey CN, *et al.* (2007) A laminin-collagen complex drives human epidermal carcinogenesis through phosphoinositol-3-kinase activation. *Cancer Res* 67:4264-4270.

Watt SA, Pourreyron C, Purdie K, Hogan C, Cole CL, Foster N, *et al.* (2011) Integrative mRNA profiling comparing cultured primary cells with clinical samples reveals PLK1 and C20orf20 as therapeutic targets in cutaneous squamous cell carcinoma. *Oncogene* Epub 2001 May 23. doi: 10.1038/onc.2011.180

Wetzels RH, Robben HC, Leigh IM, Schaafsma HE, Vooijs GP, Ramaekers FC (1991) Distribution patterns of type VII collagen in normal and malignant human tissues. *Am J Pathol* 139:451-459.

Wetzels RH, Schaafsma HE, Leigh IM, Lane EB, Troyanovsky SM, Wagenaar SS, *et al.* (1992a) Laminin and type VII collagen distribution in different types of human lung carcinoma: correlation with expression of keratins 14, 16, 17 and 18. *Histopathology* 20:295-303.

Wetzels RH, van der Velden LA, Schaafsma HE, Manni JJ, Leigh IM, Vooijs GP, *et al.* (1992b) Immunohistochemical localization of basement membrane type VII collagen and laminin in neoplasms of the head and neck. *Histopathology* 21:459-464.

Woodley DT, Krueger GG, Jorgensen CM, Fairley JA, Atha T, Huang Y, *et al.* (2003) Normal and gene-corrected dystrophic epidermolysis bullosa fibroblasts alone can produce type VII collagen at the basement membrane zone. *J Invest Dermatol* 121:1021-1028.

Woodley DT, Remington J, Huang Y, Hou Y, Li W, Keene DR, *et al.* (2007) Intravenously injected human fibroblasts home to skin wounds, deliver type VII collagen, and promote wound healing. *Mol Ther* 15:628-635.

Woodley DT, Hou Y, Martin S, Li W, Chen M (2008) Characterization of molecular mechanisms underlying mutations in dystrophic epidermolysis bullosa using site-directed mutagenesis. *J Biol Chem* 283:17838-17845.

Wooster R, Bignell G, Lancaster J, Swift S, Seal S, Mangion J, *et al.* (1995) Identification of the breast cancer susceptibility gene BRCA2. *Nature* 378:789-792.

Xie J, Murone M, Luoh SM, Ryan A, Gu Q, Zhang C, *et al.* (1998) Activating Smoothened mutations in sporadic basal-cell carcinoma. *Nature* 391:90-92.

Yamamoto K, Imakiire A, Miyagawa N, Kasahara T (2003) A report of two cases of Werner's syndrome and review of the literature. *J Orthop Surg (Hong Kong)* 11:224-233.

Yasaka N, Kawabe K, Furue M, Tamaki K, Ishibashi Y (1994) Altered expression of NU-T2-BMZ antigen and type VII collagen in basal cell epithelioma. *J Dermatol Sci* 7:136-141.

Yazdanfar A, Hashemi B (2009) Kindler syndrome: report of three cases in a family and a brief review. *Int J Dermatol* 48:145-149.

Yuen WY, Jonkman MF (2011) Risk of squamous cell carcinoma in junctional epidermolysis bullosa, non-Herlitz type: Report of 7 cases and a review of the literature. *J Am Acad Dermatol* Epub 2011 31 May. doi: 10.1016/j.jaad.2010.07.006.

4

Melanoma Cell Signalling: Looking Beyond RAS-RAF-MEK

Visalini Muthusamy and Terrence J. Piva
RMIT University
Australia

1. Introduction

Melanoma is an invasive and malignant form of skin cancer (Besaratinia and Pfeifer, 2008). It originates from melanocytes, which reside in the epidermal layer of the skin. Besides the skin, melanoma's rapidly proliferative and aggressive nature leads to its manifestation in internal organs such as brain, lung and liver (Franco-Lie et al., 2011; Lejeune et al., 1992). Ultraviolet (UV) radiation (sunlight or tanning beds) is the main carcinogen involved in melanoma development. However, the type (UVA versus UVB) and duration of UV radiation (intermittent versus chronic and childhood sun exposure) necessary for melanoma initiation remains ambiguous (Algazi et al., 2010; Besaratinia and Pfeifer, 2008; Lazovich et al., 2010; Walker, 2008). In addition, the presence of melanocytic nevi and hereditary genetic mutations predisposes individuals to melanoma (Navarini et al., 2010; Pho and Leachman, 2010; Whiteman et al., 2003). As a result of these factors, it is estimated that 132,000 melanoma skin cancers occur annually (World Health Organization [WHO], 2011). This value is set to rise by 4,500 incidences for every 10% decrease in the UV-protective ozone levels (WHO, 2011).

Prevention strategies designed to curtail the onset of melanoma and improved treatment for this evolving anomaly require urgent action. Current treatments and adjuvant therapies for melanoma includes, surgical excision, radio-, chemo- and immunotherapy (Dummer et al., 2010; Petrescu et al., 2010). However, with the recurrence of these melanomas, the spotlight is on molecular targeted therapy. Such therapies require an in depth knowledge of melanoma signalling to treat this cancer. Molecular targeted therapy has focused predominantly on the RAS-RAF-MEK [mitogen activated protein kinase (MAPK)-extracellular signal-regulated kinase (ERK) kinase] and phosphoinositide-3-kinase (PI3K)/AKT pathways (Algazi et al., 2010; Friedlander and Hodi, 2010; Held et al., 2011; Sullivan and Atkins, 2010). However, due to the complex network of signalling pathways, it has become evident that targeting single pathways to eradicate melanoma is insufficient (Table 1) (Jiang et al., 2011; Johannessen et al., 2010; Nazarian et al., 2010; Shields et al., 2007). Shields *et al.* (2007) found a distinct subset of melanoma cell lines that did not exhibit high ERK and AKT activation but had increased expression of epithelial markers like P-cadherin, E-cadherin and CD24. These epithelial-like melanoma also had a loss of p53 function, decreased microphthalmia-associated transcription factor (MITF) levels and its targeted gene expression. Recent studies have also shown that many subsets of melanoma cells exhibit resistance to B-RAF inhibitors (Jiang et al., 2011; Nazarian et al., 2010).

Alternative signalling pathways/molecules	Resistant to:	Reference
P-cadherin/E-cadherin/CD24 melanoma subgroup	ERK/AKT inhibition	(Shields et al., 2007)
C-RAF/MEK/ERK signalling	B-RAF inhibition	(Nazarian et al., 2010)
Impaired FOXO3a nuclear localisation result in reduced Bim expression	MEK1/2 inhibition	(Yang et al., 2010)
P13K/AKT signalling	B-RAF inhibition	(Jiang et al., 2011)
Amplified wild-type KIT/CDK4 signalling	B-RAF inhibition	(Smalley et al., 2008)
Platelet-derived growth factor receptor β (PDGFRβ) signalling	B-RAF inhibition	(Nazarian et al., 2010)
COT/MEK/ERK signalling	B-RAF inhibition	(Johannessen et al., 2010)
Melanoma subgroups with constitutive B-RAF and MEK activity	N-RAS inhibition	(Inamdar et al., 2010)

Table 1. Signalling pathways/molecules rendering melanoma resistance.

Melanoma resistance to chemotherapy can and has been attributed to changes in cell signalling events (Grossman and Altieri, 2001). Photodynamic therapy (PDT) and cytotoxic agents were found to enhance survivin (member of the inhibitor of apoptotic protein family) expression which desensitised these cells to apoptosis (Ferrario et al., 2007; Qiu et al., 2005). Other anti-apoptotic factors (e.g. Bcl-2, and Bcl-X_L) are also found to be highly expressed in melanoma resulting in a chemo-resistant phenotype (Grossman and Altieri, 2001; Rass and Hassel, 2009). Multi-drug resistance transporters and DNA repair mechanisms that prevent cytotoxicity induced by alkylating agents have also been implicated in chemo-resistance (Grossman and Altieri, 2001; Rass and Hassel, 2009). As such, it is imperative to address possibilities of other mutations and compensatory/alternative signalling pathways involved in melanoma development and persistence. Therefore, this review presents an overview of melanoma cell signal transduction and highlights the recent advances made in this field as well as identifying molecular targets with therapeutic potential.

2. Melanoma signalling and therapeutical targets

2.1 Common therapeutical targets

Common oncogenic mutations in melanoma have been selected for targeted therapy. Inhibitors to these mutant proteins or their downstream effectors are currently undergoing clinical evaluation. However, it has been reported that melanoma cells are able to acquire resistance to some of these drugs (Jiang et al., 2011; Nazarian et al., 2010; Paraiso et al., 2011).

2.1.1 KIT

KIT, a receptor tyrosine kinase (RTK), is involved in normal melanocyte signalling (Easty et al., 2011). It is necessary for the migration of melanocytic precursors from the neural crest and regulates the survival, development and homeostasis of melanocytes (Hou et al., 2000; Wehrle-Haller, 2003). KIT undergoes genetic alterations in chronically sun damaged, acral and mucosal melanoma subgroups (Curtin et al., 2006; Friedlander and Hodi, 2010). Some melanomas also possess amplified wild type (WT) KIT due to high copy number (Curtin et al., 2006). Its increased expression has also been observed in melanoma cells without aberrant gene amplification (Curtin et al., 2006). A gain-of-function mutation or increased kinase activity of KIT causes constitutive activity of the MAPK and PI3K pathways which may lead to a hyper-proliferative and invasive melanoma subgroup (Woodman and Davies, 2010). Therefore, it has been postulated that targeting the KIT receptor may reduce the incidence of melanoma.

Imatinib (RTK inhibitor) prevents autophosphorylation of KIT which leads to the inactivation of MAPK, JAK-STAT, PI3K/AKT and anti-apoptotic pathways (Heinrich et al., 2000; Jiang et al., 2008). Imatinib was shown to reduce proliferation in KIT mutant mucosal melanoma cell cultures (Jiang et al., 2008). Although, this inhibitor was ineffective in unamplified WT KIT melanoma, it is unclear if it can eradicate those tumours which overexpress this receptor. Smalley *et al.* (2008) found that imatinib treatment was only effective in those melanomas which had elevated levels of phosphorylated (phospho) KIT. This suggests that irrespective of its overexpression, the efficacy of imatinib in treating melanoma requires the presence of active KIT. This inhibitor has specificity towards certain KIT mutation. While it is effective against mutant KIT in the juxtamembrane domain, it is ineffective against mutations occurring in the kinase domain of these receptors. In support, V559A (juxtamembrane domain) mutated KIT in a metastatic lung melanoma patient responded to imatinib therapy (Terheyden et al., 2010). However, imatinib had no effect in D820Y (kinase domain) mutated KIT in SM3 melanoma cells but another RTK inhibitor, sunitinib, inhibited the proliferation of these cells (Ashida et al., 2009).

Some tumours have evolved imatinib resistance by creating secondary genetic mutations in KIT but their occurrence in melanoma is unknown (Lim et al., 2008). A genetic comparison between imatinib-naïve and resistant melanoma cells will be useful to identify secondary mutations generated in resistant cell lines. Mutations can occur in the extracellular, juxtamembane and kinase domains of the KIT receptor (Woodman and Davies, 2010). Double KIT mutations have been reported in those melanomas which marginally responded to imatinib treatment (Curtin et al., 2005; McDonnell et al., 2011; Torres-Cabala et al., 2009). Three indolinone compounds were found to inhibit proliferation, and induce cell cycle arrest and apoptosis in mast cells harbouring KIT juxtamembrane and kinase domain mutations (Liao et al., 2002). Other RTK inhibitors, like nilotinib and dasatinib are effective against certain multi-exon KIT mutations except for those occurring at exon 14 (T670I) (Garrido and Bastian, 2010; Schittenhelm et al., 2006). Collectively, little is known about the effectiveness of different inhibitors on patients with specific KIT mutations. Since these inhibitors do not target all mutants, a matrix of various inhibitors and their efficacy against different KIT aberrations will aid in patient selection. The weight of evidence also suggests that patient selection for KIT inhibition therapy should not solely rely on the overexpression and mutational status of this receptor (Hofmann et al., 2009; Smalley et al., 2008). It is also necessary to identify constitutive KIT activation (phosphorylated form) and their involvement in melanoma progression before administration of RTK inhibitor therapy. This information is necessary, before an evaluation of KIT as a viable therapeutic target in melanoma patients is possible.

2.1.2 N-RAS

N-RAS, a GTPase of the RAS family activates RAF proteins in the MAPK signalling cascade and is involved in regulating cellular homeostasis and stress response (Held et al., 2011; Whitwam et al., 2007). Of the RAS isoforms (K-RAS and H-RAS), N-RAS is frequently mutated at codon 61 in 15-20% of melanomas (Held et al., 2011; Karnoub and Weinberg, 2008; Platz et al., 2008; Whitwam et al., 2007). N-RAS mutations increased as the cancer progressed from radial to vertical growth phase suggesting that these mutations are involved in both melanoma development and progression (Demunter et al., 2001; Omholt et al., 2003; Rosso et al., 2009). The mutant N-RAS exists in a GTP-bound conformation due to its defective GTPase activity which prevents the hydrolysis of GTP to GDP (Karnoub and Weinberg, 2008). This constitutive activity induces persistent activation of the MAPK and PI3K pathways resulting in melanoma cell survival and proliferation (Jiang et al., 2011; Sullivan and Atkins, 2010). Eskandarpour *et al.* (2009) found that mutant N-RAS is also necessary for the invasive and migratory phenotypes of melanoma cells. Also the overexpression of RAS has been implicated in melanoma chemoresistance to cytotoxic agents (Fujita et al., 1999).

RAS undergoes post-translational modifications to facilitate its association to the plasma membrane which is necessary for its bioactivity (Nammi and Lodagala, 2000; Sebti and Hamilton, 1997). A crucial modification is the farnesylation at its carboxy-terminus catalysed by farnesyl tranferase (Nammi and Lodagala, 2000; Reiss et al., 1990; Sebti and Hamilton, 1997). N-RAS is deactivated by farnesyl transferase inhibitors (FTI) which reduce its oncogenic potential making it a viable target for melanoma therapy (Johnston, 2001; Smalley and Eisen, 2003). However, early studies found that BZA-5B (FTI) increased resistance to cisplatin (cytotoxic drug) treatment in 224 melanoma cells (Fokstuen et al., 1997). In contrast, Niessner *et al.* (2011) found that SCH66336 (Lonafarnib; FTI) together with sorafenib showed efficacy in inducing growth inhibition and apoptosis of melanoma cells through mammalian target of rapamycin (mTOR) signalling however, no changes to the upstream effector, AKT was observed. They found that the FTI did not affect RAS activity but inhibited another GTPase, RHEB, which affected the mTOR signalling pathway.

Smalley *et al.* (2003) found that SCH66336 increased melanoma chemosensitivity to cisplatin-mediated cytotoxicity through G2/M-phase cell cycle arrest. Interestingly, this was not coordinated by typical RAS-driven ERK or P13K pathways. SCH66336 alone caused G1-phase cell cycle arrest and retinoblastoma inactivation in human (Colo 853) and mouse (B16) melanoma cells resulting in low proliferation and high apoptosis levels (Smalley and Eisen, 2003). In this study, RAS activity post-FTI treatment was not observed. Therefore, it is not clear if SCH66336-induced cytotoxicity is a result of RAS inactivity or the inhibition of other farnesylated proteins. It has also been reported that the RAS mutational status did not correlate with their sensitivity to FTI which suggests that other signalling molecules are affected by these inhibitors (Niessner et al., 2011; Sebti and Hamilton, 1997; Sepp-Lorenzino et al., 1995). Although, FTI are beneficial in joint therapies to overcome drug resistance, its non-specificity to N-RAS needs to be addressed (Flaherty, 2006; Held et al., 2011; McCubrey et al., 2009). Furthermore, FTI may also be ineffective if RAS downstream targets acquire oncogenic mutations.

2.1.3 B-RAF

B-RAF is a serine threonine kinase and together with C-RAF and A-RAF belong to the RAF kinase family. In the MAPK cascade, B-RAF phosphorylates MEK which results in the activation of the ERK pathway. B-RAF mutations are prevalent in 50-60% of melanomas with the most common mutation occurring at the 600th amino acid (valine to glutamate) (Held et al., 2011; Inamdar et al., 2010). It predominantly occurs in cutaneous melanomas at sites damaged by intermittent UV exposure (Bauer et al., 2011; Puzanov and Flaherty, 2010). Mutant B-RAF is constitutively active and independent of RAS activation (Inamdar et al., 2010). Persistent B-RAF activation leads to ERK-induced melanoma survival, proliferation, angiogenesis and invasion (Inamdar et al., 2010). Therefore, the B-RAF protein has become a promising candidate for molecular targeted therapy.

The general inhibitor, Sorafenib binds to the inactive forms of B-RAF and thus, is more effective in blocking WT B-RAF then constitutively active mutant B-RAF (McCubrey et al., 2009). In contrast, PLX4720 binds to both the inactive and active forms while SB590885 only associates with active B-RAF (McCubrey et al., 2009). PLX 4720 specifically inhibits B-RAF (V600E) mutant in melanoma cells and enhances Bim_s (pro-apoptotic protein) levels to induce apoptosis (Jiang et al., 2010). Another mutant B-RAF specific inhibitor, PLX4032 sensitised melanoma cells to ionizing radiation which induced cell cycle arrest, inhibited colony formation and invasion (Sambade et al., 2011). Although, RAF inhibitors seem promising in combating melanoma growth, this therapy has met with 'roadblocks' due to the emergence of alternative signalling pathways in these cells. PLX4032 reduced tumours in melanoma patients but drug resistance occurred after the initial anti-tumour response (Nazarian et al., 2010). This was due to reactivation of C-RAF/MEK/ERK by N-RAS mutations and upregulation of the PDGFRβ-dependent survival pathways. Jiang *et al.* (2011) found that melanoma cells resistant to PLX4720 maintained high ERK levels but low MEK activity. MEK inhibition itself was shown to be ineffective in overcoming PLX4720 resistance but serum starvation, PI3K/AKT and ERK inactivation reduced melanoma cell viability. Another route of resistance evident in melanoma patients relapsing from RAF or MEK inhibition therapy was that of COT-mediated ERK activation which was independent of RAS/RAF signalling (Johannessen et al., 2010).

ATP-competitive RAF inhibitors were found to inhibit ERK activation in B-RAF mutant cells but increased the proliferation of cells in RAS/RAF WT tumours (Hatzivassiliou et al., 2010). This could be due to the induction of WT B-RAF/C-RAF homo- or heterodimers after inhibitor treatment which allows signalling to continue via the uninhibited subunit of the dimer (Hatzivassiliou et al., 2010; Poulikakos et al., 2010). It is suggested that by increasing RAF inhibitor concentrations, both subunits of the dimer can be inactivated negating downstream signalling (Poulikakos et al., 2010). In addition, protein kinase D3 blockade in conjunction with RAF or MEK inhibition can prevent the reactivation of the MAPK pathway and thereby decrease the survival of resistant melanoma cell lines (Chen et al., 2011). On the whole, further research is needed to determine other modes of overcoming RAF inhibitor resistance. This also highlights the necessity to target downstream effectors of B-RAF/N-RAS and other compensatory survival pathways in melanoma.

2.1.4 Phosphoinositide-3-kinase/AKT

The PI3K/AKT pathway is activated by N-RAS and/or RTK which directs cell growth, proliferation, differentiation and survival (Held et al., 2011; Sullivan and Atkins, 2010). There are three classes of P13K and this dictates their substrate specificity (Aziz et al., 2009). P13K has several downstream targets such as AKT, mTOR, FOXO and nuclear factor-κB (NFκB) (Held et al., 2011). Phosphatase and tensin homolog (PTEN) dephosphorylates phosphatidylinositol 3,4,5-trisphosphate (PIP_3) thus preventing AKT activation and blocking PI3K signalling. As a result of mutant N-RAS, PTEN depletion/inactivation and/or constitutive activation of receptors, the PI3K pathway is permanently activated leading to malignant transformation of melanocytes (Held et al., 2011). Constitutive PI3K activity was associated with radiation resistant melanoma cells as treatment with LY294002 (PI3K inhibitor) sensitised melanoma cells to radiation and apoptosis (Krasilnikov et al., 1999). PI3K-dependent matrix metalloproteinase expression has also been implicated in vasculogenic mimicry in highly aggressive melanomas (Hess et al., 2003).

In melanoma therapy, besides PI3K, AKT and mTOR are also potential targets because of their involvement in tumorigenesis (Ko and Fisher, 2011; Sullivan and Atkins, 2010).

Govindarajan *et al.* (2007) showed that AKT overexpressing WM35 melanoma cells had high levels of vascular endothelial growth factor (VEGF; pro-angiogenic) and reactive oxygen species (ROS) *in vitro* and when implanted into nude mice, generated highly invasive and angiogenic tumours *in vivo*. Although, AKT overexpression and mutations have been reported, it is the activity of phospho-AKT that drives melanoma development (Stahl et al., 2004; Sullivan and Atkins, 2010). Approximately, 43-60% of those melanomas examined, had deregulated AKT signalling (Stahl et al., 2004). In a phase two study, using everolimus (mTOR inhibitor) and bevacizumab (angiogenic inhibitor), 53% of the melanoma patients had reduced tumour measurements, 12% of which were significant (Hainsworth et al., 2010). However, it was found that the RAD001 (mTOR inhibitor) induced a PI3K-dependent feedback loop activating the ERK pathway in some human cancers (Carracedo et al., 2008). Therefore, it is critical that the dual inhibition of the MAPK and PI3K pathways be used in treating these melanomas.

PI-103, a dual PI3K/mTOR inhibitor promoted *in vivo* tumour growth via inhibiting apoptosis and immunosurveillance in FVB/N WT mice transplanted with 37-31E-F3 melanoma cells (Lopez-Fauqued et al., 2010). In these mice, the combination of sorafenib (B-RAF inhibitor) and PI-103 increased the tumour volume compared to that seen for sorafenib alone (Lopez-Fauqued et al., 2010). Unlike the immunocompetent FVB/N WT mice, PI-103 was effective in reducing tumour growth in immunocompromised BALB/c nude mice. This data suggests that the immune status of the mouse models can also affect efficacy of PI-103 treatment. Although, the outcomes of this study could be specific to the type of melanoma cells, mouse models and PI3K inhibitor that were used, there is the possibility of risks associated with treating patients with different immune profiles or melanoma patients under immunotherapy in combination with signal transduction inhibition [for more information see Shada *et al.* (2010)]. Some of these PI3K/AKT/mTOR inhibitors are still undergoing clinical trials (Ko and Fisher, 2011; Sullivan and Atkins, 2010).

2.2 New therapeutical targets

In this section, potential signalling molecules and lesser known therapeutical targets undergoing clinical trials are discussed (Figure 1). The inhibition of these targets may help overcome drug resistance in melanoma (Hatzivassiliou et al., 2010; Jiang et al., 2011; Nazarian et al., 2010; Paraiso et al., 2011).

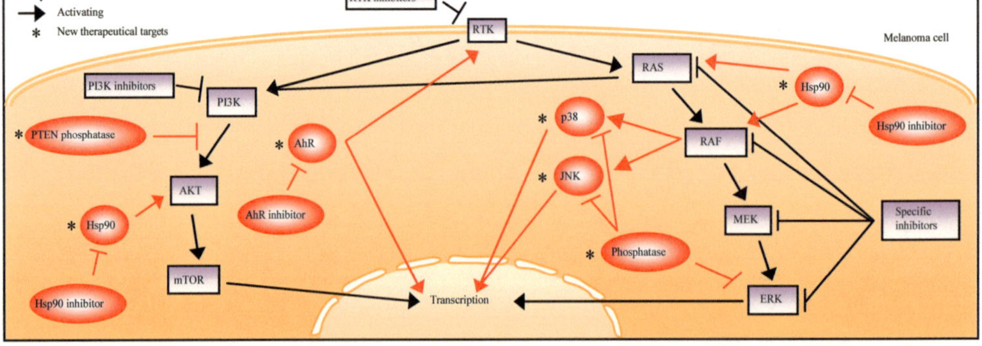

Fig. 1. A schematic diagram depicting common and new therapeutical targets in melanoma.

2.2.1 Aryl hydrocarbon receptor

Aryl hydrocarbon receptors (AhR) are cytosolic transcription factors which are triggered in response to environmental toxicants (e.g. dioxins and polychlorinated biphenyls) (Schmidt and Bradfield, 1996). After ligand binding, the AhR complex translocates into the nucleus where it dimerises with the AhR nuclear translocator while its co-factors [e.g. heat shock protein 90 (Hsp90)] dissociate to initiate transcription of target genes. It can also be activated independent of ligand binding but the mode of action is not clear (Schmidt and Bradfield, 1996). In the skin, UV radiation produces 6-formylindolo[3,2-*b*]carbazole (FICZ), an AhR ligand derived from tryptophan which can stimulate this pathway in response to stress (Fritsche et al., 2007). Fritsche *et al.* (2007) found that AhR-knockdown HaCaT keratinocytes do not possess phosoho-ERK1/2 activity due to inhibition of EGFR internalisation, which suggested that AhR is also involved in EGFR activation in these cells. It is unclear if the same occurs in melanocytes but the high levels of phospho-ERK in melanoma cells suggest a role for Ah receptors.

Environmental toxins can initiate melanogenesis by triggering the AhR signalling pathway in melanocytes (Jux et al., 2011; Luecke et al., 2010). Luecke *et al.* (2010) showed that 2,3,7,8-tetrachlorodibenzo-*p*-dioxin (TCDD), activated the AhR signalling pathway and induced tyrosinase activity, which correlated with an increase in melanin content in melanocytes. They also found that UVB radiation induced AhR-dependent pigmentation albeit weaker than that stimulated by TCDD. Since AhR-deficient mice displayed pigmented skin and fur, this transcription factor was not necessary for constitutive melanogenesis but is involved in eliciting responses initiated by exogenous stimuli (Luecke et al., 2010). In accordance, Jux *et al.* (2011) found that AhR expressed in normal murine melanocytes were involved in both cell proliferation and UV-induced skin pigmentation. Moreover, AhR-deficient melanocytes expressed low levels of c-KIT (overexpressed in some melanoma tumours) than WT melanocytes. On the whole, there is evidence to suggest that melanocytes express functional AhR which can be activated by UV radiation (Jux et al., 2011; Luecke et al., 2010).

Melanoma cells express AhR mRNA which corresponds to its intracellular protein content (Villano et al., 2006). Interestingly, these levels corresponded to increasing invasiveness of melanoma cells but were lower than that seen in melanocytes. In the highly invasive A2058 melanoma cells, the expression of AhR target genes, CYP1A1 and CYP1B1 was increased by TCDD which is a known stimulator of this signalling pathway (Villano et al., 2006). The use of AhR antagonist abrogated CYP1 expression in A2058 cells which suggests that this signalling pathway is functional in these tumour cells. Furthermore, TCDD-dependent increase in matrix metalloproteinase expression was found to aid in the metastasis of A2058 melanoma cells (Villano et al., 2006). In addition, Roman *et al.* (2009) found that both tumour volume and vasculature were decreased when B16F10 melanoma cells were transplanted onto $AhR^{-/-}$ mice, compared to $AhR^{+/+}$ mice. This decrease in angiogenesis was mediated by the downregulation of hypoxia-inducible factor-1α (HIF-1α)-dependent VEGF expression. As UV radiation can activate the AhR pathway in melanoma, it is conceivable that hyperactivation of this pathway can direct angiogenesis and metastasis of these cells (Jux et al., 2011; Kramer et al., 2005; Villano et al., 2006). Currently, further investigation is required to further our understanding of the AhR signalling pathway in melanoma.

2.2.2 Heat shock protein 90

B-RAF, N-RAS, C-RAF and p53 are some of the client proteins of Hsp90 (Heath et al., 2011; Mehta et al., 2011). Hsp90 is involved in maintaining the conformation, stability and cellular localisation of its client proteins (Powers and Workman, 2006). It also acts as a molecular chaperone for proteins involved in invasion/metastasis, angiogenesis and survival (Powers and Workman, 2006). Conjunctival melanoma tissues expressed higher levels of Hsp90 than did nevi (Westekemper et al., 2011). More importantly, those tumours which recurred locally had increased Hsp90 levels compared to recurrence-free conjunctival melanoma tumours. This suggests that Hsp90 plays a role in the metastatic progression of melanoma. Hsp90 inhibition correlated with modulations to the phospholipid metabolism and growth arrest induced by 17-AAG (Hsp90 inhibitor) in SKMEL28 and CHL-1 melanoma cells (Beloueche-Babari et al., 2010). In hypoxic melanoma tumours, Hsp90 was implicated in Bcl-2-dependent stabilisation of HIF-1α, which was found to regulate VEGF and promote tumour angiogenesis. Thus, the inhibition of Hsp90 will destabilise HIF-1α and may reduce the vascularisation of melanoma tumours. Since Hsp90 interacts with several oncognenic proteins involved in melanoma, disrupting their interaction may reduce the stability of these pro-tumour proteins (Powers and Workman, 2006).

In melanoma and breast cancer cells, survivin induced PDT resistance (Ferrario et al., 2007). PDT increased survivin expression and phosphorylation both *in vitro* (BA mouse breast cancer cells) and *in vivo* (C3H mice transplanted with BA cells). Treatment with 17-AAG and PDT reduced both phospho-survivin and –AKT levels. Additionally, there was an increase in poly (ADP-ribose) polymerase cleavage and Bcl-2 protein degradation which resulted in BT-474 (human breast cancer) cell death post-17-AAG/PD therapy. Likewise, in YUSAC2/T34A-C4 melanoma cells, forced expression of phospho-survivin led to reduced apoptosis after PDT treatment, while the reverse occurred when dominant-negative survivin was expressed. Qiu *et al.* (2005) also found that survivin desensitised melanoma cells to betulinic acid-induced cytotoxicity. Betulinic acid caused an increase in EGFR activation, phospho-ERK, phospho-AKT and survivin levels in melanoma cells. The blockade of EGFR caused a decrease in both AKT and survivin expression which resulted in cell death. Therefore, high ERK/AKT activity in combination with increased survivin levels lead to melanoma cell survival (Ferrario et al., 2007; Qiu et al., 2005). Since, both survivin and AKT are Hsp90 client proteins and have been implicated in PDT- and chemo-resistant melanoma cells, targeting Hsp90 may have beneficial effects (Qiu et al., 2005).

Mehta *et al.* (2011) found that Hsp90 inhibitors suppressed proliferation, colony formation and transformation of melanoma cells irrespective of their B-RAF mutational status. However, Hsp90 inhibitors (PF-4470296 and PF-3823863) degraded mutant but not WT B-RAF protein and reduced the activation of MEK/ERK in B-RAF mutant A2058 melanoma cells (Mehta et al., 2011). These inhibitors also induced the degradation of C-RAF, AKT, ErbB2 and cMET (involved in tumour progression) in both mutant (A2058) and WT (MeWo) BRAF melanoma cell lines. In *in vivo* studies, PF-3823863 induced tumour growth inhibition in both A2058 and MeWo melanoma xenografts. Although, PF-4470296 and PF-3823863 are effective in treating both WT and mutant B-RAF melanomas, the mechanism involved seems to be different; unlike mutant B-RAF, WT B-RAF is not depleted but other oncogenic client proteins responsible for tumour survival and growth are affected. However, Banerji *et al.* (2008) found 17-AAG to be ineffective when administered to two melanoma patients with WT N-RAS/B-RAF (1-1.5 months to progression) compared to one with mutant N-RAS (and WT B-RAF; 49 months to progression) and another with mutant B-RAF (and WT N-RAS; 15 months to progression). In the same study, two other patients with mutant B-RAF (and WT N-RAS) only had 1.5-2 months of stabilised disease before the tumour progressed. This study had a small number of test subjects and only one patient had mutant N-RAS which makes the results inconclusive. Nevertheless, data on a patient's mutational status corresponding to Hsp90 inhibition will assist in the use of such inhibitors similar to the application of B-RAF (section 2.1.3) and KIT inhibitors (section 2.1.1) as discussed earlier.

Montaqut *et al.* (2008) found that AZ628 (B-RAF inhibitor)-resistant melanoma cells had elevated levels of C-RAF that was responsible for the survival of these cells. Treatment with geldanamycin sensitised these cells to apoptosis by inhibiting Hsp90. This suggests that a combined application of RAF and Hsp90 inhibitors may improve treatment outcomes of melanoma patients. In a phase I clinical trial, the combination of sorafenib (B-RAF inhibitor) and tanespimycin (17-AAG) showed clinical efficacy in four out of six melanoma patients (Vaishampayan et al., 2010). When 17-DMAG (Hsp90 inhibitor) was co-treated with imatinib mesylate (RTK inhibitor), a synergistic anti-proliferative effect was seen in uveal melanoma cells (WT B-RAF) (Babchia et al., 2008). Imatinib inhibits specific KIT mutations and secondary mutations have arised in imatinib-resistant tumours (Lim et al., 2008; Terheyden et al., 2010). Since KIT is a client protein of Hsp90, the inhibition of this heat shock protein may destabilise KIT irrespective of different receptor domain mutations thereby improving imatinib's efficacy. On the whole, Hsp90 inhibitors would augment the effectiveness of other oncogenic protein (e.g. B-RAF, KIT) inhibitors in these patients.

Gaspar *et al.* (2009) identified a possible mechanism of resistance which may occur in melanoma treated with 17-AAG. After continuous drug exposure, a 17-AAG-resistant melanoma cell line, WM266.4-RA6 was developed. This resistance was found to occur via downregulation of NAD(P)H/quinone oxidoreductase (NQO1) as ES936 (NQO1 inhibitor) reduced 17-AAG sensitivity in the non-resistant WM266.4 parental line. This suggests that 17-AAG efficacy relies on NQO1 upregulation in these cells (Gaspar et al., 2009; Siegel et al., 2011). Although, the same resistance occurred in glioblastoma cells, other structurally dissimilar Hsp90 inhibitors (VER-49009 and NVP-AUY922) were also shown to be effective (Gaspar et al., 2009). In another study, NVP-AUY922 inhibited proliferation in WM266.4 (mutant B-RAF), SKMEL2 (mutant N-RAS; high NQO1) and SKMEL5 (mutant BRAF; low NQO1) melanoma cells in an NQO1-independent manner (Eccles et al., 2008). Although, the efficacy of its inhibiton in WT/mutant B-RAF or N-RAS is still ambiguous, Hsp90 has a broad spectrum of targets and its inhibition will affect multiple signalling pathways in tumours irrespective of their mutational status. Furthermore, Hsp90's role in both the RAS/RAF/MEK and PI3K/AKT pathways which are common oncogenic pathways in melanoma makes it a promising target. Currently, some of these Hsp90 inhibitors are undergoing clinical trials.

2.2.3 p38 MAPK and JNK

Besides ERK, p38 MAPK and c-Jun NH_2-terminal kinase (JNK) belong to the MAPK family (Muthusamy and Piva, 2010). UV-induced activation of p38 and JNK in normal skin cells were either pro- or anti-apoptotic depending on the cell type, UV type and dose used (Muthusamy and Piva, 2010). Unlike ERK, p38 and JNK pathways have not been frequently linked to melanoma incidences. However, there is evidence to suggest that these pathways may play a role in synergistic or additive effects together with chemotherapeutic agents to elicit cytotoxicity in melanoma cells (Keuling et al., 2010; Selimovic et al., 2008; Shieh et al., 2010).

Melanoma cells resistant to ABT-737 die when they are co-treated with the p38 inhibitor, SB202190 (Keuling et al., 2010). The combination of ABT-737 and SB202190, enhanced caspase-dependent apoptosis in four melanoma cell lines harbouring different mutations. In contrast, the use of either SB203580 (p38 inhibitor) or SP600125 (JNK inhibitor) abolished Taxol-mediated apoptosis, ROS generation and decreased uncoupling protein 2 (UCP2) levels in A375 and BLM melanoma cells (Selimovic et al., 2008). Therefore, Taxol affects melanoma cells by upregulating these (p38 and JNK) pathways which in turn regulates the membrane potential, intracellular UCP2 and ROS levels. The JNK pathway was found to mediate doxycycline-induced cell death via ROS generation and apoptosis signal-regulating kinase 1 (ASK1) activation in A2058 melanoma cells (Shieh et al., 2010). Imatinib mesylate, a RTK inhibitor, mediated apoptosis and induced high levels of phospho-JNK and p38 in B16F0 melanoma cells (Chang et al., 2011). In this study, SP600125 was shown to enhance apoptosis in the imatinib mesylate-treated melanoma cells.

p38 was implicated in aiding melanoma transendothelial migration in co-cultures with human vascular endothelial cells (HUVEC) (Khanna et al., 2010). When A2058 melanoma cells were co-cultured with HUVEC, the latter's vascular endothelial (VE)-cadherin junctions were disrupted and gap formations occurred allowing migration of melanoma cells. Neutralisation of soluble factors (IL8, IL1β) released from A2058 melanoma cells abrogated the p38 pathway in HUVEC and prevented VE-cadherin disassembly and gap formation which was also affirmed by the inhibition of p38 in these cells. In contrast, downregulation of Ras association domain family 1, isoform A (RASSF1A)/ASK1/p38 in part, was involved in melanoma development. RASSF1A levels were lower in melanoma tissues compared to benign and normal melanocytes (Yi et al., 2011). Expression of RASSF1A in RASSF1A-deficient A375 melanoma cells induced an anti-proliferative and pro-apoptotic effect which coincided with decreased tumorigenic potential of these cells as well as an increase in ASK1 and p38 levels.

Collectively, the roles of p38 and JNK in melanoma development, apoptosis or chemoresistance needs to be tested on a case by case basis as it seems to vary with different cytotoxic agents and cell types. Forced expression of active p38/JNK or its inhibition may be useful in enhancing the efficacy of chemotherapeutic agents in inducing apoptosis in tumour cells. In order to prevent disruption of normal cellular homeostasis, it is imperative to identify melanoma-specific treatment vehicles.

2.2.4 Phosphatases

Phosphatases regulate cell signal transduction by dephosphorylating phospho-proteins resulting in either their activation or deactivation (Bermudez et al., 2010; Haagenson and Wu, 2010). Protein tyrosine phosphatases (PTP) and serine/threonine phosphatases (S/TP) dephosphorylate tyrosine and serine/threonine residues, respectively (Hamilton and Bernhard, 2009). Phosphatases in the nucleus are involved in controlling cell cycle progression and other nuclear processes (Bollen and Beullens, 2002). The MAPK signalling pathway has several MAPK phosphatases (MKP) regulating the activity of each kinase. The dual specificity phosphatases (DSP) target MAPK at both tyrosine and threonine residues (Bermudez et al., 2010). In some human cancers, these phosphatases are either overexpressed or suppressed leading to deregulated cell signalling (Haagenson and Wu, 2010).

PTEN is a phosphatase that removes phospho-groups in both lipids and proteins (Hamilton and Bernhard, 2009), and is deleted/inactivated in some melanomas (Paraiso et al., 2011). PTEN dephosphorylates AKT and inhibits cell survival and its loss enables melanoma cells to overcome B-RAF inhibition via the AKT survival pathway (Paraiso et al., 2011). In PLX4720 (B-RAF inhibitor)-treated $PTEN^{+/+}$ melanoma cells, AKT signalling was inhibited and Bim-mediated apoptosis was enhanced compared to $PTEN^{-/-}$ cells (Paraiso et al., 2011). Stewart *et al.* (2002) found no mutations in PTEN coding regions but the protein levels were low or undetectable in five melanoma cell lines (WM35, WM134, A375, A375-S2, MeWo). When PTEN adenoviral vectors (Ad-PTEN) were transfected into these cells, there was an increase in AKT dephosphorylation, apoptosis and growth inhibtion. A decrease in cell migration/invasive property and a corresponding increase in E-cadherin levels were also observed. These data emphasise the role PTEN phosphatase plays in melanoma.

Chen *et al.* (2010) found that high levels of phospho-myristoylated alanine-rich C-kinase substrates (MARCKS) and their upstream activator, protein kinase Cα (PKC) were responsible for metastasis of B16F10 melanoma cells. In weakly motile F1 melanoma cells, phospho-MARCKS were undetectable but PKC levels were still high which suggests that an inhibitory mechanism exists to maintain low phospho-MARCKS levels in these cells. When the F1 cells were treated with okadaic acid (protein phosphatase inhibitor; inhibits PP1 and 2A) the phosphorylation of MARCKS increased while the addition of a PKC inhibitor abolished these levels (Chen and Rotenberg, 2010; Clarke et al., 1993). This study suggests that there is a ratio between PKC and protein phosphatase levels which determines the amount of phospho-MARCKS present in these cells and this may affect their motility. Therefore, it is possible that in metatstatic melanoma cells, high levels of protein kinases may override the effect of protein phosphatases or these phosphatases may be either suppressed or lost.

McArdle *et al.* (2003) observed that advanced melanoma had greater phosphotyrosine residues than did early stage lesions. Microarray analysis of metastatic melanoma cell lines (WM9, WM39, WM852) showed a 32% difference in total phosphatase gene expression compared to normal melanocytes. In some of these cells, DSP, PTP, S/TP and acid/alkaline phosphatases were downregulated when compared to naevus and melanocytes (McArdle et al., 2005). Of the DSP identified, DSP10 (MKP5) was lower in all three melanoma cell lines tested while DSP5 expression was decreased. DSP10 is a cytoplasmic and nuclear phosphatase which dephosphorylates p38 and JNK while DSP5 is localised to the nucleus and inactivates ERK (Bermudez et al., 2010). It was speculated that since DSP10 maps to chromosome 10q25, it might be downregulated/deleted as it is in the same region as PTEN (chromosome 10q23.3) which is often lost in some melanomas (McArdle et al., 2005). The low levels of PTP in conjunction with amplified phosphotyrosine levels may prevent inactivation of crucial kinases that drives melanoma metastasis.

In contrast, some melanoma cell lines have higher total PTP activity than do melanocytes. Since, only total PTP was measured irrespective of subcellular localisation, type and function, it is possible that those which were upregulated may be pro-tumorigenic. Sun *et al.* (2011) found that the PP1 catalytic subunit β isoform was significantly overexpressed in human melanoma compared to nevi samples. DSP4 (MKP2) which dephosphorylates MAPK was found to be upregulated in melanoma cell lines (Teutschbein et al., 2010). It is possible that their increase could compensate for the high levels of ERK produced in these cells. Laurent *et al.* (2011) found that overexpression of PTP4A3 in uveal melanoma cell lines correlated to a high degree of cell migration and invasisveness *in vivo*. Another phosphatase, PP2A was involved in tumour cell migration as its inhibition by cytostatin upregulated those cytokines involved in augmenting natural killer cell levels and activity *in vivo* which resulted in reduced mice B16 melanoma pulmonary metastasis (Kawada et al., 2003). In another study, MKP1 (DSP1) expression was found to be higher in melanoma tissue samples (~six-fold) than in melanocytes (Kundu et al., 2010). Tyrosine phosphatase inhibitor-3 inhibited MKP1 activity and had a synergistic effect with interferon α2b to inhibit WM9 melanoma cell growth (Kundu et al., 2010). MKP1 has been associated with chemoresistance in other human cancers (lung and breast cancer) but it is not known if the same occurs in melanoma (Haagenson and Wu, 2010).

Tang *et al.* (1999) observed a greater expression of cyclin-dependent kinase 2 (CDK), CDK6 and CDC25A in metastatic melanomas than in benign nevi. CDC25A is a tyrosine phosphatase that dephosphorylates/activates CDK, allowing entry into the cell cycle and as such may be involved in melanoma proliferation (Tang et al., 1999). Koma *et al.* (2004) found that deltagamma 1 (Δγ1) (truncated variant of PP2A B65γ regulatory subunit) confers radioresistance to metastatic melanoma cells. When F10 cells were transfected with Δγ1, there was a decrease in radiation-induced p53 protein levels, BAX transactivation and apoptosis *in vivo*. This is due to Δγ1-mediated dephosphorylation of MDM2 which targets p53 for degradation and as a result prevents the production of p53-inducible apoptotic factors. It is conceivable that the transition from benign to metastatic melanoma may also be aided by progressive mutations occurring in these phosphatases.

Although, microarray and global gene expression data is useful to elucidate those phosphatases regulated in melanoma, there seems to be a lack of functional studies conducted in these tumours. Data on the mutational status of phosphatases in melanoma is limited. Nevertheless, the existing data creates a compelling argument that these proteases may prove to be a valuable tool in targeting phospho-proteins that regulate pro-tumour activities in these cells. As phosphatase inhibitors can promote tumour activity, it is necessary to delineate the specific roles played by these phosphatases in melanoma (Fujiki and Suganuma, 2009).

3. Conclusion

On the whole, it has been shown from numerous studies that melanomas cannot be treated using a single agent. This is partly due to the presence of melanoma subgroups harbouring one or more mutations; KIT only, N-RAS only, B-RAF only, KIT and N-RAS, and KIT and B-RAF mutant melanomas (Curtin et al., 2006). In addition, a cocktail of inhibitors and new therapeutical targets are necessary to prevent drug resistance due to activation of alternative/compensatory signalling. Although, joint therapies have recently been suggested, a cocktail of drugs may induce systemic toxicities and other anomalies, and as such requires more pre-clinical studies on effective dosages. In conclusion, the RAS-RAF-MEK pathway still remains a promising target for therapy but the identification of new molecular targets might enhance the efficacy of existing treatments. This would allow for melanoma therapy to 'strike from all angles' in terms of oncogenic mutations, survival pathways, metastasis and angiogenesis.

4. References

Algazi, A. P., Soon, C. W., and Daud, A. I. 2010. Treatment of cutaneous melanoma: current approaches and future prospects. *Cancer Management and Research*;2:197-211.

Ashida, A., Takata, M., Murata, H., Kido, K., and Saida, T. 2009. Pathological activation of KIT in metastatic tumors of acral and mucosal melanomas. *International Journal of Cancer*;124(4):862-868.

Aziz, S. A., Davies, M., Pick, E., Zito, C., Jilaveanu, L., Camp, R. L., Rimm, D. L., Kluger, Y., and Kluger, H. M. 2009. Phosphatidylinositol-3-kinase as a therapeutic target in melanoma. *Clinical Cancer Research*;15(9):3029-3036.

Babchia, N., Calipel, A., Mouriaux, F., Faussat, A. M., and Mascarelli, F. 2008. 17-AAG and 17-DMAG-induced inhibition of cell proliferation through B-Raf downregulation in WT B-Raf-expressing uveal melanoma cell lines. *Investigative Ophthalmology and Visual Science*;49(6):2348-2356.

Banerji, U., Affolter, A., Judson, I., Marais, R., and Workman, P. 2008. BRAF and NRAS mutations in melanoma: potential relationships to clinical response to HSP90 inhibitors. *Molecular Cancer Therapeutics*;7(4):737-739.

Bauer, J., Buttner, P., Murali, R., Okamoto, I., Kolaitis, N. A., Landi, M. T., Scolyer, R. A., and Bastian, B. C. 2011. BRAF mutations in cutaneous melanoma are independently associated with age, anatomic site of the primary tumor, and the degree of solar elastosis at the primary tumor site. *Pigment Cell & Melanoma Research*;24(2):345-351.

Beloueche-Babari, M., Arunan, V., Jackson, L. E., Perusinghe, N., Sharp, S. Y., Workman, P., and Leach, M. O. 2010. Modulation of melanoma cell phospholipid metabolism in response to heat shock protein 90 inhibition. *Oncotarget*;1(3):185-197.

Bermudez, O., Pages, G., and Gimond, C. 2010. The dual-specificity MAP kinase phosphatases: critical roles in development and cancer. *American Journal of Physiology - Cell Physiology*;299(2):C189-202.

Besaratinia, A., and Pfeifer, G. P. 2008. Sunlight ultraviolet irradiation and BRAF V600 mutagenesis in human melanoma. *Human Mutation*;29(8):983-991.

Bollen, M., and Beullens, M. 2002. Signaling by protein phosphatases in the nucleus. *Trends in Cell Biology*;12(3):138-145.

Carracedo, A., Ma, L., Teruya-Feldstein, J., Rojo, F., Salmena, L., Alimonti, A., Egia, A., Sasaki, A. T., Thomas, G., Kozma, S. C., Papa, A., Nardella, C., Cantley, L. C., Baselga, J., and Pandolfi, P. P. 2008. Inhibition of mTORC1 leads to MAPK pathway activation through a PI3K-dependent feedback loop in human cancer. *Journal of Clinical Investigation*;118(9):3065-3074.

Chang, S. P., Shen, S. C., Lee, W. R., Yang, L. L., and Chen, Y. C. 2011. Imatinib mesylate induction of ROS-dependent apoptosis in melanoma B16F0 cells. *Journal of Dermatological Science*;62(3):183-191.

Chen, J., Shen, Q., Labow, M., and Gaither, L. A. 2011. Protein kinase D3 sensitizes RAF inhibitor RAF265 in melanoma cells by preventing reactivation of MAPK signaling. *Cancer Research*;71(12):4280-4291.

Chen, X., and Rotenberg, S. A. 2010. PhosphoMARCKS drives motility of mouse melanoma cells. *Cellular Signalling*;22(7):1097-1103.

Clarke, P. R., Siddhanti, S. R., Cohen, P., and Blackshear, P. J. 1993. Okadaic acid-sensitive protein phosphatases dephosphorylate MARCKS, a major protein kinase C substrate. *FEBS Letters*;336(1):37-42.

Curtin, J. A., Busam, K., Pinkel, D., and Bastian, B. C. 2006. Somatic activation of KIT in distinct subtypes of melanoma. *Journal of Clinical Oncology*;24(26):4340-4346.

Curtin, J. A., Fridlyand, J., Kageshita, T., Patel, H. N., Busam, K. J., Kutzner, H., Cho, K. H., Aiba, S., Brocker, E. B., Leboit, P. E., Pinkel, D., and Bastian, B. C. 2005. Distinct sets of genetic alterations in melanoma. *New England Journal of Medicine*;353(20):2135-2147.

Demunter, A., Stas, M., Degreef, H., De Wolf-Peeters, C., and Van Den Oord, J. J. 2001. Analysis of N- and K-ras mutations in the distinctive tumor progression phases of melanoma. *Journal of Investigative Dermatology*;117(6):1483-1489.

Dummer, R., Hauschild, A., Guggenheim, M., Jost, L., and Pentheroudakis, G. 2010. Melanoma: ESMO Clinical Practice Guidelines for diagnosis, treatment and follow-up. *Annals of Oncology*;21 Suppl 5:v194-197.

Easty, D. J., Gray, S. G., O'Byrne, K. J., O'Donnell, D., and Bennett, D. C. 2011. Receptor tyrosine kinases and their activation in melanoma. *Pigment Cell & Melanoma Research*;24(3):446-461.

Eccles, S. A., Massey, A., Raynaud, F. I., Sharp, S. Y., Box, G., Valenti, M., Patterson, L., De Haven Brandon, A., Gowan, S., Boxall, F., Aherne, W., Rowlands, M., Hayes, A., Martins, V., Urban, F., Boxall, K., Prodromou, C., Pearl, L., James, K., Matthews, T. P., Cheung, K. M., Kalusa, A., Jones, K., Mcdonald, E., Barril, X., Brough, P. A., Cansfield, J. E., Dymock, B., Drysdale, M. J., Finch, H., Howes, R., Hubbard, R. E., Surgenor, A., Webb, P., Wood, M., Wright, L., and Workman, P. 2008. NVP-AUY922: a novel heat shock protein 90 inhibitor active against xenograft tumor growth, angiogenesis, and metastasis. *Cancer Research*;68(8):2850-2860.

Eskandarpour, M., Huang, F., Reeves, K. A., Clark, E., and Hansson, J. 2009. Oncogenic NRAS has multiple effects on the malignant phenotype of human melanoma cells cultured in vitro. *International Journal of Cancer*;124(1):16-26.

Ferrario, A., Rucker, N., Wong, S., Luna, M., and Gomer, C. J. 2007. Survivin, a member of the inhibitor of apoptosis family, is induced by photodynamic therapy and is a target for improving treatment response. *Cancer Research*;67(10):4989-4995.

Flaherty, K. T. 2006. Chemotherapy and targeted therapy combinations in advanced melanoma. *Clinical Cancer Research*;12(7 Pt 2):2366s-2370s.

Fokstuen, T., Rabo, Y. B., Zhou, J. N., Karlson, J., Platz, A., Shoshan, M. C., Hansson, J., and Linder, S. 1997. The Ras farnesylation inhibitor BZA-5B increases the resistance to cisplatin in a human melanoma cell line. *Anticancer Research*;17(4A):2347-2352.

Franco-Lie, I., Iversen, T., Robsahm, T. E., and Abdelnoor, M. 2011. Incidence trends of melanoma of the skin compared with other localisations, in the Norwegian population, 1956-2005. *Annals of Oncology*;22(6):1443-1450.

Friedlander, P., and Hodi, F. S. 2010. Advances in targeted therapy for melanoma. *Clinical Advances in Hematology and Oncology*;8(9):619-635.

Fritsche, E., Schafer, C., Calles, C., Bernsmann, T., Bernshausen, T., Wurm, M., Hubenthal, U., Cline, J. E., Hajimiragha, H., Schroeder, P., Klotz, L. O., Rannug, A., Furst, P., Hanenberg, H., Abel, J., and Krutmann, J. 2007. Lightening up the UV response by identification of the arylhydrocarbon receptor as a cytoplasmatic target for ultraviolet B radiation. *Proceedings of the National Academy of Sciences of the United States of America*;104(21):8851-8856.

Fujiki, H., and Suganuma, M. 2009. Carcinogenic aspects of protein phosphatase 1 and 2A inhibitors. *Progress in Molecular and Subcellular Biology*;46:221-254.

Fujita, M., Norris, D. A., Yagi, H., Walsh, P., Morelli, J. G., Weston, W. L., Terada, N., Bennion, S. D., Robinson, W., Lemon, M., Maxwell, I. H., and Yohn, J. J. 1999. Overexpression of mutant ras in human melanoma increases invasiveness, proliferation and anchorage-independent growth in vitro and induces tumour formation and cachexia in vivo. *Melanoma Research*;9(3):279-291.

Garrido, M. C., and Bastian, B. C. 2010. KIT as a therapeutic target in melanoma. *Journal of Investigative Dermatology*;130(1):20-27.

Gaspar, N., Sharp, S. Y., Pacey, S., Jones, C., Walton, M., Vassal, G., Eccles, S., Pearson, A., and Workman, P. 2009. Acquired resistance to 17-allylamino-17-demethoxygeldanamycin (17-AAG, tanespimycin) in glioblastoma cells. *Cancer Research*;69(5):1966-1975.

Govindarajan, B., Sligh, J. E., Vincent, B. J., Li, M., Canter, J. A., Nickoloff, B. J., Rodenburg, R. J., Smeitink, J. A., Oberley, L., Zhang, Y., Slingerland, J., Arnold, R. S., Lambeth, J. D., Cohen, C., Hilenski, L., Griendling, K., Martinez-Diez, M., Cuezva, J. M., and Arbiser, J. L. 2007. Overexpression of Akt converts radial growth melanoma to vertical growth melanoma. *Journal of Clinical Investigation*;117(3):719-729.

Grossman, D., and Altieri, D. C. 2001. Drug resistance in melanoma: mechanisms, apoptosis, and new potential therapeutic targets. *Cancer and Metastasis Reviews*;20(1-2):3-11.

Haagenson, K. K., and Wu, G. S. 2010. Mitogen activated protein kinase phosphatases and cancer. *Cancer Biology & Therapy*;9(5):337-340.

Hainsworth, J. D., Infante, J. R., Spigel, D. R., Peyton, J. D., Thompson, D. S., Lane, C. M., Clark, B. L., Rubin, M. S., Trent, D. F., and Burris, H. A., 3rd. 2010. Bevacizumab and everolimus in the treatment of patients with metastatic melanoma: a phase 2 trial of the Sarah Cannon Oncology Research Consortium. *Cancer*;116(17):4122-4129.

Hamilton, J., and Bernhard, E. J. 2009. Cell signalling and radiation survival: the impact of protein phosphatases. *International Journal of Radiation Biology*;85(11):937-942.

Hatzivassiliou, G., Song, K., Yen, I., Brandhuber, B. J., Anderson, D. J., Alvarado, R., Ludlam, M. J., Stokoe, D., Gloor, S. L., Vigers, G., Morales, T., Aliagas, I., Liu, B., Sideris, S., Hoeflich, K. P., Jaiswal, B. S., Seshagiri, S., Koeppen, H., Belvin, M., Friedman, L. S., and Malek, S. 2010. RAF inhibitors prime wild-type RAF to activate the MAPK pathway and enhance growth. *Nature*;464(7287):431-435.

Heath, E. M., Kaufman, K. L., and Christopherson, R. I. 2011. B-RAF: A contributor to the melanoma phenotype. *International Journal of Biochemistry and Cell Biology*;43(1):29-32.

Heinrich, M. C., Griffith, D. J., Druker, B. J., Wait, C. L., Ott, K. A., and Zigler, A. J. 2000. Inhibition of c-kit receptor tyrosine kinase activity by STI 571, a selective tyrosine kinase inhibitor. *Blood*;96(3):925-932.

Held, L., Eigentler, T. K., Meier, F., Held, M., Rocken, M., Garbe, C., and Bauer, J. 2011. Oncogenetics of melanoma: basis for molecular diagnostics and therapy. *Journal der Deutschen Dermatologischen Gesellschaft*. (In Press)

Hess, A. R., Seftor, E. A., Seftor, R. E., and Hendrix, M. J. 2003. Phosphoinositide 3-kinase regulates membrane Type 1-matrix metalloproteinase (MMP) and MMP-2 activity during melanoma cell vasculogenic mimicry. *Cancer Research*;63(16):4757-4762.

Hofmann, U. B., Kauczok-Vetter, C. S., Houben, R., and Becker, J. C. 2009. Overexpression of the KIT/SCF in uveal melanoma does not translate into clinical efficacy of imatinib mesylate. *Clinical Cancer Research*;15(1):324-329.

Hou, L., Panthier, J. J., and Arnheiter, H. 2000. Signaling and transcriptional regulation in the neural crest-derived melanocyte lineage: interactions between KIT and MITF. *Development*;127(24):5379-5389.

Inamdar, G. S., Madhunapantula, S. V., and Robertson, G. P. 2010. Targeting the MAPK pathway in melanoma: why some approaches succeed and other fail. *Biochemical Pharmacology*;80(5):624-637.

Jiang, C. C., Lai, F., Tay, K. H., Croft, A., Rizos, H., Becker, T. M., Yang, F., Liu, H., Thorne, R. F., Hersey, P., and Zhang, X. D. 2010. Apoptosis of human melanoma cells induced by inhibition of B-RAFV600E involves preferential splicing of bimS. *Cell Death Disease*;1(9):e69.

Jiang, C. C., Lai, F., Thorne, R. F., Yang, F., Liu, H., Hersey, P., and Zhang, X. D. 2011. MEK-Independent Survival of B-RAFV600E Melanoma Cells Selected for Resistance to Apoptosis Induced by the RAF Inhibitor PLX4720. *Clinical Cancer Research*;17(4):721-730.

Jiang, X., Zhou, J., Yuen, N. K., Corless, C. L., Heinrich, M. C., Fletcher, J. A., Demetri, G. D., Widlund, H. R., Fisher, D. E., and Hodi, F. S. 2008. Imatinib targeting of KIT-mutant oncoprotein in melanoma. *Clinical Cancer Research*;14(23):7726-7732.

Johannessen, C. M., Boehm, J. S., Kim, S. Y., Thomas, S. R., Wardwell, L., Johnson, L. A., Emery, C. M., Stransky, N., Cogdill, A. P., Barretina, J., Caponigro, G., Hieronymus, H., Murray, R. R., Salehi-Ashtiani, K., Hill, D. E., Vidal, M., Zhao, J. J., Yang, X., Alkan, O., Kim, S., Harris, J. L., Wilson, C. J., Myer, V. E., Finan, P. M., Root, D. E., Roberts, T. M., Golub, T., Flaherty, K. T., Dummer, R., Weber, B. L., Sellers, W. R., Schlegel, R., Wargo, J. A., Hahn, W. C., and Garraway, L. A. 2010. COT drives resistance to RAF inhibition through MAP kinase pathway reactivation. *Nature*;468(7326):968-972.

Johnston, S. R. 2001. Farnesyl transferase inhibitors: a novel targeted therapy for cancer. *The Lancet Oncology*;2(1):18-26.

Jux, B., Kadow, S., Luecke, S., Rannug, A., Krutmann, J., and Esser, C. 2011. The aryl hydrocarbon receptor mediates UVB radiation-induced skin tanning. *Journal of Investigative Dermatology*;131(1):203-210.

Karnoub, A. E., and Weinberg, R. A. 2008. Ras oncogenes: split personalities. *Nature Reviews Molecular Cell Biology*;9(7):517-531.

Kawada, M., Kawatsu, M., Masuda, T., Ohba, S., Amemiya, M., Kohama, T., Ishizuka, M., and Takeuchi, T. 2003. Specific inhibitors of protein phosphatase 2A inhibit tumor metastasis through augmentation of natural killer cells. *International Immunopharmacology*;3(2):179-188.

Keuling, A. M., Andrew, S. E., and Tron, V. A. 2010. Inhibition of p38 MAPK enhances ABT-737-induced cell death in melanoma cell lines: novel regulation of PUMA. *Pigment Cell & Melanoma Research*;23(3):430-440.

Khanna, P., Yunkunis, T., Muddana, H. S., Peng, H. H., August, A., and Dong, C. 2010. p38 MAP kinase is necessary for melanoma-mediated regulation of VE-cadherin disassembly. *American Journal of Physiology - Cell Physiology*;298(5):C1140-1150.

Ko, J. M., and Fisher, D. E. 2011. A new era: melanoma genetics and therapeutics. *Journal of Pathology*;223(2):241-250.

Koma, Y. I., Ito, A., Watabe, K., Kimura, S. H., and Kitamura, Y. 2004. A truncated isoform of the PP2A B56gamma regulatory subunit reduces irradiation-induced Mdm2 phosphorylation and could contribute to metastatic melanoma cell radioresistance. *Histology and Histopathology*;19(2):391-400.

Kramer, H. J., Podobinska, M., Bartsch, A., Battmann, A., Thoma, W., Bernd, A., Kummer, W., Irlinger, B., Steglich, W., and Mayser, P. 2005. Malassezin, a novel agonist of the aryl hydrocarbon receptor from the yeast Malassezia furfur, induces apoptosis in primary human melanocytes. *ChemBioChem*;6(5):860-865.

Krasilnikov, M., Adler, V., Fuchs, S. Y., Dong, Z., Haimovitz-Friedman, A., Herlyn, M., and Ronai, Z. 1999. Contribution of phosphatidylinositol 3-kinase to radiation resistance in human melanoma cells. *Molecular Carcinogenesis*;24(1):64-69.

Kundu, S., Fan, K., Cao, M., Lindner, D. J., Tuthill, R., Liu, L., Gerson, S., Borden, E., and Yi, T. 2010. Tyrosine phosphatase inhibitor-3 sensitizes melanoma and colon cancer to biotherapeutics and chemotherapeutics. *Molecular Cancer Therapeutics*;9(8):2287-2296.

Laurent, C., Valet, F., Planque, N., Silveri, L., Maacha, S., Anezo, O., Hupe, P., Plancher, C., Reyes, C., Albaud, B., Rapinat, A., Gentien, D., Couturier, J., Sastre-Garau, X., Desjardins, L., Thiery, J. P., Roman-Roman, S., Asselain, B., Barillot, E., Piperno-Neumann, S., and Saule, S. 2011. High PTP4A3 phosphatase expression correlates with metastatic risk in uveal melanoma patients. *Cancer Research*;71(3):666-674.

Lazovich, D., Vogel, R. I., Berwick, M., Weinstock, M. A., Anderson, K. E., and Warshaw, E. M. 2010. Indoor tanning and risk of melanoma: a case-control study in a highly exposed population. *Cancer Epidemiology, Biomarkers and Prevention*;19(6):1557-1568.

Lejeune, F. J., Lienard, D., Sales, F., and Badr-El-Din, H. 1992. Surgical management of distant melanoma metastases. *Seminars in Surgical Oncology*;8(6):381-391.

Liao, A. T., Chien, M. B., Shenoy, N., Mendel, D. B., Mcmahon, G., Cherrington, J. M., and London, C. A. 2002. Inhibition of constitutively active forms of mutant kit by multitargeted indolinone tyrosine kinase inhibitors. *Blood*;100(2):585-593.

Lim, K. H., Huang, M. J., Chen, L. T., Wang, T. E., Liu, C. L., Chang, C. S., Liu, M. C., Hsieh, R. K., and Tzen, C. Y. 2008. Molecular analysis of secondary kinase mutations in imatinib-resistant gastrointestinal stromal tumors. *Medical Oncology*;25(2):207-213.

Lopez-Fauqued, M., Gil, R., Grueso, J., Hernandez-Losa, J., Pujol, A., Moline, T., and Recio, J. A. 2010. The dual PI3K/mTOR inhibitor PI-103 promotes immunosuppression, in vivo tumor growth and increases survival of sorafenib-treated melanoma cells. *International Journal of Cancer*;126(7):1549-1561.

Luecke, S., Backlund, M., Jux, B., Esser, C., Krutmann, J., and Rannug, A. 2010. The aryl hydrocarbon receptor (AHR), a novel regulator of human melanogenesis. *Pigment Cell & Melanoma Research*;23(6):828-833.

Mcardle, L., Bergin, O., Fallowfield, M. E., Dervan, P. A., and Easty, D. J. 2003. Tyrosine phosphate in melanoma progression. *British Journal of Dermatology*;149(2):289-295.

Mcardle, L., Rafferty, M. M., Satyamoorthy, K., Maelandsmo, G. M., Dervan, P. A., Herlyn, M., and Easty, D. J. 2005. Microarray analysis of phosphatase gene expression in human melanoma. *British Journal of Dermatology*;152(5):925-930.

Mccubrey, J. A., Steelman, L. S., Abrams, S. L., Chappell, W. H., Russo, S., Ove, R., Milella, M., Tafuri, A., Lunghi, P., Bonati, A., Stivala, F., Nicoletti, F., Libra, M., Martelli, A. M., Montalto, G., and Cervello, M. 2009. Emerging Raf inhibitors. *Expert Opinion on Emerging Drugs*;14(4):633-648.

Mcdonnell, K., Betz, B., Fullen, D., and Lao, C. D. 2011. V559A and N822I double KIT mutant melanoma with predictable response to imatinib? *Pigment Cell & Melanoma Research*;24(2):390-392.

Mehta, P. P., Kung, P. P., Yamazaki, S., Walls, M., Shen, A., Nguyen, L., Gehring, M. R., Los, G., Smeal, T., and Yin, M. J. 2011. A novel class of specific Hsp90 small molecule inhibitors demonstrate in vitro and in vivo anti-tumor activity in human melanoma cells. *Cancer Letters*;300(1):30-39.

Montagut, C., Sharma, S. V., Shioda, T., Mcdermott, U., Ulman, M., Ulkus, L. E., Dias-Santagata, D., Stubbs, H., Lee, D. Y., Singh, A., Drew, L., Haber, D. A., and Settleman, J. 2008. Elevated CRAF as a potential mechanism of acquired resistance to BRAF inhibition in melanoma. *Cancer Research*;68(12):4853-4861.

Muthusamy, V., and Piva, T. J. 2010. The UV response of the skin: a review of the MAPK, NFκB and TNFα signal transduction pathways. *Archives for Dermatological Research*;302(1):5-17.

Nammi, S., and Lodagala, D. S. 2000. Ras farnesyltransferase inhibition: a novel and safe approach for cancer chemotherapy. *Acta Pharmacologica Sinica*;21(5):396-404.

Navarini, A. A., Kolm, I., Calvo, X., Kamarashev, J., Kerl, K., Conrad, C., French, L. E., and Braun, R. P. 2010. Trauma as triggering factor for development of melanocytic nevi. *Dermatology*;220(4):291-296.

Nazarian, R., Shi, H., Wang, Q., Kong, X., Koya, R. C., Lee, H., Chen, Z., Lee, M. K., Attar, N., Sazegar, H., Chodon, T., Nelson, S. F., Mcarthur, G., Sosman, J. A., Ribas, A., and Lo, R. S. 2010. Melanomas acquire resistance to B-RAF(V600E) inhibition by RTK or N-RAS upregulation. *Nature*;468(7326):973-977.

Niessner, H., Beck, D., Sinnberg, T., Lasithiotakis, K., Maczey, E., Gogel, J., Venturelli, S., Berger, A., Mauthe, M., Toulany, M., Flaherty, K., Schaller, M., Schadendorf, D., Proikas-Cezanne, T., Schittek, B., Garbe, C., Kulms, D., and Meier, F. 2011. The farnesyl transferase inhibitor lonafarnib inhibits mTOR signaling and enforces sorafenib-induced apoptosis in melanoma cells. *Journal of Investigative Dermatology*;131(2):468-479.

Omholt, K., Platz, A., Kanter, L., Ringborg, U., and Hansson, J. 2003. NRAS and BRAF mutations arise early during melanoma pathogenesis and are preserved throughout tumor progression. *Clinical Cancer Research*;9(17):6483-6488.

Paraiso, K. H., Xiang, Y., Rebecca, V. W., Abel, E. V., Chen, A., Munko, A. C., Wood, E., Fedorenko, I. V., Sondak, V. K., Anderson, A. R., Ribas, A., Dalla Palma, M., Nathanson, K. L., Koomen, J. M., Messina, J. L., and Smalley, K. S. 2011. PTEN loss confers BRAF inhibitor resistance to melanoma cells through the suppression of BIM expression. *Cancer Research*;71(7):2750-2760.

Petrescu, I., Condrea, C., Alexandru, A., Dumitrescu, D., Simion, G., Severin, E., Albu, C., and Albu, D. 2010. Diagnosis and treatment protocols of cutaneous melanoma: latest approach 2010. *Chirurgia*;105(5):637-643.

Pho, L. N., and Leachman, S. A. 2010. Genetics of pigmentation and melanoma predisposition. *Giornale Italiano di Dermatologia e Venereologia*;145(1):37-45.

Platz, A., Egyhazi, S., Ringborg, U., and Hansson, J. 2008. Human cutaneous melanoma; a review of NRAS and BRAF mutation frequencies in relation to histogenetic subclass and body site. *Molecular Oncology*;1(4):395-405.

Poulikakos, P. I., Zhang, C., Bollag, G., Shokat, K. M., and Rosen, N. 2010. RAF inhibitors transactivate RAF dimers and ERK signalling in cells with wild-type BRAF. *Nature*;464(7287):427-430.

Powers, M. V., and Workman, P. 2006. Targeting of multiple signalling pathways by heat shock protein 90 molecular chaperone inhibitors. *Endocrine-Related Cancer*;13 Suppl 1:S125-135.

Puzanov, I., and Flaherty, K. T. 2010. Targeted molecular therapy in melanoma. *Seminars in Cutaneous Medicine and Surgery*;29(3):196-201.

Qiu, L., Wang, Q., Di, W., Jiang, Q., Schefeller, E., Derby, S., Wanebo, H., Yan, B., and Wan, Y. 2005. Transient activation of EGFR/AKT cell survival pathway and expression of survivin contribute to reduced sensitivity of human melanoma cells to betulinic acid. *International Journal of Oncology*;27(3):823-830.

Rass, K., and Hassel, J. C. 2009. Chemotherapeutics, chemoresistance and the management of melanoma. *Giornale Italiano di Dermatologia e Venereologia*;144(1):61-78.

Reiss, Y., Goldstein, J. L., Seabra, M. C., Casey, P. J., and Brown, M. S. 1990. Inhibition of purified p21ras farnesyl:protein transferase by Cys-AAX tetrapeptides. *Cell*;62(1):81-88.

Roman, A. C., Carvajal-Gonzalez, J. M., Rico-Leo, E. M., and Fernandez-Salguero, P. M. 2009. Dioxin receptor deficiency impairs angiogenesis by a mechanism involving VEGF-A depletion in the endothelium and transforming growth factor-beta overexpression in the stroma. *Journal of Biological Chemistry*;284(37):25135-25148.

Rosso, R., Romagosa, Y., and Kirsner, R. S. 2009. Progression of NRAS and BRAF mutations in cutaneous melanoma. *Journal of Investigative Dermatology*;129(6):1318.

Sambade, M. J., Peters, E. C., Thomas, N. E., Kaufmann, W. K., Kimple, R. J., and Shields, J. M. 2011. Melanoma cells show a heterogeneous range of sensitivity to ionizing radiation and are radiosensitized by inhibition of B-RAF with PLX-4032. *Radiotherapy and Oncology*;98(3):394-399.

Schittenhelm, M. M., Shiraga, S., Schroeder, A., Corbin, A. S., Griffith, D., Lee, F. Y., Bokemeyer, C., Deininger, M. W., Druker, B. J., and Heinrich, M. C. 2006. Dasatinib (BMS-354825), a dual SRC/ABL kinase inhibitor, inhibits the kinase activity of wild-type, juxtamembrane, and activation loop mutant KIT isoforms associated with human malignancies. *Cancer Research*;66(1):473-481.

Schmidt, J. V., and Bradfield, C. A. 1996. Ah receptor signaling pathways. *Annual Review of Cell and Developmental Biology*;12:55-89.

Sebti, S. M., and Hamilton, A. D. 1997. Inhibition of Ras prenylation: a novel approach to cancer chemotherapy. *Pharmacology and Therapeutics*;74(1):103-114.

Selimovic, D., Hassan, M., Haikel, Y., and Hengge, U. R. 2008. Taxol-induced mitochondrial stress in melanoma cells is mediated by activation of c-Jun N-terminal kinase (JNK) and p38 pathways via uncoupling protein 2. *Cellular Signalling*;20(2):311-322.

Sepp-Lorenzino, L., Ma, Z., Rands, E., Kohl, N. E., Gibbs, J. B., Oliff, A., and Rosen, N. 1995. A peptidomimetic inhibitor of farnesyl:protein transferase blocks the anchorage-dependent and -independent growth of human tumor cell lines. *Cancer Research*;55(22):5302-5309.

Shada, A. L., Molhoek, K. R., and Slingluff, C. L., Jr. 2010. Interface of signal transduction inhibition and immunotherapy in melanoma. *Cancer Journal*;16(4):360-366.

Shieh, J. M., Huang, T. F., Hung, C. F., Chou, K. H., Tsai, Y. J., and Wu, W. B. 2010. Activation of c-Jun N-terminal kinase is essential for mitochondrial membrane potential change and apoptosis induced by doxycycline in melanoma cells. *British Journal of Pharmacology*;160(5):1171-1184.

Shields, J. M., Thomas, N. E., Cregger, M., Berger, A. J., Leslie, M., Torrice, C., Hao, H., Penland, S., Arbiser, J., Scott, G., Zhou, T., Bar-Eli, M., Bear, J. E., Der, C. J., Kaufmann, W. K., Rimm, D. L., and Sharpless, N. E. 2007. Lack of extracellular signal-regulated kinase mitogen-activated protein kinase signaling shows a new type of melanoma. *Cancer Research*;67(4):1502-1512.

Siegel, D., Shieh, B., Yan, C., Kepa, J. K., and Ross, D. 2011. Role for NAD(P)H:quinone oxidoreductase 1 and manganese-dependent superoxide dismutase in 17-(allylamino)-17-demethoxygeldanamycin-induced heat shock protein 90 inhibition in pancreatic cancer cells. *Journal of Pharmacology and Experimental Therapeutics*;336(3):874-880.

Smalley, K. S., Contractor, R., Nguyen, T. K., Xiao, M., Edwards, R., Muthusamy, V., King, A. J., Flaherty, K. T., Bosenberg, M., Herlyn, M., and Nathanson, K. L. 2008. Identification of a novel subgroup of melanomas with KIT/cyclin-dependent kinase-4 overexpression. *Cancer Research*;68(14):5743-5752.

Smalley, K. S., and Eisen, T. G. 2003. Farnesyl transferase inhibitor SCH66336 is cytostatic, pro-apoptotic and enhances chemosensitivity to cisplatin in melanoma cells. *International Journal of Cancer*;105(2):165-175.

Stahl, J. M., Sharma, A., Cheung, M., Zimmerman, M., Cheng, J. Q., Bosenberg, M. W., Kester, M., Sandirasegarane, L., and Robertson, G. P. 2004. Deregulated Akt3 activity promotes development of malignant melanoma. *Cancer Research*;64(19):7002-7010.

Stewart, A. L., Mhashilkar, A. M., Yang, X. H., Ekmekcioglu, S., Saito, Y., Sieger, K., Schrock, R., Onishi, E., Swanson, X., Mumm, J. B., Zumstein, L., Watson, G. J., Snary, D., Roth, J. A., Grimm, E. A., Ramesh, R., and Chada, S. 2002. PI3 kinase blockade by

Ad-PTEN inhibits invasion and induces apoptosis in RGP and metastatic melanoma cells. *Molecular Medicine*;8(8):451-461.

Sullivan, R. J., and Atkins, M. B. 2010. Molecular targeted therapy for patients with melanoma: the promise of MAPK pathway inhibition and beyond. *Expert Opinion on Investigational Drugs*;19(10):1205-1216.

Sun, D., Zhou, M., Kowolik, C. M., Trisal, V., Huang, Q., Kernstine, K. H., Lian, F., and Shen, B. 2011. Differential expression patterns of capping protein, protein phosphatase 1, and casein kinase 1 may serve as diagnostic markers for malignant melanoma. *Melanoma Research.* (In Press)

Tang, L., Li, G., Tron, V. A., Trotter, M. J., and Ho, V. C. 1999. Expression of cell cycle regulators in human cutaneous malignant melanoma. *Melanoma Research*;9(2):148-154.

Terheyden, P., Houben, R., Pajouh, P., Thorns, C., Zillikens, D., and Becker, J. C. 2010. Response to imatinib mesylate depends on the presence of the V559A-mutated KIT oncogene. *Journal of Investigative Dermatology*;130(1):314-316.

Teutschbein, J., Haydn, J. M., Samans, B., Krause, M., Eilers, M., Schartl, M., and Meierjohann, S. 2010. Gene expression analysis after receptor tyrosine kinase activation reveals new potential melanoma proteins. *BMC Cancer*;10:386.

Torres-Cabala, C. A., Wang, W. L., Trent, J., Yang, D., Chen, S., Galbincea, J., Kim, K. B., Woodman, S., Davies, M., Plaza, J. A., Nash, J. W., Prieto, V. G., Lazar, A. J., and Ivan, D. 2009. Correlation between KIT expression and KIT mutation in melanoma: a study of 173 cases with emphasis on the acral-lentiginous/mucosal type. *Modern Pathology*;22(11):1446-1456.

Vaishampayan, U. N., Burger, A. M., Sausville, E. A., Heilbrun, L. K., Li, J., Horiba, M. N., Egorin, M. J., Ivy, P., Pacey, S., and Lorusso, P. M. 2010. Safety, efficacy, pharmacokinetics, and pharmacodynamics of the combination of sorafenib and tanespimycin. *Clinical Cancer Research*;16(14):3795-3804.

Villano, C. M., Murphy, K. A., Akintobi, A., and White, L. A. 2006. 2,3,7,8-tetrachlorodibenzo-p-dioxin (TCDD) induces matrix metalloproteinase (MMP) expression and invasion in A2058 melanoma cells. *Toxicology and Applied Pharmacology*;210(3):212-224.

Walker, G. 2008. Cutaneous melanoma: how does ultraviolet light contribute to melanocyte transformation? *Future Oncology*;4(6):841-856.

Wehrle-Haller, B. 2003. The role of Kit-ligand in melanocyte development and epidermal homeostasis. *Pigment Cell Research*;16(3):287-296.

Westekemper, H., Karimi, S., Susskind, D., Anastassiou, G., Freistuhler, M., Steuhl, K. P., Bornfeld, N., Schmid, K. W., and Grabellus, F. 2011. Expression of HSP 90, PTEN and Bcl-2 in conjunctival melanoma. *British Journal of Ophthalmology*;95(6):853-858.

Whiteman, D. C., Watt, P., Purdie, D. M., Hughes, M. C., Hayward, N. K., and Green, A. C. 2003. Melanocytic nevi, solar keratoses, and divergent pathways to cutaneous melanoma. *Journal of the National Cancer Institute*;95(11):806-812.

Whitwam, T., Vanbrocklin, M. W., Russo, M. E., Haak, P. T., Bilgili, D., Resau, J. H., Koo, H. M., and Holmen, S. L. 2007. Differential oncogenic potential of activated RAS isoforms in melanocytes. *Oncogene*;26(31):4563-4570.

Woodman, S. E., and Davies, M. A. 2010. Targeting KIT in melanoma: a paradigm of molecular medicine and targeted therapeutics. *Biochemical Pharmacology*;80(5):568-574.

World Health Organization, (2011). Ultraviolet radiation and the INTERSUN Programme, 17.06.2011, Available from http://www.who.int/uv/faq/skincancer/en/index1.html

Yang, J. Y., Chang, C. J., Xia, W., Wang, Y., Wong, K. K., Engelman, J. A., Du, Y., Andreeff, M., Hortobagyi, G. N., and Hung, M. C. 2010. Activation of FOXO3a is sufficient to reverse mitogen-activated protein/extracellular signal-regulated kinase kinase inhibitor chemoresistance in human cancer. *Cancer Research*;70(11):4709-4718.

Yi, M., Yang, J., Chen, X., Li, J., Li, X., Wang, L., Tan, Y., Xiong, W., Zhou, M., Mccarthy, J. B., Li, G., Xiang, B., and Xie, H. 2011. RASSF1A suppresses melanoma development by modulating apoptosis and cell-cycle progression. *Journal of Cellular Physiology*;226(9):2360-2369.

5

Merkel Cell Polyomavirus: A Causal Factor in Merkel Cell Carcinoma

Marijke Van Ghelue[1] and Ugo Moens[2]
[1]*Department of Medical Genetics, University Hospital Northern-Norway, Tromsø, Norway*
[2]*University of Tromsø, Faculty of Health Sciences, Department of Medical Biology, Tromsø, Norway*

1. Introduction

The RNA viruses hepatitis C virus and human T-cell lymphotropic virus type I (or human T-cell leukaemia virus type 1), and the DNA viruses hepatitis B virus, high-risk human papillomaviruses, human herpes virus-8 (Kaposi's sarcoma-associated herpes virus) and Epstein Barr virus are acknowledged as carcinogenic to humans. Human polyomaviruses have oncogenic potentials in cell cultures and animal models, but their role in human cancer remains controversial. In 2008, a new polyomavirus member discovered in Merkel cell carcinoma tissue was concordantly named Merkel cell polyomavirus (MCPyV). Subsequent epidemiologic studies have shown that viral DNA is present in approximately 80% of Merkel cell carcinomas investigated and MCPyV positive Merkel cell carcinoma have a higher virus load than non-malignant tissues. In addition, the patients have higher viral antibody levels than controls. Moreover, the viral genome seems monoclonally integrated in the primary tumour and in metastatic cells, and expresses a truncated version of the major oncoprotein, large T-antigen. This C-terminal truncated large T-antigen retains its DnaJ and retinoblastoma binding domains, which are necessary for transformation of cells *in vitro*, but lacks its DNA helicase activity so that it cannot sustain viral DNA replication. These observations suggest that MCPyV can contribute to Merkel cell carcinoma pathogenesis and may therefore add a new virus to the list of human cancer viruses. Here we present information on the biology of polyomaviruses with special focus on MCPyV, review the role of MCPyV in Merkel cell carcinoma, and discuss the molecular mechanisms by which this virus may induce cancer.

2. Merkel cell carcinoma

Merkel cells, originally described by Friedrich Sigmund Merkel in 1875, are believed to migrate during development from the neural crest to the basal layer of the epidermal cells near the end of axons and the outer root sheet of hair follicles [Szeder et al., 2003; Calder & Smoller, 2010]. These cells are especially dense in the skin of the limbs and face, and around hair follicles, but they are also present in oral mucus membranes [Lacour et al., 1991]. Their role remains incompletely understood, but they may function as mechanoreceptors or chemoreceptors [Mahrle & Orfanos, 1974]. This was recently supported by phenotypic observations in conditional knock out mice deficient in expressing the transcription factor Atoh1 [Van Keymeulen et al., 2009]. These mice lacked Merkel cells and *ex vivo* skin/nerve preparations of these animals demonstrated complete loss of the characteristic neurophysiologic responses normally mediated by Merkel cell-neurite complexes. Merkel cells are therefore required for the proper encoding of Merkel receptor responses, suggesting that these cells form an indispensible part of the somatosensory system [Maricich et al., 2009]. Although data suggest that Merkel cells may have a neural crest origin [reviewed in Moll et al., 2005; Boulais & Misery, 2007, The Rockville MCC group, 2009], they also express the epithelial marker cytokeratin 20 (CK20) [Southgate et al., 1999], indicating an epithelial origin. In 1972, Toker described an unusual form of skin cancer as trabecular carcinoma of the skin [Toker, 1972]. Later, these carcinomas were shown to derive from Merkel cells and this type of cancer was therefore renamed Merkel cell carcinoma (MCC) [Gould et al., 1985]. Whether MCC arises from normal Merkel cells is still controversial [The Rockville MCC group, 2009]. Currently, MCC is thought to originate from a primitive totipotent stem cell with the ability to differentiate along divergent histological phenotypes [Calder & Smoller, 2010].

MCC is a rare but aggressive skin cancer of neuroendocrine origin with propensity for local recurrence and regional lymph node metastasis. MCC is most common on the head and neck (approximately 50% of the cases) and the extremities (40% of the patients), and the remaining cases occur on the trunk and on genitalia [Pectasides et al., 2006; Lemos & Nghiem, 2007; Heymann, 2008; Becker et al., 2009; Pulitzer et al., 2009]. MCC is heterogeneous clinically, morphologically and in expression of neuroendocrine, epithelial and oncogenic markers. Histological characterization of the MCC is based on demonstration of cytoplasmic neurosecretory granules of Merkel cell by electron microscopy and positive immunohistochemical staining for cytokeratins CK20, Cam 5.2, CD56, and neuroendocrine markers such as chromogranin A, synaptophysin and neuron-specific enolase [Heymann, 2008]. Classic MCC cell lines grow as non-adherent, clustered cells, while variant MCC cells grow as adherent cells [Leonard et al., 1995]. Comparing the gene expression profile between these two distinct MCC subtypes revealed higher transcript levels of genes encoding signal transduction proteins in classic MCC, while variant MCC possessed elevated transcription of cell cycle genes [Van Gele et al., 2004].

MCC is extremely unusual before the age of 50 (~5% of the cases) and people at risk include those with fair skin, excessive UV-light exposure and immunosuppressed patients. The median age at presentation is 76 years for women and 74 years for men and there is a slight male predominance [Calder & Smoller, 2010]. The majority of the patients are white (94.9%) and chronically immunosuppressed individuals are 10 to 15 times more likely to develop MCC than age-matched controls. Moreover, this malignancy is more lethal in immunodeficient patients than in immunocompetent individuals [Engels et al., 2008; Houben et al., 2009; Becker et al., 2009; Pulitzer et al., 2009; The Rockville MCC group, 2009; Wong & Wang, 2010; Calder & Smoller, 2010]. The incidence rate is 0.44 cases per 100,000 individuals in the USA and 0.15 cases per 100,000 individuals in Japan. The number of MCC cases has tripled the last 15 years [Hodgson, 2005; Nakajima et al., 2009]. The reason for this may be ageing of the population and improved diagnosis. So far, no optimal therapeutic regime exists so that surgical excision of the primary tumour and lymph node dissection, followed by postoperational radiation therapy is the standard practice. Although MCC is claimed to be an aggressive cancer, a retrospective study on almost 4,000 patients has shown that the 10-year relative survival rate is 57% [Albores-Saavedra et al., 2009].

The molecular mechanisms that drive the pathogenesis of MCC remain incompletely understood. Aberrant DNA methylation of the promoters of the cyclin-dependent protein kinase inhibitor p14^{ARF} and the tumour suppressor RASSF1A is believed to be important in MCC tumorigenesis [Lassacher et al., 2008]. Heterozygous loss of chromosome 10q23, which contains the tumour suppressor *PTEN*, overexpression of the anti-apoptotic proteins Bcl-2 and survivin, and of the L-*myc* proto-oncogene have frequently been observed in MCC, while expression levels of the p53 family member p63 correlates with the aggressiveness of the cancer [Kennedy et al., 1996; Feinmesser et al., 1999; Van Gele et al., 2001; Asioli et al., 2007; Kim & McNiff, 2008; Paulson et al., 2009]. However, the role of these events in MCC has to be established. The recent discovery of the presence of a new polyomavirus in most MCC may have shed some light on the enigma what may be a major cause of MCC.

3. Human polyomaviruses

Members of the *Polyomaviridae* family are characterized by a double-stranded circular DNA genome surrounded by a viral protein structure, referred to as capsid. They lack, however, a host-cell derived lipid structure known as the envelope. The virus particles are about 45 nm in diameter and the viral genome is approximately 5,000 base-pairs [Imperiale & Major, 2007]. The first member of this family was isolated in from mice 1953. The name polyomavirus ("poly" for many and "oma" for cancer) refers to the virus' ability to induce different types of tumours when injected in mice [reviewed in Stoner & Hübner, 2001]. The oncogenic properties of mouse polyomavirus encouraged scientists in their search to isolate other polyomaviruses, including human polyomaviruses. In 1960, the second member of this family was isolated from monkey kidney cells used for producing poliovirus vaccine. This virus was named simian virus 40 (SV40) and could transform cell culture, including human cells and induce tumours in animal models [Vilchez & Butel, 2004]. In 1971, two independent research groups reported the isolation of the first human polyomaviruses. One virus was detected in the urine of a kidney transplant recipient with the initials B.K., while the other human polyomavirus was isolated from the brain of a Hodgkin lymphoma patient with the initials J.C. who suffered from progressive multifocal leukoencephalopathy (PML). These viruses were named as BK virus (BKV) and JC virus (JCV), respectively [Gardner et al., 1971; Padgett et al., 1971]. The International Committee on Taxonomy of Viruses recommends using the abbreviations BKPyV and JCPyV, respectively [Johne et al., 2011].

SV40 and lymphotropic polyomavirus (LPyV), another monkey virus also seem to infect the human population, but with a much lower incidence than BKPyV and JCPyV. Whereas up to 90%, respectively 60% of the adults have antibodies against BKPyV, respectively JCPyV. SV40 and LPyV infections are less common with only 2% of the human population showing specific anti-SV40 antibodies and 15% possessing anti-LPyV antibodies [Knowles, 2006; Carter et al., 2009; Kean et al., 2009]. The latter number may be overestimated because recently a new human polyomavirus (HPyV9) that is closely related to LPyV has been isolated so that the seropositivity to LPyV may be partially explained by cross-reactivity with HPyV9 [Scuda et al., 2011]. Human polyomaviruses establish a life-long latent infection in immunocompetent hosts, while immunocompromised individuals such as autoimmune patients and AIDS patients or immunosuppressive treatment such as in bone marrow and renal transplant patients may lead to reactivation of the viruses. Reactivation of BKPyV can lead to nephropathy or hemorrhagic cystitis, while JCPyV is the causative agent of progressive multifocal leukoencephalopathy [Jiang et al., 2009].

For many years, occurrence of the known human polyomaviruses in individuals was monitored mostly by PCR and serological methods. In recent years, mainly by use of novel methodology, several new polyomaviruses have been isolated. They include KIPyV, WUPyV, HPyV6, HPyV7, trichodysplasia spinulosa-associated polyomavirus (TSPyV), and HPyV9 [Allander et al., 2007; Gaynor et al., 2007; Schowalter et al., 2010; van der Meijden et al., 2010; Scuda et al., 2011; reviewed in Moens et al., 2010 and Moens et al., 2011]. Their role in human pathologies remains unknown, except for TSPyV which may be the etiological factor in trichodysplasia spinulosa, a rare skin disease exclusively found in immunocompromised patients and characterized by the development of follicular papules and keratin spines known as spicules [van der Meijden et al., 2010; Matthews et al., 2011].

Another new polyomavirus was isolated in Merkel cell carcinoma tissue, hence its name Merkel cell polyomavirus or MCPyV [Feng et al., 2008]. Whereas, the role of human polyomaviruses in cancer remains a matter of dispute despite their oncogenic properties in cell culture and in animal models, as well as the presence of viral nucleic acid sequences and proteins in cancer tissue, MCPyV is considered as an etiological factor in MCC [Abend et al., 2009; Maginnis & Atwood, 2009; Gjoerup & Chang, 2010]. This virus and its role in MCC is the focus of this review.

4. Molecular biology of human polyomaviruses

The viral genome of human polyomaviruses can be divided into three functional regions: the early region encoding large T-antigen (LT-ag) and small t-antigen (st-ag), the late region encoding the capsid proteins VP1, VP2 and VP3, and the non-coding control region encompassing the origin of replication and promoter sequences that control transcription of the viral genes (Figure 1). LT-ag is required for viral DNA replication and regulates the expression of the viral genes, while st-ag has an auxiliary role for LT-ag. The early region of some human polyomaviruses encodes alternative proteins whose functions are incompletely understood. The late regions of BKPyV, JCPyV and SV40 also contain an ORF for the agnoprotein that is required for efficient virus propagation in cell culture [Carswell & Alwine, 1986; Khalili et al., 2005; Sariyer et al., 2006; Johannessen et al., 2008; Suzuki et al., 2010]. No corresponding ORF seems to be present in the other human polyomaviruses [Yoshiike & Takemoto, 1986; Allander et al., 2007; Gaynor et al., 2007; Feng et al., 2008; Schowalter et al., 2010; van der Meijden et al., 2010; Scuda et al., 2011]. The reason why agnoprotein seems to be abundant in the human polyomaviruses LPyV, KIPyV, WUPyV, MCPyV, HPyV6, HPyV7, TSPyV and HPyV, but not in SV40, BKPyV and JCPyV remains mysterious, but it may be because of different life cycle strategies or host cell tropism. SV40 encodes a fifth late protein, referred to as VP4. This protein enhances lysis of the host cell and facilitates release of mature virus particles [Daniels et al., 2007]. KIPyV, WUPyV, MCPyV, TSPyV, HPyV6, HPyV7, and HPyV9 all lack a VP4-like open reading frame (ORF).

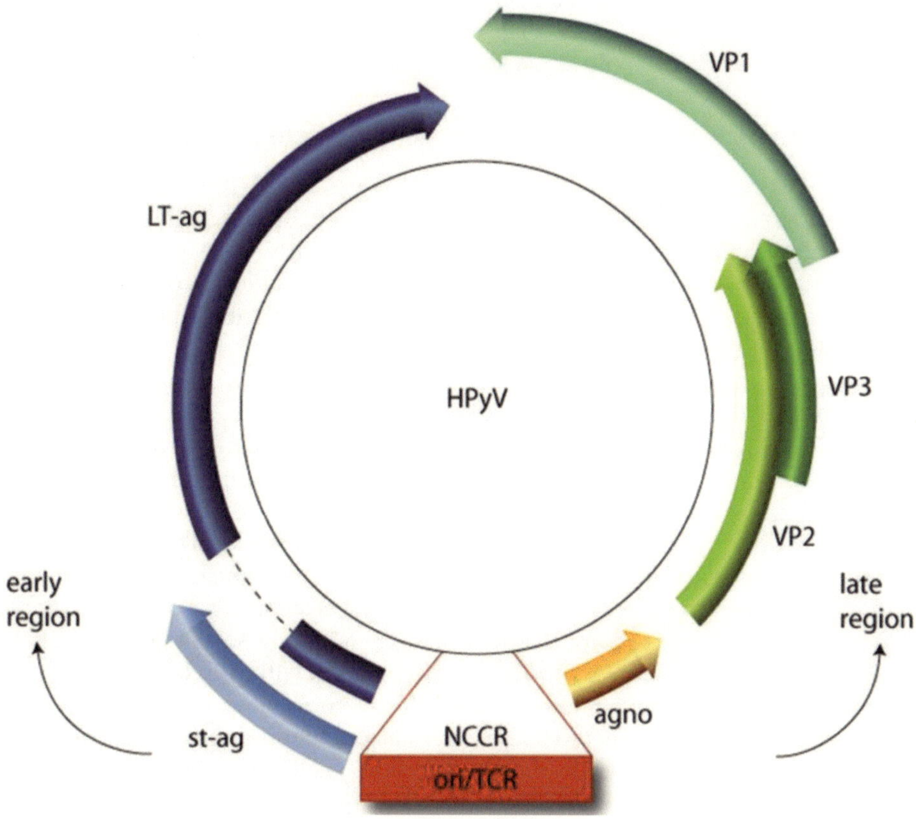

Fig. 1. Genomic organization of human polyomaviruses. The open reading frame encoding agnoprotein (agno) is not present in all human polyomaviruses. See text for details.

BKPyV and JCPyV contain a putative VP4 ORF with the N-terminal MVRQVAxREG amino acid sequence (x= E in BKPyV and Q in JCPyV), which is reminiscent of SV40 VP4 (MVRQVANREG), while LPyV has a putative ORF with the N-terminal motif MRQA at the corresponding site. However, VP4 expression by BKPyV, JCPyV and LPyV has not been confirmed.

The genomes of SV40, BKPyV, JCPyV and MCPyV encode a miRNA that down-regulates LT-ag expression levels [Sullivan et al., 2005; Seo et al., 2008]. Cells expressing SV40 miRNA are less susceptible to cytotoxic T cells and trigger less cytokine expression than cells infected with an SV40 mutant lacking miRNA. Hence, miRNA-mediated downregulation of LT-ag levels may allow the virus to escape the immune system [Sullivan et al., 2005]. BKPyV and JCPyV miRNA can also reduce the protein levels of LT-ag by preventing mRNA translation or targeting it for destruction. Whether this also affects cytotoxic T cells responses remains unknown. Recent findings by Bauman and colleagues shed light on the molecular mechanism by which these viruses can evade the immune system and remain latent. They demonstrated that JCPyV- and BKPyV-encoded miRNA target the stress-induced ligand ULBP3, which is recognized by the natural killer cell receptor NKG2D. Consequently, viral miRNA downregulation results in reduced

NKG2D-destruction of BKPyV/JCPyV infected cells by natural killer cells [Bauman et al., 2011]. This miRNA-mediated evasion of the immune system may allow the viruses to establish a latent infection. MCPyV also encodes a miRNA that is antisense to LT-ag mRNA and consequently can reduce the levels of LT-ag [Seo et al., 2009].

5. Mechanisms by which human polyomaviruses cause cellular transformation

Infection of cultured cell lines, including human, with SV40, BKPyV, JCPyV and LPyV leads to transformation, while transgenic animals expressing early gene products or animals infected with these viruses can develop tumours [Moens et al., 2007b; Gjoerup and Chang, 2010]. The oncogenic properties of these viruses are primarily attributed to the action of LT-ag, but also st-ag and agnoprotein possess oncogenic potentials.

LT-ag is a multifunctional protein that is mandatory for viral DNA replication. It contains several functional domains performing different roles (Figure 2). LT-ag binds as an hexamer to G(G/A)GGC motifs at the viral origin of replication and forms a complex with the cellular replication proteins DNA polymerase α/primase, replication protein A, and topoisomerase. LT-ag has also DNA helicase activity that helps unwinding the double-stranded DNA during replication [reviewed in Simmons et al., 2004]. It can bind the tumour suppressors p53 and the retinoblastoma (pRb) family members, thereby forcing the cell into the S phase. This is pivotal for the virus because the virus depends completely on the host cell's DNA replication machinery. LT-ag contains a so-called pRb pocket with the consensus motif LXCXE that is required for interaction with pRb family members. The pRb family members control S phase progression by controlling the expression of E2F-responsive genes. E2F is a family of transcription factors that transcribes genes controlling cell cycle progression and DNA replication such as cyclins, cyclin-dependent kinases, dihydrofolate reductase, thymidine kinase, DNA polymerase I, c-Myc, c-Myb, but also genes whose products are involved in DNA repair, differentiation and apoptosis. Another LT-ag domain that plays a crucial role in regulating the activity of pRb is the DnaJ domain. This N-terminal located region binds Hsc70, a chaperone with weak intrinsic ATPase activity. The DnaJ domain stimulates Hsc70's ATPase activity and this DnaJ/Hsc70 interaction influences viral DNA replication, transactivation of the viral promoters and viral assembly. Additionally, it is critical for oncogenic transformation via functional inactivation of the pRb family members. The energy generated by DnaJ domain-mediated hydrolysis of ATP is used to split pRb/E2F complexes [Moens et al., 2007a; Moens et al., 2007b; Gjoerup and Chang, 2010]. The C-terminal domain of LT-ag is involved in binding the tumour suppressor p53. The p53 protein represses cell cycle proliferation and angiogenesis, stimulates apoptosis and is involved in controlling DNA repair [Vogelstein et al., 2000; Vousden et al., 2009]. Several other properties of LT-ag can contribute to neoplastic transformation. It has been shown that LT-ag stimulates telomerase activity, inhibits apoptosis, activates signalling pathways triggering cell cycle progression, interferes with DNA repair and chromosome fidelity, promotes angiogenesis, perturbs protein turn-over, and affects gene expression by interfering with transcription, DNA methylation, chromatine structure. Hence, prolonged LT-ag expression may lead to uncontrolled cell cycle progression, inhibition of angiogenesis and apoptosis, and accumulation of DNA damage [reviewed in Moens et al., 2007a; Moens et al., 2007b; Gjoerup and Chang, 2010].

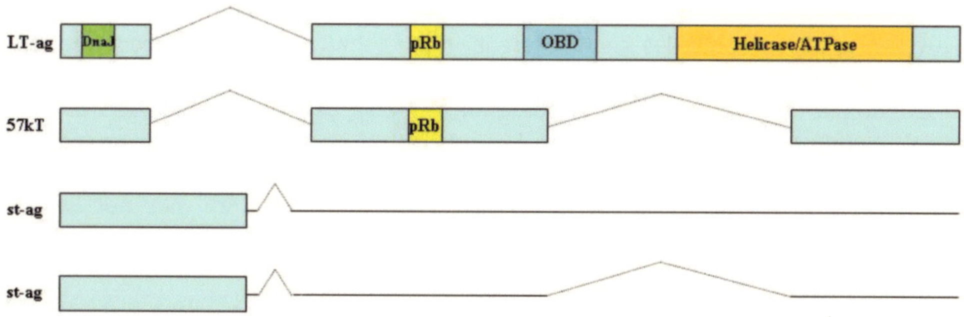

Fig. 2. Functional domains of the human polyomavirus LT-ag and the different splicing products generated from transcription of the early region of MCPyV. These transcripts encode LT-ag, the truncated variant 57kT and two different mRNAs for st-ag. See text for details.

St-ag seems to exert an auxiliary function in LT-ag-mediated transformation. St-ag shares the N-terminal ~80 amino acids with LT-ag and therefore contains the DnaJ domain, but unlike LT-ag, it lacks the pRb pocket. The major contribution of st-ag in the oncogenic process is through inactivation of protein phosphatase 2A (PP2A). The unique C-terminal part of st-ag binds to the A-subunit of the trimeric PP2A holoenzyme, leading to inhibition of the catalytic activity. St-ag mediated inactivation of PP2A can activate signalling pathways, alter gene expression, inhibit apoptosis/prolongation of cell survival, change protein stability, stimulate telomerase activity, disrupt the cytoskeleton and induce chromosome instability [Moens et al., 2007b].

The agnoprotein of JCPyV can arrest cells in G2/M phase probably through upregulated expression of the cyclin-dependent kinase inhibitor $p21^{Waf1/Cip1}$ [Darbinyan et al., 2002]. JCPyV agnoprotein can interact with the Ku70, which is a component of the non-homologous end joining (NHEJ) DNA repair complex, leading to inhibition of NHEJ DNA repair [Darbinyan et al., 2004]. Thus, agnoprotein may contribute to transformation through interference with the cell cycle and DNA repair.

Similar studies with the newly discovered human polyomaviruses are lacking, but as these viruses also encode LT-ag and st-ag, it is assumed that they may possess similar oncogenic properties.

6. Merkel cell polyomavirus (MCPyV): Molecular biology

In 2008, Feng and colleagues detected two sequences with highest homology to the LT-ags of LPyV and BKPyV in MCC transcriptomes consisting of >380,000 cDNA sequences obtained by pyrosequencing [Feng et al., 2008]. The authors succeeded in cloning and sequencing the entire genome of two variants of this virus, which turned out to be a novel polyomavirus. This new polyomavirus was commonly found in MCC samples and accordingly named Merkel cell polyomavirus (MCPyV). The MCPyV variant 350 (accession number EU375803) and variant 339 (accession number EU375804) diverge by 191 base-pairs inserted in the LT-ag of MCPyV339, 5 base-pairs inserted in the MCPyV 339 non-coding region, and additional 41 nucleotides substitutions dispersed throughout their genomes

[Feng et al., 2008]. The genetic organization of MCPyV (Figure 3) resembles that of other polyomaviruses, except for the absence of an open reading frame encoding agnoprotein. The early region of MCPyV encodes three different proteins that are translated from differently spliced transcripts. The LT-ag and st-ag share the N-terminal 79 amino acids, but diverge in their C-terminal domain. The 57kT is identical to LT-ag except for a deletion in the C-terminal region of the protein (Figure 2). The late region encodes the capsid proteins VP1 and VP2, but the VP2 ORF lacks the conserved Met-Ala-Leu motif that forms the start of VP3 in other human polyomaviruses. This may suggest that MCPyV may not encode a functional VP3 [Pastrana et al., 2009]. However, an open reading frame encoding a putative VP3 starting with Met-Thr-Ile is present in both MCC and non-MCC isolates suggesting that a functional VP3 is expressed [Feng et al., 2008; Carter et al., 2009; Schowalter et al., 2010; Touzé et al., 2011]. MCPyV also encodes a viral miRNA that can downregulate the levels of LT-ag [Seo et al., 2009].

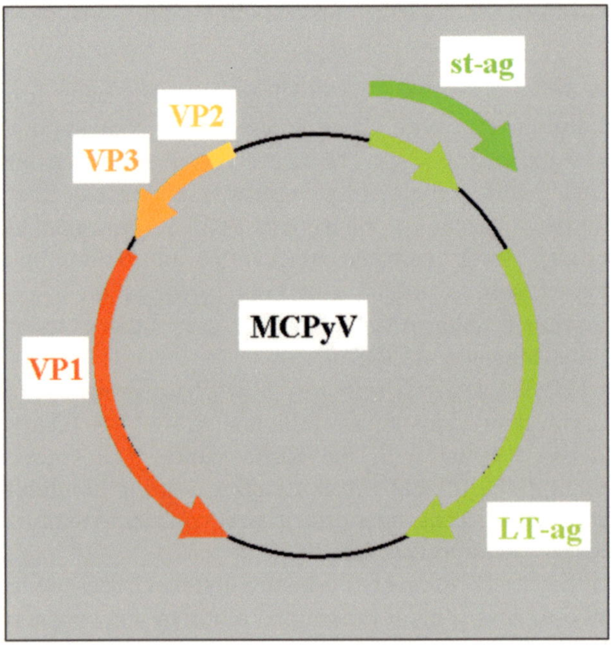

Fig. 3. Genomic organization of MCPyV. The early region encodes for LT-ag, st-ag and 57kT (not shown), while the late region encodes the capsid proteins VP1, VP2 and VP3.

Although originally isolated from MCC, MCPyV infection is probably not restricted to Merkel cells in the skin because these cells make up <1% of the cells in the epidermis, yet MCPyV virions are being shed from the skin at high numbers [Schowalter et al., 2010]. These findings strongly suggest that more common cells in the epidermis like keratinocytes and/or melanocytes may be involved in the production of virions. The presence of MCPyV in keratinocytes has not been investigated, while MCPyV DNA was not detected in melanocytes [Giraud et al., 2008; Mogha et al., 2010]. Hence, a role for these two cell types as reservoirs for MCPyV remains unclear. Other cell types in the skin may function as reservoir because MCPyV DNA is present in eyebrow hairs, skin lesions and warts from immunocompetent and immunosuppressed patients [Wieland et al., 2009; Schowalter et al., 2010; van der Meijden et al., 2010; Mertz et al., 2010a; Foulongne et al., 2010a].

7. MCPyV: Route of infection, cell tropism and transmission

The route of infection of MCPyV is not know, but viral DNA is found in nasal swabs, oral cavity, mouth wash, tonsil biopsies, and oesophagus from healthy individuals, signifying an oral route of infection [Bialasiewicz et al., 2009; Dworkin et al., 2009; Goh et al., 2009; Kantola et al., 2009; Sharp et al., 2009; Loyo et al., 2010; Babakir-Mina et al., 2010]. The primary target cells and the host cells that can function as reservoir are not known, but the virus seems to be common in healthy skin, skin lesions, eyebrow hairs, and warts, indicating a dermatotropism of this virus [Wieland et al., 2009; van der Meijden et al., 2010; Mertz et al., 2010a; Faust et al., 2011; Wieland et al., 2011]. MCPyV DNA is also found in blood, gall bladder, appendix, liver, lung, lymphoid, and intestine tissue [Feng et al., 2008; Sharp et al., 2009; Goh et al., 2009; Shuda et al., 2009; Foulongne et al., 2010a; Husseiny et al., 2010; Loyo et al., 2010; Toracchio et al., 2010; Campello et al., 2011; Pancaldi et al., 2011; reviewed in Moens et al., 2010 and Gjoerup and Chang, 2010]. Another study has suggested that MCPyV may persist in and spread through inflammatory monocytes [Mertz et al., 2010b].

To expound the cell tropism, Erickson and colleagues identified the MCPyV receptor by using purified VP1 pentamers and liposomes. They found that MCPyV pentamers bound strongly ganglioside GT1b, very weakly GD1b (i.e. the receptor for BKPyV), and not GM1 (i.e. the receptor for SV40) and GD1a (i.e. the mouse polyomavirus receptor). This indicates that GT1b is a putative receptor for MCPyV and that MCPyV has different host cell targets than the other HPyV [Erickson et al., 2009]. The binding of MCPyV pentamers to its target receptor may be more complicated. GT1b is abundant in neuronal cell membranes, yet MCPyV DNA seems absent in cerebrospinal fluid and brain and central nervous system tumours [Feng et al., 2008; Barzon et al., 2009; Busam et al., 2009; Giraud et al., 2009]. Moreover, MCPyV pentamers could bind to HeLa (human cervical cancer carcinoma cells) and HEK29T (adenovirus transformed human embryonal kidney cells that express SV40 LT-ag) cells, which may not be genuine target cells as no MCPyV has been detected in cervical tissue nor in the kidneys so far. Moreover, MCPyV viruria is rare, indicating that the kidneys may not be an *in vivo* reservoir [Feng et al., 2008; Giraud et al., 2008; Duncavage et al., 2009a; Katano et al., 2009; Sastre-Garau et al., 2009]. The use of pentamers that may acquire a different conformation than intact virus particles and the requirement of a co-receptor may explain infection of none bona fide host cells.

The way of transmission of MCPyV is also unknown, but the faecal-oral route has been suggested because MCPyV DNA can be detected in samples from the gastrointestinal tract and in urban sewage [Feng et al., 2008; Bofill-Mas et al., 2010; Loyo et al., 2010; Campello et al., 2011]. Moreover, the average viral DNA load in aero-digestive tract is 100 fold higher than the respiratory and genitourinary tract [Loyo et al., 2010]. The results should be interpreted with caution because a limited number of patients were tested. Other studies failed to detect MCPyV DNA in colon adenocarcinoma and in stool samples, jeopardizing a faecal-oral route of transmission [Kantola et al., 2009; Sastre-Garau et al., 2009]. The virus may also spread through respiratory droplets or blood as viral sequences are detected in nasopharyngeal aspirates, nose swabs and blood, but proof for this way of transmission is lacking. Moreover, the prevalence of MCPyV in these samples is lower than in MCC [Dworkin et al., 2009; Helmbold et al., 2009; Kantola et al., 2009; Sharp et al., 2009; Shuda et al., 2009; Tolstov et el., 2009; Mertz et al., 2010b; Babakir-Mina et al., 2010; Loyo et al., 2010; Pancaldi et al., 2011]. Direct contact is most probably the mode of transmission because MCPyV DNA is frequently detected in benign skin, healthy individuals are chronically infected with MCPyV, and the virus seems to be continuously shed from the skin [Feng et al., 2008; Dworkin et al., 2009; Helmbold et al., 2009; Wieland et al., 2009; Mertz et al., 2010b; Foulongne et al., 2010b; Loyo et al., 2010; Schowalter et al., 2010]. Schowalter and collaborators collected skin swab samples with approximately 3 months interval from 16 volunteers. All samples tested MCPyV DNA positive and contained ~$2x10^6$ genome equivalents/ml of gradient material. [Schowalter et al., 2010]. Efficient horizontal spreading of MCPyV through skin-to-skin contact may also explain the high seroprevalence in the human population (see next section). The absence of MCPyV antibodies in children less than 1 year old argues against vertical transmission [Tolstov et al., 2009].

8. MCPyV seroprevalence

PCR-based studies have demonstrated that MCPyV infection is common in the normal population and that different tissues can harbour viral DNA [reviewed in Moens et al., 2011]. Serological studies demonstrate that MCPyV infection is widespread in man (Table 1). Of 41 MCC patients (age 42-86 years; 27 men and 14 women) tested, 36 (88%) had MCPyV VP1 antibodies. Tumour material of 31 MCC patients was available for MCPyV DNA analysis and viral DNA was detected in 24 specimens. Of these 24 patients, 22 (92%) had MCPyV VP1 antibodies [Carter et al., 2009]. The authors tested 76 age-and sex-matched controls and found that 40 (53%) were seropositive, showing that there was a significant difference ($p<0.001$) between the MCC patients and the 76 controls for the presence of MCPyV antibodies. The same group analyzed another 451 randomly selected women whose age varied between younger than 30 years and >70 years and found that 271 (60%) were seropositive. No significant differences were observed with increasing age. The seroprevalences for the age groups <30, 30-39, 40-49, 50-59, 60-69 and <70 were 60%, 54%, 66%, 61%, 66% and 58%, respectively. This indicates that most viral infection must have occurred before the age of 30 and that the prevalence was stable at older ages [Carter et al., 2009]. Although this second control group existed exclusively of women, there was no significant difference with the first control group. Thus, the presence of MCPyV VP1 antibodies does not seem to be gender-dependent. Carter and his colleagues found that antibodies in serum samples reacted strongly with VP1 from MCPyV strain w162, while little or no reactivity was found against VP1 from strain 350, although these VP1s differ only by four amino acids [Carter et al., 2009]. Hence, caution must be taken when performing serological studies because the amino acid composition of VP1 in the assay may affect the reactivity of the circulating MCPyV VP1 antibodies in the serum of the patient and therefore the outcome of the test. Kean and co-workers also reported a differential seroreactivity to MCPyV isolates 350 and 339 [Kean et al., 2009]. In their study, 1501 adult healthy blood donors (age >21 yrs) were tested and 379 individuals (25%) had antibodies that reacted with MCPyV strain 350 recombinant VP1, while 692 blood donors (46%) possessed antibodies that recognized strain 339 recombinant VP1. The difference was less in a paediatric cohort <21years of age. Of 721 children examined, 164 (23%) were seropositive for MCPyV strain 350 and 247 (34%) for strain 339. The authors did not detect differences in seroprevalence in respect to gender, nor was there a significant difference in seropositivity between children and adults. This indicates that primary infection occurs during early childhood. However, for MCPyV strains, there was a tendency to increased seropositivity in elderly individuals.

MCPyV positive MCC	Non MCC subjects	ag§	reference
88% (n=41; age 42-86 yrs)	53% (n=76; age <75 yrs) 60% (n=451; age 24-77 yrs)	VP1	Carter et al., 1999
	46% (n=1501; age >21 yrs) 34% (n=721; age < 21 yrs)	VP1	Kean et al., 1999
100% (n=21; age 14-95 yrs)	88% (n=48; age 47-75 yrs)	VP1	Pastrana et al., 2009
100% (n=21; age 14-95 yrs)*	64% (n=116; age >18 yrs) 63% (n=100; age > 47 yrs) 74% (n=50; age nm#)	VP1	Tolstov et al., 2009
not tested	11% (n=217; age 0-13 years) 37% (n=71; age 6-11 years)	VP1	Chen et al., 2011
91% (n=139; age 31-91 yrs)	66% (n=530; age-matched)	VP1	Paulson et al., 2010
100% (n=51; age 37-91 yrs)	85% (n=82; age 22-83 years)	VP1	Touzé et al..,2011
not tested	65% (n=434; age 29-97 years)	VP1	Faust et al., 2011
average VP1 seropositivity: 95% (n=252)	**average VP1 seropositivity: 57% (n=4397)**		
26% (n=205; age 31-96 yrs)	2% (n=530; age-matched)	LT-ag	Paulson et al., 2010
41% (n=205; age 31-96 yrs)	1% (n=530; age-matched)	st-ag	Paulson et al., 2010

§antigen; *same patients as in Pastrana et al., 2009; #nm= not mentioned.

Table 1. Seropositivity against MCPyV VP1, LT-ag and st-ag in MCC and non MCC subjects.

The average seropositivity for strain 350 in individuals <70 years is 23%, while 40% of persons older then 70 had antibodies. Similarly, 38% of the tested persons younger than 70 were seropositive for MCPyV strain 339 VP1, while 61% of those older than 70 years were seropositive [Kean et al., 2009]. In another study, the presence of MCPyV neutralizing antibodies in sera was determined. All (n=21) MCC patients (age 14-95 years) whose tumours were MCPyV DNA positive had specific MCPyV antibodies with a geometric mean titre of 160,000 in the assay used. While 42/48 (88%) sera of blood donors (age 47-75 years) also contain MCPyV specific antibodies, the mean titre was ~60 times lower. Similarly, low titres were found in 3 out of 6 MCC patients negative for MCPyV, while the other two patients had no detectable levels of MCPyV antibodies [Pastrana et al., 2009]. This was confirmed by the work of two other groups. Tolstov and collaborators found that IgG levels against the capsid proteins of MCPyV were higher in MCPyV positive MCC patients than in MCPyV negative patients, blood donors and systemic lupus erythematosus (SLE) patients

[Tolstov et al., 2009]. All of their 21 MCPyV positive MCC patients had significantly higher MCPyV specific IgG antibodies than antibody levels found in 3/6 (50%) MCPyV negative MCC patients, in 107/166 (64%) blood donors, in 63/100 (63%) commercial donors and in 37/50 (74%) SLE patients. The IgM levels in all patient groups were comparable [Tolstov et al., 2009]. French MCPyV positive MCC patients had on average 15-fold higher anti-VP1 antibody titres than controls [Touzé et al., 2011]. One obvious explanation for the higher MCPyV-specific antibody titres in MCPyV positive MCC patients is that VP1 is expressed on the cell surface of the tumour cells. However, immunohistochemical staining of 10 MCC tumour cells that had previously shown to express MCPyV LT-ag was negative for VP1, suggesting that VP1 is not expressed in MCC [Pastrana et al., 2009]. Touzé and colleagues were also unable to detect VP1 in 21 MCPyV positive MCC samples obtained from 16 patients [Touzé et al., 2011]. This indicates that tumour cells do not produce VP1 (due to integrational interruption of the late region) or do so at levels undetectable by immunohistochemical staining. Another reason for the higher antibody levels in MCPyV positive MCC patients could be their immunocompromised condition such that a delayed immune response upon primary infection may have resulted in much higher virus load inducing higher titres. Another possibility is that MCPyV may establish a persistent infection in other cell types than Merkel cells in these patients or that unusually high immunogenic MCPyV strains are circulating in these patients [Pastrana et al., 2009]. The fact that a substantial number of individuals of healthy controls and other patient groups displayed MCPyV VP1 antibody titres in the same range as MCPyV positive MCC patients argues against this [Pastrana et al., 2009; Tolstov et al., 2009]. This also implies that not everybody with high MCPyV specific antibody titres develops MCC.

Pastrana and colleagues observed a gradual age-related decline in MCPyV antibody titres for the MCPyV positive MCC patients, but the number in each age category was limited [Pastrana et al., 2009]. This was in contrast with the findings of Tolstov and co-workers in 150 Langerhans cell histiocytosis patients whose age ranged from 1 month to 72 years old. The authors measured an age-dependent increase of MCPyV-specific IgG antibodies with approximately 40% of the patients younger than 50 years old having antibodies; this number increased to 80% in patients older than 50 years [Tolstov et al., 2009]. The reason for the opposite results by the two groups remains unknown, but may be due to different assays, different patient groups, or the limited number of individuals examined. Interestingly, none of the six Langerhans cell histiocytosis patients who were less then 1 year old had MCPyV antibodies, arguing against vertical transmission of the virus [Tolstov et al., 2009]. A serological study with 217 Finnish children suffering from acute lower respiratory tract infection confirmed that MCPyV infection probably occurs after the age of one [Chen et al., 2011]. IgG antibodies immunoreactive with VP1 strain 339 were present in sera from 2 out of 51 (4%) children less than 1 year old, while 9% (n=140) of children between 1 and 4 years of age were seropositive. Seroprevalence increased to 35% (n=26) in the age category 4-13 years. The overall seroprevalence was 11% (24/217). Serum samples obtained 5-8 years later were available for 72 of these 217 children. The initial (at age 0-3 years) MCPyV VP1 IgG positivity rate of 6% in these children rose to 37% (26/71) during the follow-up. Notably, of the 67 children whose first sample was seronegative, 22 (33%) were seropositive for their follow-up sample. The same authors also examined 158 children age 1-4 years who had inflammation of the middle ear. Six of them (4%) were seropositive, while 3 years later, 29 (18%) had VP1 antibodies. While in the group of children with acute lower respiratory tract infection no significant gender differences were observed, seroprevalence, seroconversion and antibody titres were higher (p=0.08, p=0.08 and p=0.1, respectively) [Chen et al., 2011]. Another study confirmed the higher prevalence and higher titres of VP1 antibodies in sera from MCC patients compared to control subjects. While 91% (n=134) of the MCC patients were seropositive, 66% (n=530) of the controls had anti-VP1 antibodies [Paulson et al., 2010]. The authors included an additional 66 sera from MCC patients and tested for the presence of antibodies against LT-ag and st-ag. While 2% (respectively 1%) control subjects had antibodies against LT-ag (respectively st-ag), 26% (respectively 41%) of the MCC patients were seropositive for LT-ag (respectively st-ag). Interestingly, higher MCPyV DNA load in MCC tumours is associated with higher LT-/st-ag antibody titres and patients with advanced disease had significantly higher titres. These results suggest that LT-ag/st-ag antibodies may serve as a clinically useful MCC disease marker [Paulson et al., 2010].

In conclusion, seroprevalence and antibody titres in MCPyV positive MCC patients are higher than in control subjects, but MCPyV infection is very common in the adult population. Results from independent groups revealed that 46-88% of the non MCC adults (approximately 4,400 subjects) had MCPyV antibodies [Carter et al., 2009; Kean et al., 2009; Pastrana et al., 2009; Tolstov et al., 2009; Paulson et al., 2010; Touzé et al., 2011; Faust et al., 2011]. Serological studies also indicate that primary infection is acquired early in life and that seropositivity inclines with age. MCPyV DNA was amplified in a nasopharyngeal aspirate from a ~2 month old baby [Bialasiewicz et al., 2009], and the prevalence of MCPyV DNA in these samples increase from 0.6% in children <15 years (n=340) to 8.5% in adults ≥15 years of age [Goh et al., 2009]. These findings are in agreement with the age-related occurrence of MCPyV antibodies.

9. MCPyV and MCC: Genoprevalence

After the original isolation of MCPyV in MCC, a large number of studies have been performed world-wide to look for viral DNA in MCC. Results from these studies show that approximately 80% of the examined MCC samples contain MCPyV DNA, hence strongly suggesting MCPyV as a candidate etiological agent in the development of MCC (Table 2). Although MCC occurs most commonly in the skin, it is also detected in sun-protected sites such as the oral and nasal mucosa, vulva, and penis. In a case report, MCPyV DNA and LT-ag expression were demonstrated in a patient with nasopharyngeal MCC, both in the primary tumour and in a lymph node metastasis, showing that MCPyV may also be an etiological factor in these types of MCC [Wu et al., 2010]. MCPyV seems to be distributed globally, but the rates of MCPyV DNA positive MCCs in European (80%; n=865), North America (72%; n=254) and Asia (76%; n=58) are higher than in Australia (24%; n=21; **Table 2**). However, only a limited number of cases were examined in Asia and in Australian [Garenski et al., 2009; Katano et al., 2009; Nakajima et al., 2009; Woo et al., 2010]. Studies that tested 10 or more subjects, gave a prevalence that varies between 54-88% for North-America, 64-100% for Europe, 55-79% for Asia, and 24% for Australia.

Recently, an immuno-histochemistry study confirmed that only 19 of 104 (18%) MCC samples from Australian patients had detectable LT-ag expression [Paik et al., 2011]. It is speculated that owing to increased sun exposure in Australia, viral pathogenesis could be a less important cofactor in MCC. Sun exposure may drive MCC through an alternative, virus-independent oncogenic pathway [Garenski et al., 2009; Paik et al., 2011].

N#	prevalence	region	country	reference
10	8 (80%)	LT, VP1	USA	Feng et al., 2008
13	7 (54%)	LT, VP1	USA	Ridd et al., 2008
53	45 (85%)	LT	Germany	Becker et al., 2009
5	2 (40%)	LT	the Netherlands	Wetzels et al., 2009
31	24 (77%)	LT	USA	Carter et al., 2009
17	15 (88%)	LT	USA	Busam et al., 2009
23	17 (74%)	st	USA	Bhatai et al., 2009
9	8 (89%)	LT, VP1	France	Foulongne et al., 2008
50	43 (86%)	LT	Germany	Houben et al., 2010
91	84 (92%)	LT	Germany	Helmbold et al., 2009
14	11 (79%)	LT, VP1	Japan	Nakajima et al., 2009
7	6 (86%)	LT, VP1	USA	Loyo et al., 2010
1	1 (100%)	LT, VP1	Switzerland	Mertz et al., 2010
39	30 (77%)	LT, VP1	Germany	Kassem et al., 2008
34	30 (88%)	LT	Germany	Wieland et al., 2009
5	5 (100%)	LT	Germany	Wieland et al., 2009
1	1 (100%)	LT, VP1	Switzerland	Mertz et al., 2010
114	91 (80%)	LT, VP1	Finland	Sihto et al., 2009
10	7 (70%)	LT, VP2,	USA	Shuda et al., 2009
1	1 (100%)	LT	USA	Duncavage et al., 2009
29	22 (76%)	LT	USA	Duncavage et al., 2009
5	5 (100%)	LT	Finland	Koljonen et al., 2009
16	11 (69%)	LT	North America	Garenski et al., 2009
21	5 (24%)	LT	Australia	Garenski et al., 2009
33	21 (64%)	LT, st	Germany	Andres et al., 2009+2010
11	6 (55%)	LT, st, VP1-3	Japan	Katano et al., 2009
22	13 (59%)	LT	USA	Paulson et al., 2009
27	19 (70%)	LT, VP1	USA	Tolstov et al., 2009
32	21 (66%)	LT, VP, NCCR	France	Touzé et al., 2009
10	10 (100%)	LT, st, VP1	France	Sastre-Garau et al., 2009
7	5 (89%)	LT, VP1	Hungary	Varga et al., 2009
2	2 (100%)	LT1, LT3	USA	Wu et al., 2010
9	8 (89%)	LT1, LT3, VP1	France	Foulongne et al., 2008
33	31 (94%)	LT3, VP1	France	Laude et al., 2010
68	51 (75%)	VP1	France	Touzé et al.,2011
27	19 (70%)	LT	USA	Paulson et al., 2011
32	24 (75%)	LT and VP1	Germany	Werling et al., 2011
9	8 (89%)	LT1,VP1	Italy	Paolini et al., 2011
26	20 (77%)	LT, VP1	Japan	Kuwamoto et al., 2011
87	67 (77%)	LT	Finland	Waltari et al., 2010
44	29 (66%)	LT, VP1	Germany	Handschel et al., 2010
6	4 (67%)	LT	USA	Lewis et al., 2010
13	7 (54%)	LT, VP1	USA	Ridd et al., 2009
7	7 (100%)	LT	South Korea	Woo, 2010
3	2 (67%)	LT	Germany	Schmitt et al., 2011
91	71 (78%)	LT	Finland	Sihto et al., 2011
Σ=1198	**924 (77%)**			

Table 2. Prevalence of MCPyV DNA in MCC.#N=number of patients.

There is a slighter overall incidence of MCC among women than among men, while other studies found the opposite [Kaae et al., 2010; Calder & Smoller, 2010]. Not all studies that have examined the presence of MCPyV DNA in MCC have specified the distribution of positive and negative samples among male and female patients. A compilation of published data reveals that the rate of MCPyV DNA positive MCCs in men is 78% (n=130), which is similar to women (75%; n=83). However, the investigation of only a limited number of patients urges the caution interpretation of the results [Becker et al., 2009; Wetzels et al., 2009; Bhatai et al., 2010; Foulongne et al, 2008; Nakajima et al., 2009; Mertz et al., 2010 a; Sihto et al., 2009; Koljonen et al., 2009; Katano et al., 2009; Paulson et al., 2009; Varga et al., 2009; Wu et al., 2010; Woo et al., 2010]. Only Sihto and colleagues screened a relative large cohort (80 men and 34 women) and they found that 84% of their male MCC patients were positive for MCPyV DNA against 71% for the female MCC patients [Sihto et al., 2009]. A recent study by the same group on a Finnish cohort showed the opposite tendency [Sihto et al., 2011]. They found that the presence of LT-ag was associated with the female gender, but 70% (63/91) of their patients were female.

10. Mechanisms for MCPyV-induced MCC

10.1 Expression of truncated LT-ag

One of the criteria for a causal role of a virus in cancer is the requirement of expression of part of the viral genome to maintain the transformed state of the cell. This was originally proven by studies with Rous sarcoma virus carrying a temperature-sensitive mutation in the v-*src* gene and later confirmed for SV40 in a transgenic mouse model that allowed timely regulated doxycycline-dependent expression of LT-ag [Kawai & Hanafusa; 1971; Friis et al., 1980; Ewald et al., 1996]. At the non-permissive temperature, the mutant Rous sarcoma virus was unable to induce or maintain morphological transformation of chick embryo cells, while cell transformation appeared when cultures were shifted to a permissive temperature [Kawai & Hanafusa; 1971; Friis et al., 1980]. Turning on expression of SV40 LT-ag at birth, induced cellular transformation by 4 months of age. Silencing LT-ag for 3 weeks reversed the hyperplasia state. However, turning off LT-ag 7 months after birth did not abolish the hyperplasia, indicating that LT-ag was no longer required to maintain the transformed state [Ewald et al., 1996]. The observations that MCPyV positive MCC express LT-ag and that MCPyV positive MCC patients have much higher LT-ag seropositivity than non-MCC patients may indicate that the presence of this oncoprotein is involved in MCC [Shuda et al., 2009; Busam et al., 2009; Paulson et al., 2010; Houben et al, 2011; see Table 1]. This assumption is supported by results from knockdown studies in MCPyV positive MCC cell lines and a xeno-transplantation model, which illustrated that continuous expression of LT-ag and st-ag is required for cell proliferation and tumour progression [Houben et al., 2010; Houben et al., 2011].

Unexpectedly, MCPyV positive tumours express truncated LT-ag due to nonsense mutations or frame shift mutations generating premature stop codons (Figure 4; [Feng et al., 2008; Shuda et al., 2009; Duncavage et al., 2009a; Laude et al., 2010]). The mutation does not affect st-ag, but truncated LT-ag and 57kT become indistinguishable. The truncated LT-ag and 57kT proteins retain the DnaJ region and pRb-binding pocket, but lack the origin of replication- and the p53-binding domains, and the domains with helicase and ATPase activity. The fact that truncated LT-ag in MCC still can bind pRb and that loss of pRb is not a frequent occurrence in MCC suggests that inactivation of pRb through LT-ag binding is essential for MCPyV-mediated MCC tumorigenesis [Houben et al., 2009]. This prompted Houben and co-workers to examine the importance of LT-ag:pRb interaction in MCC. Specific knock down of LT-ag resulted in a marked growth inhibition and accumulation of MCPyC positive MCC cells in G1 phase of the cell cycle. The transformed phenotype was rescued by ectopic expression of LT-ag with an intact pRb motif, but not by LT-ag with a mutated pRb binding site [Houben et al., 2011]. These observations suggest that the LT-ag:pRb interaction is essential for tumour development.

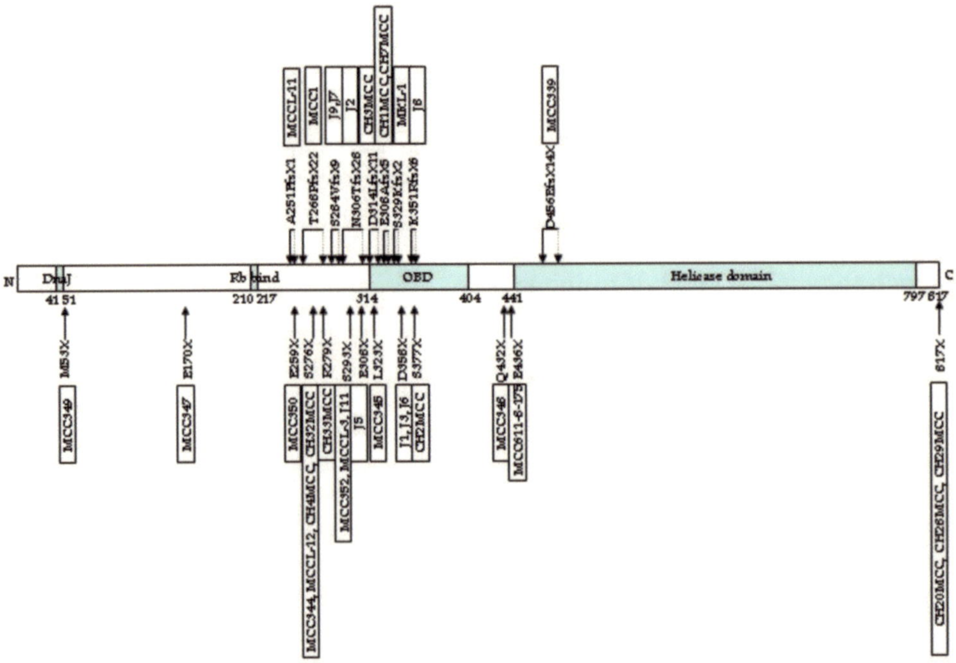

Fig. 4. Mutations causing truncation of LT-ag that have been reported in MCC [Feng et al., 2008; Fisher et al., 2010; Laude et al., 2010; Nakamura et al., 2010; Schrama et al., 2010 and MCC611-8-175 Genbank ACJ05659.1]. The arrows in the lower part of the figure represent the sites where nonsense mutations have occurred. The mutation of the amino acid into the corresponding nonsense codon (indicated by X) is given. The double arrows at the top part of the figure symbolize the site of the mutation that causes the frame shift (first arrow) and the introduction of a stop codon due to this frame shift (second arrow). The X followed by a number indicates how many codons downstream of the frameshift a stopcodon is introduced. The functional DnaJ, pRb binding, origin binding domain (ODB) and helicase domains are indicated and the numbers beneath the domains represent the amino acid residues of the beginning and the end of the respective domains. The name of the reported strain is encompassed in a rectangle.

Skin MCPyV isolates obtained from 14 different healthy subjects encoded full-length open reading frames for predicted viral proteins, including LT-ag [Schowalter et al., 2010]. Thus, in contrast to MCC, normal skin tissue seems to be infected with MCPyV encoding full-length LT-ag. Sequencing a full-length MCPyV genome from a Kaposi's sarcoma case revealed that the LT-ag gene would produce a truncated form of the protein [Katano et al.,

2009]. This example illustrates that expression of truncated LT-ag is not restricted to MCC, but can occur in other malignancies. Whether MCPyV infection is a risk for Kaposi's sarcoma remains elusive.

The truncated LT-ag mutant proteins identified in MCC are deprived of their DNA helicase activity and consequently unable to sustain viral DNA replication [Shuda et al., 2009]. This may prevent virus production and eventually lysis of the infected cells and is thus incompatible with expansion of the virus-infected cell [Houben et al., 2009]. Replication deficient MCPyV may persist in the host cell without causing destruction of the infected cell. The truncated LT-ag, however, retains its oncogenic potentials and this may lead to transformation of the infected cell. This finding is reminiscent with early observations that revealed that replication-deficient SV40 or SV40 encoding LT-ag defective in origin-binding displayed elevated transforming potentials compared to wild-type virus [reviewed in zur Hausen, 2008b]. Furthermore, studies with transgenic mice expressing SV40 LT-ag showed that a C-terminal truncated LT-ag variant that still can bind pRb, but lacks its helicase domain retains its transforming property [Rathi et al., 2009]. Hence, expression of a SV40 truncated LT-ag mutant with similar functions as MCPyV LT-ag variants described in MCC induced hyperplasia and eventually dysplasia. This observation suggests that a similar mechanism may be operational in MCPyV positive MCC.

10.2 Mutations in st-ag in MCC

So far, no mutations in st-ag expressed in MCC have been reporter. One normal skin isolate (9b) had a single base-pair insertion in the C-terminal part of st-ag causing a premature stop codon resulting in truncation of the last 15 amino acids, but the functional implication for this mutation has not been examined [Schowalter et al., 2010]. The corresponding residues in SV40 st-ag are not necessary for the interaction with PP2A, suggesting that this MCPyV st-ag mutant still can interact with PP2A [Mateer et al., 1998]. Interestingly, the transcript levels of st-ag, but not LT-ag or VP1 in the skin of a healthy woman containing episomal MCPyV DNA increased following solar UV-irradiation administration [Mogha et al., 2010]. Because the LT-ag and st-ag transcripts are generated from the same unspliced precursor, a post-transcriptional mechanism may be operational such as at the splicing level to generate different amounts of LT- and st-ag transcripts. Alternatively UV-light may activate pathways that control the decay of LT-ag and st-ag mRNA differently [Bollig et al., 2002].

10.3 Polymorphism in the non-coding control region (NCCR)

Previous studies with the human polyomaviruses BKPyV and JCPyV revealed that variation in the NCCR affects their transforming properties [Moens et al., 1995; Ricciardiello et al., 2001]. Thus, increased promoter activity of MCPyV variants may result in enhanced levels of the oncoproteins LT-ag, 57kT and st-ag or/and stimulate the expression of cellular genes in the vicinity of integrated viral genome. Mutations that increase the intrinsic activity of the MCPyV NCCR may affect the oncogenic potential of the virus and therefore be a hallmark for MCC-derived virus isolates. So far, the genomes of tumour-derived MCPyV and isolates from non MCC patients display little variation in their NCCR [Feng et al., 2008; Touzé et al., 2009; Kwun et al., 2009; Pastrana et al., 2009]. The tumour-derived MCPyV isolate MCC350 contains the 5 base-pair deletion GAGTT in its regulatory region compared to the MCC339 strain [Feng et al., 2008]. This deletion was also detected in MCPyV isolates from 5 out of 7 French MCC patients [Touzé et al., 2009], in the MCVw156 strain and the TKS MCPyV DNA isolated from a from Kaposi's sarcoma. The latter had a 25 base pair tandem repeat in its NCCR duplicating a motif that stimulates transcription and *in vitro* replication of SV40 and JCPyV [Martin et al., 1985; Katano et al., 2009]. However, an isolate (isolate 16b) obtained from skin swabs of a healthy person contained the same duplication, showing that this feature is not restricted to MCPyV present in malignant tissue [Schowalter et al., 2010]. So far, there is no indication that a specific NCCR is associated with MCPyV in MCC.

10.4 Integrational inactivation

Chromosomal integration is a characteristic of viruses causing cancer in humans [Matsuoka & Jeang, 2007; zur Hausen, 2009; Tsai & Chung, 2010]. Integration may cause disruption of genes, creating viral-cellular fusion proteins or altered expression of cellular proto-oncogenes or tumour suppressor genes. These events might be oncogenic. MCPyV genomes are clonally integrated into the DNA of the primary MCC tumour cells and their metastatic cells, suggesting that integration occurred before clonal expansion [Feng et al., 2008; Duncavage et al., 2009a]. The viral DNA seems to be integrated at different locations within the cellular genome in different MCC tumours and MCC cell lines examined [Feng et., 2008; Sastre-Garau et al., 2009; Laude et al., 2010]. The first report on MCPyV in MCC showed integration on chromosome 3p14.2, in intron 1 of the receptor tyrosine phosphatase type G (*PTPRG*) gene, a gene identified as a putative tumour suppressor gene [Feng et al., 2008]. Table 3 summarizes other identified integration sites. The functional implication in tumorigenesis is not known because no altered gene expression related to MCPyV insertion was monitored [Sastre-Garau et al., 2009]. The virus host junction can occur in VP1, NCCR, and in the 3' part of LT-ag [Feng et al., 2008; Sastre-Garau et al., 2009; Laude et al., 2010].

insertion	putative target gene	link to cancer	reference
2q32.3	not determined		Sastre-Garau et al., 2009
3p14.2	receptor tyrosine phosphatase type G	tumour suppressor	Feng et al., 2008
3q26.33	ATP1-1B		Sastre-Garau et al., 2009
4q13.1	SRD5A2L2		Sastre-Garau et al., 2009
5q35.1	TLX3		Sastre-Garau et al., 2009
6q23.3	IL20RA	lung carcinogenesis	Sastre-Garau et al., 2009
6p24	GDP-mannose 4,6 dehydratase	fucosylation in colon cancer	Laude et al., 2010
8q24.21	MYC	Proto-oncogene	Sastre-Garau et al., 2009
9q33	DENN/MADD domain containing 1A isoform 1		Laude et al., 2010
11p15	Parvin-α,	adhesion and motility	Laude et al., 2010
11p15	TEF-1/TEAD1		Laude et al., 2010
12q23.1	AX747640		Sastre-Garau et al., 2009
15q14	ATP binding domain 4 isoform 2		Laude et al., 2010
20q11.21	SNTA1		Sastre-Garau et al., 2009
Yq12	not determined		Sastre-Garau et al., 2009

Table 3. Chromosomal integration sites of MCPyV.

Several groups reported that MCPyV DNA is not exclusively integrated in MCC, but may also exist episomal. Wetzels and her colleagues could demonstrate the presence of viral particles in one of their MCC samples by electron microscopy, suggesting non-integrated viral DNA. Wetzels did not examine whether integrated viral DNA was present in the MCC sample that contains virus particles [Wetzels et al., 2009]. Sastre-Garau and co-workers characterized one MCC case where the tumour cells contained both integrated and episomal MCPyV DNA [Sastre-Garau et al., 2009]. Laude and co-workers also found MCC containing MCPyV encoding full-length LT-ag. They reported the coexistence of integrated concatemers or latent episomes of MCPyV genome and truncated integrated viral sequences in five MCC cases [Laude et al., 2010]. The presence of virions indicates active viral replication and therefore a LT-ag that can sustain viral DNA replication, i.e. LT-ag that possesses helicase activity. Because integration and truncated LT-ag expression are hallmarks of MCPyV-positive MCC, it is possible that in MCC containing only episomal viral DNA, that the virus was merely a fortuitous co-inhabitant of the tumour cells.

10.5 MyCPyV and cellular miRNA expression

Viral infections can cause altered expression patterns of miRNA in the host cell because viral-encoded miRNA or/and viral proteins can target cellular miRNA/targetome pathways, thereby contributing to the oncogenic properties of viruses [Skalsky & Cullen, 2010; Lin & Flemington, 2011]. MiRNA are generated by RNA polymerase II and HPyV LT-ag and st-ag have been shown to affect the expression of many genes, including RNA polymerase II transcribed genes [Moens et al., 1997; Klein et al., 2005; Deeb et al., 2007]. It is not known whether MCPyV infection or expression of its LT-ag or/and st-ag results in altered expression of cellular miRNA, but SV40 st-ag enhances expression of miR-27a in a PP2A-dependent manner and contributes to the malignant transformation of human bronchial epithelial cells. The transcript encoding the cell-cycle progression protein Fbxw7 was a target for miR-27a. Thus, promotion of cell growth through the suppression of Fbxw7 by st-ag-induced miR-27a overexpression may play a role in malignant transformation [Wang et al., 2011]. Profiling miRNA in MCPyV positive and negative MCC may indicate whether altered cellular miRNA expression is a co-mechanism in MCC pathogenesis.

11. Therapy

Currently, there is no specific treatment for MCC. Local excision of the tumour combined with radiation therapy and chemotherapy is the most common protocol [Tai, 2008; Ramahi et al., 2011]. Because of the high association rate of MCPyV with MCC, antiviral-specific therapy may form an attractive therapy for MCC. Although a few clinical trials with MCC were started or are in progress [ClinicalTrials.gov], none of them are specifically aimed at targeting MCPyV. Vaccination is an encouraging possibility in light of the success with the oncoviruses such as hepatitis B virus and high-risk human papillomaviruses. To begin to explore the idea of a MCPyV vaccine, Pastrana and her collaborators immunized mice with virus-like particles (VLP) composed of MCPyV VP1 and VP2. All vaccinated animals generated strong neutralizing antibodies. In fact the titres were comparable to the titres of animals challenged with human papillomavirus VLP and higher than animals injected with JCPyV VLP. Thus, MCPyV VLP appears to be a strong immunogen and thus a promising vaccine candidate [Pastrana et al., 2009]. One case report describes that subcutaneous administration of 3,000,000 IU of interferon-β (IFN-β) per day to a Japanese 62-year-old woman with MCPyV positive MCC resulted into a beneficial response after 3 weeks with complete remission that continued for more than 8 years [Nakajima et al., 2009]. IFN-α could induce apoptosis of MCC-1 cell lines *in vitro*, but its effect on patients was not tested [Krasagakis et al., 2008]. These results suggest that interferons may be useful in MCC therapy. Other feasible approaches are disruptor molecules, antiviral drugs and RNA interference. Continuous expression of LT-ag with an intact pRb binding site is required to maintain the transformed phenotype of MCC. Molecules disrupting pRb:LT-ag interactions may possess low off-target effects and therefore be an attractive strategy for future MCC therapy [Houben et al., 2011]. Similarly, disruptors of the Dna J domain may be applied. Antiviral drugs that interfere with the different stages of the life cycle of MCPyV may prevent virus spread after primary infection, but no such drugs are currently available and it is very unrealistic to establish the time point of primary infection in individuals. SiRNA-mediated knock down of MCPyV LT-ag expression may be another therapeutic approach. Eliminating LT-ag expression in MCCs may therefore be sufficient to reverse the malignant cell to a more benign cell or trigger cell death as demonstrated in MCC cell lines [Houben et al., 2010]. It was shown that JCPyV- and BKPyV-encoded miRNA target ULBP3, a ligand for the natural killer cell receptor NKG2D, thereby protecting BKPyV/JCPyV infected cells from destruction [Bauman et al., 2011]. It is not known whether MCPyV miRNA exerts the same function, but if so, anti-miRNA against the MCPyV-encoded miRNA will maintain the ULBP3 expression levels in viral infected cells and will stimulate their elimination by natural killer cells.

12. Conclusions and future perspectives

Several findings underscore a causal role for MCPyV in MCC. The viral genome load and prevalence of MCPyV DNA are significantly higher in MCC than in other MCPyV infected tissues, in contrast to non-MCC tissue, the viral genome in MCC is integration and expresses truncated LT-ag that cannot sustain viral replication, but still interacts with pRb. In accordance with other tumour viruses, there seems to be a very long incubation time between viral infection and development of the tumour because primary infection can occur in early childhood, but MCC is extremely unusual before the age of 50. These observations suggest that additional events (e.g. skin exposure to UV-light, gender, perturbation of the immune system, co-infection other viruses, ethnicity, mutations in cellular genome) are required for MCC-induced malignancy. The absence of MCPyV in about 20% of MCC indicates the existence of MCPyV-independent pathogenic pathways in this malignancy. This is supported by the finding that MCPyV seems to be associated with classic, but not variant MCC cell lines and that MCC display chromosomal abnormalities with loss of heterozygocity of chromosome 1p being the most common [Shuda et al., 2008; Leonard et al., 2000]. Alternatively, MCPyV may initiate neoplastic events, but the continuous presence of the virus is not required explaining why no traces of the virus can be detected in some of the MCC ('hit-and-run' hypothesis). The fact that MCPyV DNA is detected in many different tissues both in healthy individuals and in different patient groups raises the question whether MCPyV may be involved in other malignancies or diseases. The connection of MCPyV DNA in other tissues is not as strong as MCPyV and MCC and the state of the viral genome (episomal or integrated) and the mutational analysis of LT-ag have not been meticulously examined [reviewed in Moens et al., 2010]. World-wide studies are warranted to determine the possible association of MCPyV with other malignant and non-malignant diseases. Other important information that should be acquired includes determining the integration sites and the consequences on viral and cellular gene expression, and does miRNA expression pattern in MCPyV positive versus MCPyV negative MCC differ and if so, are these differences provoked by the virus and are they contributing to MCC pathogenesis? Besides these cancer-related issues, other fundamental issues such as route of infection, cell tropism and transmission need to be studied.

13. References

Abend, J.R.; Jiang, M. & Imperiale, M.J. (2009). BK virus and human cancer: innocent until proven guilty. *Seminars in Cancer Biology*, Vol. 19, No. 4 (August 2004), pp. 252-260, ISSN 1044-579X

Albores-Saavedra, J.; Batich, K.; Chable-Montero, F.; Sagy, N.; Schwartz, A.M. & Henson, D.E. (2009). Merkel cell carcinoma demographies, morphology, and survival based on 3870 cases: a population based study. *Journal of Cutaneous Pathology*, Vol. 37, No. 1 (January 2009), pp. 20-27, ISSN 0303-6987

Allander, T.; Andreasson, K.; Gupta, S.; Bjerkner, A.; Bogdanovic, G.; Persson, M.A.; Dalianis, T., Ramqvist, T. & Andersson, B. (2007). Identification of a third human polyomavirus. *Journal of Virology*, Vol. 81, No. 8, (April 2007), pp. 4130-4136 ISSN 0022-538X

Andres, C.; Belloni, B.; Puchta, U.; Sander, C.A. & Flaig, M.J. (2010). Prevalence of MCPyV in Merkel cell carcinoma and non-MCC tumors. *Journal of Cutaneous Pathology*, Vol. 37, No. 1, (January 2010), pp. 28-34, ISSN 0303-6987

Andres, C.; Belloni, B. & Flaig, M.J. (2011). Value of Merkel cell Polyomavirus DNA Detection in Routine Pathology. *American journal of dermatopathology*, Vol. 33, No. 3 (May 2011), pp. 329-330, ISSN 0193-1091

Asioli, S.; Righi, A.; Volante, M.; Eusebi, V. & Bussolati, G. (2007). P63 expression as a new prognostic marker in Merkel cell carcinoma. *Cancer*, Vol. 110, No.3 (Augustus 2007), pp. 640.647, ISSN 1097-0142

Babakir-Mina, M.; Ciccozzi, M.; Lo Presti, A.; Greco, F.; Perno, C.F. & Ciotti, M. (2010). Identification of Merkel cell polyomavirus in the lower respiratory tract of Italian patients. *Journal of Medical Virology*, Vol. 82, No. 3 (March 2010), pp. 505-509, ISSN 1096-9071

Barzon, L.; Squarzon, L.; Militello, V.; Trevisan, M.; Porzionato, A.; Macchi, V.; De Caro, R. & Palù, G. (2009). WU and KI polyomaviruses in the brains of HIV-positive patients with and without progressive multifocal leukoencephalopathy. *Journal of Infectious Diseases*, Vol. 200, No. 11 (December 2009), pp. 1755-1758, ISSN 0022-1899

Bauman, Y.; Nachmani, D.; Vitenshstein, A.; Tsukerman, P.; Drayman, N.; Stern-Ginossar, N.; Lankry, D.; Gruda, R. & Mandelboim, O. (2011). An identical miRNA of the human JC and BK polyomaviruses targets the stress-induced lignad ULBP3 to escape immune elimination. *Cell Host Microbe*, Vol. 9, No. 2 (February 2011), pp. 93-102, ISSN 1931-3128

Becker, J.C.; Schrama, D. & Houben, R. (2009). Merkel cell carcinoma. *Cellular and Molecular Life Sciences*, Vol. 66, No. 1 (January 2009), pp. 1-8, ISSN 1420-682X

Bhatia, K.; Goedert, J.J.; Modali, R.; Preiss, L. & Ayers, L.W. (2010). Immunological detection of viral large T antigen identifies a subset of Merkel cell carcinoma tumors with higher viral abundance and better clinical outcome. *International Journal of Cancer*, Vol. 127, No. 6 (September 2010), pp. 1493-1496, ISSN 1097-0215

Bialasiewicz, S.; Lambert, S.B.; Whiley, D.M.; Nissen, M.D. & Sloots, T.P. (2009). Merkel cell polyomvirus DNA in respiratory speciments from children and adults. *Emerging Infectious Diseases*, Vol. 15, No. 3 (March 2009), pp. 492-494, ISSN 1080-6059

Bofill-Mas, S.; Rodriguez-Manzano, J.; Calgua, B.; Carratala, A. & Girones, R. (2010). Newly descrive human polyomaviruses Merkel cell, KI and WU are present in urban sewage and may represent potential enviromental contaminants. *Virology Journal*, Vol.7(June 2010), pp. 141-146, ISSN 1743-422X

Bollig, F.; Winzen, R; Kracht, M.; Ghebremedhin, B.; Ritter, B.; Wilhelm, A.; Resch, K. & Holtmann, H. (2002). Evidence for general stabilization of mRNAs in response to UV light. *European Journal of Biochemistry*, Vol. 269, No. 3 (December 2002), pp. 5830-5839, ISSN 0014-2956

Boulais, N. & Misery, L. (2007). Merkel cells. *Journal of the American Academy of Dermatology*, 57, No. 1 (July 2007), pp. 147-165, ISSN 0190-9622

Busam, K.J.; Jungbluth, A.A.; Rekthman, N.; Coit, D.; Pulitzer, M.; Bini, J.; Arora, R.; Hanson, N.C.; Tassello, J.A.; Frosina, D.; Moore, P. & Chang, Y. (2009). Merkel cell polyomavirus expression in Merkel cell carcinomas and its absence in combined tumors and pulmonary neuroendocrine carcinomas. *The American Journal of Surgical Pathology*, Vol. 33, No. 9 (September 2009), pp. 1378-1385, ISSN 01475185

Calder, K.B. & Smoller, B.R. (2010). New insights into Merkel cell carcinoma. *Advances in Anatomic Pathology*, Vol. 17, No. 3 (May 2010), pp. 155-161, ISSN 1072-4109

Campello, C.; Comar, M.; D'Agaro, P.; Minicozzi, A.; Rodella, L. & Poli, A. (2011). A molecular case-control study of the Merkel cell polyomavirus in colon cancer. *Journal of Medical Virology*, Vol. 83, No. 4 (April 2011), pp. 721-724, ISSN 1096-9071

Carter, J.J.; Paulson, K.G.; Wipf, G.C.; Miranda, D.; Madeleine, M.M.; Johnson, L.G.; Lemos, B.D.; Lee, S.; Warcola, A.H.; Iyer, J.G.; Nghiem, P. & Galloway, D.A. (2009) Association of Merkel Cell polyomavirus-specific antibodies with Merkel cell carcinoma. *Journal of the National Cancer Institute*, Vol. 1001, No. 21 (November 2009), pp.1510-1522 ISSN 0027-8874

Carswell, S. & Alwine, J.C. (1986). Simian virus 40 facilitates perinuclear-nuclear localization of VP1, the major capsid protein. *Journal of Virology*, Vol. 204, No. 1 (July 1986), pp. 1055-1061, ISSN 0022-538X

Chen, T.; Hedman, L.; Mattila, P.S.; Jartti, T.; Ruuskanenc O.; Söderlund-Venermoa, M. & Hedman K. (2011). Serological evidence of Merkel cell polyomavirus primary infections in childhood. *Journal of Clinical Virology*, Vol. 50 No. 2 (February 2011), pp. 125–129, ISSN 1386-6532

ClinicalTrials.gov

Daniels, R.; Sadowicz, D. & Hebert, D.N. (2007). A very late viral protein triggers the release of SV40. *PloS Pathogens*, Vol. 3, No. 7 (July 2007), pp. e98, ISSN 1553-7366

Darbinyan, A.; Darbinian, N.; Safak, M.; Radhakrishnan, S.; Giordano, A. & Khalili, A. (2002). Evidence for dysregulation of cell cycle by human polyomavirus, JCV, late auxiliary protein. *Oncogene*, Vol. 21, No. 36 (Augustus 2002), pp. 5574-5581, ISSN 0950-9232

Darbinyam, A.; Siddiqui, K.M.; Slonina, D.; Darbinian, N.; Amini, S.; White, M.K. & Khalili, K. (2004). Role of JC virus agnoprotein in DNA repair. *Journal of Virology*, Vol. 78, No. 16 (Augustus 2004), pp. 8593-8600, ISSN 0022-538X

DeCaprio, J.A. (2009). Does detection of Merkel cell polyomavirus in Merkel cell carcinoma provide prognostic information? *Journal of the National Cancer Institute*, Vol. 101, No. 13 (July 2009), pp. 905-907, ISSN 0027-8874

Deeb, K.K.; Michalowska, A.M.; Yoon, C.Y.; Krummey, S.M.; Hoenerhoff, M.J.; Kavanaugh, C.; Li, M.C.; Demayo, F.J.; Linnoila, I.; Deng, C.X.; Lee, E.Y.H.P.; Medina, D.; Shih, J.H. & Green, J.E. (2007). Identification of an integrated SV40 T7t-antigen cancer signature in aggressive human breast, prostate, and lung carcinomas with poor prognosis. *Cancer Research*, Vol. 67, No. 17 (September 2007), pp. 8065-8080, ISSN 1538-7445

Duncavage, E.J.; Le, B.M.; Wang, D. & Pfeifer, J.D. (2009a). Merkel cell polyomavirus: a specific marker for merkel cell carcinoma in histologically similar tumors. *American Journal of Surgical Pathohology*, Vol. 33, No. 12 (December 2009), pp. 1771-1777, ISSN 01475185

Duncavage, E.J.; Zehnbauer, B.A. & Pfeifer, J.D. (2009b). Prevalence of Merkel cell polyomavirus in Merkel cell carcinoma. *Modern Pathology*, Vol.22, No. 4, (April 2009), pp.516-521, ISSN 0893-3952

Dworkin, A.M.; Tseng, S.Y.; Allain, D.C.; Iwenofu, O.H.; Peters, S.B. & Toland, A.E. (2009). Merkel cell polyomavirus in cutaneous squamous cell carcinoma of immunocompetent individuals. *Journal of Investigative Dermatology*, Vol. 129, No. 12 (December 2009), pp. 2868-2874, ISSN 0022-202X

Ewald, D.; Li, M.; Efrat, S.; Auer, G.; Wall, R.J.; Furth, P.A. & Hennighausen L. (1996). Time-Sensitive Reversal of Hyperplasia in Transgenic Mice Expressing SV40 T Antigen. *Science*, Vol. 273, No. 5280 (September 1996), pp. 1384-1386, ISSN 0036-8075

Engels, E.A.; Biggar, R.J.; Hall, H.I.; Cross, H.; Crutchfield, A.; Finch, J.L.; Grigg, R.; Hylton, T.; Pawlish, K.S.; McNeel, T.S. & Goedert, J.J. (2008). Cancer risk in people infected with human immunodeficiency virus in the United States. *International Journal of Cancer*, Vol. 123, No. 1 (July 2008), pp. 187-194, ISSN 1097-0215

Erickson, K.D.; Garcea, R.L. & Tsai, B. (2009). Ganglioside GT1b is a putative host cell receptor for the Merkel cell polyomavirus. *Journal of Virology*, Vol. 83, No. 19 (October 2009), pp. 10275-10279, ISSN 0022-538X

Faust, H.; Pastrana, D.V.; Buck, C.B.; Dillner, J. & Ekström, J. (2011). Antibodies to Merkel cell polyomavirus correlate to presence of viral DNA in the skin. *Journal of Infectious Diseases*, Vol. 203, No. 8 (April 2011), pp. 1096-1100, ISSN 0022-1899

Feinmesser, M.; Halpern, M.; Fenig, E.; Tsabari, C.; Hodak, E.; Sulkes, J.; Brenner, B. & Okon, E. (1999). Expression of the apoptosis-related oncogenes bcl-2, bax, and p53 in Merkel cell carcinoma. Can they predict treatment response and clinical outcome? *Human Pathology*, Vol. 30, No. 11 (November 1999), pp. 1367-1372, ISSN 0046-8177

Feng, H.; Shuda, M.; Chang, Y. & Moore, P.S. (2008). Clonal integration of a polyomavirus in human Merkel cell carcinoma. *Science*, Vol. 319, No. 5866 (February 2008), pp. 1096-1100, ISSN 0036-8075

Fischer, N.; Brandner, J.; Fuchs, F.; Moll, I. & Grundhoff, A. (2010) Detection of Merkel cell polyomavirus (MCPyV) in Merkel cell carcinoma cell lines: cell morphology and growth phenotype do not reflect presence of the virus. *International Journal of Cancer*, Vol. 126, No. 9 (May 2010), pp. 2133–2142, ISSN 1097-0215

Foulongne, V.; Kluger, N.; Dereure, O.; Brieu, N.; Guillot, B. & Segondy, M. (2008). Merkel cell polyomavirus and Merkel cell carcinoma, France. *Emerging Infectious Diseases*. Vol. 14, No. 9 (September 2008), pp. 1491-1493, ISSN 1080-6059

Foulongne, V. ; Kluger, N. ; Dereure, O. ; Mercier, G. ; Molès, J.P. ; Guillot, B. & Segondy, M. (2010a). Merkel cell polyomavirus in cutaneous swabs. *Emerging Infectious Diseases*, Vol. 16, No. 4 (April 2010), pp. 685-687, ISSN 1080-6059

Foulongne, V.; Dereure, O.; Kluger, N.; Molès, J.P.; Guillot, B. & Segondy, M. (2010b). Merkeld cell polyomavirus DNA detection in lesional and nonlesional skin from patients with Merkel cell carcinoma or other skin diseases. *British Journal of Dermatology*, Vol. 162, No. 1 (January 2010), pp. 59-63, ISSN 0007-0963

Friis, R.R.; Jockusch, B.M.; Boschek, C.B.; Ziemiecki, A.; Rübsamen, H. & Bauer, H. (1980). Transformation-defective, temperature-sensitive mutants of Rous sarcoma virus have areversibly defective src-gene product. *Cold Spring Harbor Symposia on Quantitative Biology*, Vol. 44, No. 2, pp. 1007-1012, ISSN 0091-7451

Gardner, S.D.; Field, A.M.; Coleman, D.V. & Hulme, B. (1971). New human papovavirus (B.K.) isolated from urine after renal transplantation. *Lancet* Vol.1, No. 7712, (June 1971), pp. 1253-1257, ISSN 0140-6736

Garneski, K.M.; Warcola, A.H.; Feng, Q.; Kiviat, N.B.; Leonard, J.H. & Nghiem, P. (2009). Merkel cell polyomavirus is more frequently present in North American than Australian Merkel cell carcinoma tumors. *Journal of Investigative Dermatology*, Vol. 129 No. 1 (January 2009), pp. 246-248, ISSN 0022-202X

Gaynor, A.M.; Nissen, M.D.; Whiley D.M.; Mackay, I.M.; Lambert S.B.; Wu, G.; Brennan, D.C.; Storch, G.A.; Sloots, T.P. & Wang, D. (2007). Identification of a novel polyomavirus from patients with acute respiratory tract infections. *PLoS Pathogens*, Vol. 3, No. 5 (May 2007), pp. e64, ISSN 1553-7366

Giraud, G.; Ramqvist, T.; Ragnarsson-Olding, B. & Dalianis, T. (2008). DNA from BK virus and JC virus and from KI, WU, and MC polyomaviruses as well as from SV40 is not detected in non-UV-light associated primary malignant melanomas of mucous membranes. *Journal of Clinical Microbiology*, Vol. 46, No. 11 (November 2008), pp. 3595-3598, ISSN 0095-1137

Giraud, G.; Ramqvist, T.; Pastrana, D.V.; Pavot, V.; Lindau, C.; Kogner, P.; Orrego, A.; Buck, C.B.; Allander, T.; Holm, S.; Gustavsson, B. & Dalianis, T. (2009). DNA from KI, WU and Merkel cell polyomaviruses is not detected in childhood central nervous system tumours or neuroblastomas. *PLoS One*, Vol. 4, No. 12 (December 2009), pp. e8239; ISSN 1932-6203.

Gjoerup, O. & Chang, Y. (2010). Update on human polyomaviruses and cancer. *Advances in Cancer Research*, Vol. 106, No. pp. 1-51, ISSN 0065-230X

Goh, S.; Lindau, C.; Tiveljung-Lindell, A. & Allander, T. (2009). Merkel cell polyomavirus in respiratory tract secretions. *Emerging Infectious Diseases*, Vol. 15, No. 3 (March 2009), pp. 489-491, ISSN 1080-6059

Gould, V.E.; Moll, R.; Moll, I.; Lee, I. & Franke, W.W. (1985). Neuroendocrine (Merkel) cells of the skin: hyperplasias, dysplasias, and neoplasms. *Laboratory Investigation*, Vol. 52, No. 4 (April 1985), pp. 334-353, ISSN 0023-6837

Handschel, J.; Müller, D.; Depprich, R.A.; Ommerborn, M.A.; Kübler, N.R.; Naujoks, C.; Reifenberger, J.; Schäfer, K.L. & Braunstein, S. (2010). The new polyomavirus (MCPyV) does not affect the clinical course in MCCs. *International Journal of Oral and Maxillofacial Surgery*, Vol. 39, No. 11, (November 2010), pp. 1086-1090, ISSN 0901-5027

Helmbold, P.; Lahtz, C.; Enk, A.; Herrmann-Trost, P.; Marsch W.C.; Kutzner, H. & Dammann, R.H. (2009). Frequent occurrence of RASSF1A promoter hypermethylation and Merkel cell polyomavirus in Merkel cell carcinoma. *Molecular Carcinogenesis*, Vol. 48, No. 10 (October 2009), pp. 903-909, ISSN 1098-2744

Heymann, W.R. (2008). Merkel cell carcinoma: insights into pathogenesis. *Journal of the American Academy of Dermatology*, Vol. 59, No. 3 (September 2008), pp. 503-504, ISSN 0190-9622

Hodgson, N.C. (2005). Merkel cell carcinoma: changing incidence trends. *Journal of Surgical Oncology*, Vol. 89, No. 1 (January 2005), pp. 1-4, ISSN 1591-1063

Houben, R.; Schrama, D. & Becker, J.C. 2009. Molecular pathogenesis of Merkel cell carcinoma. *Experimental Dermatology*, Vol. 18, No.3 (March 2009), pp. 193-198, ISSN 0906-6705

Houben, R.; Shuda, M.; Weinkam, R.; Schrama, D.; Feng, H.; Chang, Y.; Moore, P.S. & Becker, J.C. (2010). Merkel cell polyomavirus-infected Merkel cell carcinoma cells require expression of viral T antigens. *Journal of Virology*, Vol. 84, No. 14 (July 2010), pp. 7064-7072, ISSN 0022-538X

Houben, R.; Adam, C.; Baeurle, A.; Hesbacher, S.; Grimm, J.; Angermeyer, S.; Henzel, K.; Hauser, S.; Elling, R.; Bröcker, E.B.; Gaubatz, S.; Becker, J.C. & Schrama, D. (2011). An intact retinoblastoma protein binding site in Merkel cell polyomavirus large T antigen is required for promoting growth of Merkel cell carcinoma cells. *International Journal of Cancer*, March 16 [Epub ahead of print].

Husseiny, M.I.; Anastasi, B.; Singer, J. & Lacey, S.F. (2010). A comparative study of Merkel cell, BK and JC polyomavirus infections in renal transplant recipients and healthy subjects. *Journal of Clinical Virology*, Vol. 49, No. 2 (October 2010), pp. 137-140, ISSN 1386-6532

Imperiale, M.J. & Major EO. (2007). Polyomaviridae, In: *Fields Virology*, 5th edition; Knipe, D.M., Howley, P.M., Griffin, D.E., Lamb, R.A., Martin, M.A., Roizman, B., & Straus, S.E., pp. 2263-2298, Lippincott Williams and Wilkins, ISBN 10:02-7817-6060-7, Philadelphia.

Jiang, M.; Abend, J.R.; Johnson, S.F. and Imperiale, M.J. 2009. The role of polyomaviruses in human diseases. *Virology*, Vol. 384, No. 2, (February 2009), pp. 266-273 ISSN 0042-6822

Johannessen, M.; Myhre, M.R.; Dragset, M.; Tümmler, C. & Moens, U. (2008). Phosphorylation of human polyomavirus BK agnoprotein at Ser-11 is mediated by PKC and has an important regulative function. *Virology*, Vol. 379, No. 1 (September 2008), pp. 97-109, ISSN 0042-6822

Johne, R.; Buck, C.B.; Allander, T.; Atwood, W.J.; Garcea, R.L.; Imperiale, M.J.; Major, E.O.; Ramqvist, T. & Norkin, L.C. (2011). Taxonomical developments in the family Polyomaviridae. *Archives of Virology*, 12 May [Epub ahead of print], DOI 10.1007/s00705-011-1008-x, ISSN 0304-8608

Kaae, J.; Hansen, A.V.; Biggar, R.J.; Boyd, H.A.; Moore, P.S.; Wohlfart, J. & Melbye, M. (2010). Merkel cell carcinoma: incidence, mortality, and risk of other cancers. *Journal of the National Institute of Cancer*, Vol. 102, No. 11 (June 2010), pp. 793-801, ISSN 0027-8874

Kantola, K.; Sadeghi, M.; Lahtinen, A.; Koskenvuo, M.; Aaltonen, L.M.; Möttönen, M.; Rahiala, J.; Saarinen-Pihkala, U.; Riikonen, P.; Jartti, T.; Ruuskanen, O.; Söderlund-Venermo, M. & Hedman. K. (2009). Merkel cell polyomavirus DNA in tumor-free tonsillar tissues and upper respiratory tract samples: implications for respiratory transmission and latency. *Journal of Clinical Virology*, Vol. 45, No. 4 (August 2009), pp. 292-295, ISSN 1386-6532

Kassem, A.; Schöpflin, A.; Diaz, C.; Weyers, W.; Stickeler, E.; Werner, M. & Zur Hausen, A. (2008).Frequent detection of Merkel cell polyomavirus in human Merkel cell carcinomas and identification of a unique deletion in the VP1 gene. *Cancer Research*. Vol. 68, No. 13 (July 2008), pp. 5009-5013, ISSN 0008-5472

Katano, H.; Ito, H.; Suzuki, Y.; Nakamura, T.; Sato, Y.; Tsuji, T.; Matsuo, K.; Nakagawa, H. & Sata, T. (2009). Detection of Merkel cell polyomavirus in Merkel cell carcinoma and Kaposi's sarcoma. *Journal of Medical Virology*, Vol. 81, No. 11, pp. 1951-1958, ISSN 1096-9071

Kawai, S. & Hanafusa, H. (1971). The effects of reciprocal changes in temperature on the transformed state of cells infected with a rous sarcoma virus mutant. *Virology*, Vol. 46, No. 2 (November 1971), pp. 470-479, ISSN 0042-6822

Kean, J.M.; Rao, S.; Wang, M. & Garcea, R.L. (2009). Seroepidemiology of human polyomaviruses. *PLoS Pathogens*, Vol. 5, No. 3, pp. e1000363, ISSN 1553-7366

Kennedy, M.M.; Blessing, K.; King, G. & Kerr, K.M. (1996). Expression of bcl-2 and p53 in Merkel cell carcinoma. An immunohistochemical study. *American Journal of Dermatopathology*, Vol. 18, No. 3 (June 1996) pp. 273-277, ISSN 0193-1091

Khalili K, White, M.K.; Sawa, H.; Nagashima, K. & Safak, M. 2005. The agnoprotein of polyomaviruses: a multifunctional auxiliary protein. *Journal of Cellular Physiology*, Vol. 204, No. 1 (July 2005), pp. 1-7, ISSN 00219541

Kim, J. & McNiff, J.M. (2008). Nuclear expression of surviving portends a poor prognosis in Merkel cell carcinoma. *Modern Pathology*, Vol. 21, No. 6 (June 2008), pp. 764-769, ISSN 0893-3952

Klein, A.; Guhl, E.; Zollinger, R.; Tzeng, Y.J.; Wessel, R.; Hummel, M.; Graesmann, M. & Graesmann, A. (2005). Gene expression profiling: cell cycle deregulation and aneuploidy do not cause breast cancer formation in WAP-SVT/t transgenic animals. *Journal of Molecular Medicine*, Vol. 83, No. 5 (May 2005), pp. 362-376, ISSN 0946-2716

Knowles, W.A. (2006). Discovery and epidemiology of the human polyomaviruses BK virus (BKV) and JC virus (JCV). *Advances in Experimental Medicine and Biology*, Vol. 577, pp. 19-45, ISSN 0065-2598

Koljonen, V.; Kukko, H.; Pukkala, E.; Sankila, R.; Böhling, T.; Tukiainen, E.; Sihto, H. & Joensuu, H. (2009). Chronic lymphocytic leukaemia patients have a high risk of Merkel-cell polyomavirus DNA-positive Merkel-cell carcinoma. *British Journal of Cancer*, Vol. 101, No.8 (September 2010), pp. 1444-1447, ISSN 0007-0920

Krasagakis, K.; Kruger-Krasagakis, S.; Tzanakakis, G.N.; Darivianaki, K.; Stathopoulus, E.N. & Tosca, A.D. (2008). Interferon-alpha inhibits proliferation and induces apoptosis of Merkel cell carcinoma in vitro. *Cancer Investigation*, Vol. 26, No. 6 (July 2008), pp.562-568, ISSN 0735-7907

Kuwamoto, S.; Higaki, H.; Kanai, K.; Iwasaki, T.; Sano, H.; Nagata, K.; Kato, K.; Kato, M.; Murakami, I.; Horie, Y.; Yamamoto, O. & Hayashi, K. (2011). Association of Merkel cell polyomavirus infection with morphologic differences in Merkel cell carcinoma. *Human Pathology*, Vol. 42, No. 5, (May 2011), pp. 632-640, ISSN 0046-8177

Kwun, H.J.; Guastafierro, A.; Shuda, M.; Meinke, G.; Bohm, A.; Moore, P.S. & Chang, Y. (2009). The minimum replication origin of Merkel cell polyomavirus has a unique large T-antigen loading architecture and requires small t-antigen expression for optimal replication. *Journal of Virology*, Vol. 83, No. 23 (September 2009), pp. 12118-12128 ISSN 0022-538X

Lacour, J.P.; Dubois, D.; Pisani, A. & Ortonne, J.P. (1991). Anatomical mapping of Merkel cells in normal adult epidermis. *British Journal of Dermatology*, Vol. 156, No. 6 (December 1991), pp. 535-542, ISSN 1365-2133

Lassacher, A.; Heitzer, E.; Kerl, H. & Wolf, P. (2008). p14ARF Hypermethylation is common but INK4a-ARF locus or p53 mutations are rare in Merkel cell carcinoma. *Journal of Investigative Dermatology*, Vol. 128, No. 7 (July 2008), pp. 1788-1796, ISSN 0022-202X

Laude, H.C.; Jonchère, B.; Maubec, E.; Carlotti, A.; Marinho, E.; Couturaud, B.; Peter, M.; Sastre-Garau, X.; Avril, M.F.; Dupin, N. & Rozenberg, F. (2010). Distinct Merkel cell polyomavirus molecular features in tumour and non tumour specimens from patients with Merkel cell carcinoma. *PLoS Pathogens*, Vol. 6, No. 8 (Augustus 2010), pp. e10001076, ISSN 1553-7366

Lemos, B. & Nghiem, P. (2007). Merkel cell carcinoma: more deaths but still no pathway to blame. *Journal of Investigative Dermatology*, Vol. 127, No. 9 (September 2007), pp. 2100-2103, ISSN 0022-202X

Leonard, J.H.; Dash, P.; Holland, P.; Kearsley, J.H. & Bell J.R. (1995). Characterisation of four merkel cell carcinoma adherent cell lines. *International Journal of Cancer*, Vol. 60, No. 1 (January 1995), pp. 100-107, ISSN 1097-0215

Leonard, J.H.; Cook, A.L.; Nancarrow, D.; Hayward, N.; Van Gele, M.; Van Roy, N. & Speleman, F. (2000). *Cancer detection and Prevention*, Vol. 24, No. 6 (December 2000), pp. 620-627, ISSN 0361-090X

Lewis, J.S.Jr.; Duncavage, E. & Klonowski, P.W. (2010). Oral cavity neuroendocrine carcinoma: a comparison study with cutaneous Merkel cell carcinoma and other mucosal head and neck neuroendocrine carcinomas. *Oral Surgery, Oral Medicine, Oral Pathology, Oral Radiology & Endodontics*, Vol. 110, No. 2, (August 2010), pp. 209-217, ISSN 1079-2104

Lin, Z. & Flemington, E.K. (2011). miRNAs in the pathogenesis of oncogenic human viruses. *Cancer Letters*, Vol. 305, No. 2 (June 2011), pp. 186-199, ISSN 0304-3835

Loyo, M.; Guerrero-Preston, R.; Brait, M.; Hoque, M.O.; Chuang, A.; Kim, M.S.; Sharma, R.; Liégeois, N.J.; Koch, W.M.; Califano, J.A.; Westra, W.H. & Sidransky, D. (2010). Quantitative detection of Merkel cell virus in human tissues and possible mode of transmission. *International Journal of Cancer*, Vol. 126, No. 12 (June 2010), pp. 2991-2996, ISSN 1097-0215

Maginnis, M.S. & Atwood, W.J. (2009). JC virus: an oncogenic virus in animals and humans? *Seminars in Cancer Biology*, Vol. 19, No. 4 (August 2004), pp. 261-269, ISSN 1044-579X

Mahrle, G. & Orfanos, C.E. (1974). Merkel cells as human cutaneous neuroreceptor cells : Their presence in dermal neural corpuscles and in the external hair root sheath of human adult skin. *Archives für Dermatologische Forschung*, Vol. 251, No.1 (March 1974), pp. 19-26, ISSN 0340-3696

Maricich, S.M.; Wellnitz, S.A.; Nelson, A.M.; Lesniak, D.R.; Gerling, G.J.; Lumpkin, E.A. & Zoghbi, H.Y. (2009). Merkel cells are essential for light-touch responses. *Science*, Vol. 324, No. 5934 (June 2009), pp. 1580-1582, ISSN 0036-8075

Martin, J.D.; King, D.M.; Slauch, J.M. & Frisque, R.J. (1985). Differences in regulatory sequences of naturally occurring JC virus variants. *Journal of Virology*, Vol. 53, No. 1 (January 1985), pp. 306-311, ISSN 0022-538X

Mateer, S.C.; Fedorov, S.A. & Mumby, M.C. (1998). Identification of structural elements involved in the interaction of simian virus 40 small tumor antigen with protein phosphatase 2A. *Journal of Biological Chemistry*, Vol. 273, No. 52 (December 1998), pp. 35339-34635, ISSN 0021-9258

Matthews, M.R.; Wang, R.C.; Reddick, R.L.; Saldivar, V.A. & Browning, J.C. (2011). Viral-associated trichodysplasia spinulosa: a case with electron microscopic and molecular detection of the trichodysplasia spinulosa-associated human polyomavirus. *Journal of Cutaneous Pathology* Vol. 38, No. 5 (May 2011), pp.420-431, ISSN 1600-0560

Matsuoka, M. & Jeang, K.T. (2007). Human T-cell leukaemia virus type 1 (HTLV-1) infectivity and cellular transformation. *Nature Reviews Cancer*, Vol. 7, No. 4 (April 2007), pp. 270-280, ISSN 1474-175X

Mertz, K.D.; Pfaltz, M.; Junt, T.; Schmid, M.; Fernandez-Figueras, M.T.; Pfaltz, K.; Barghorn, A. & Kempf. W. (2010a). Merkel cell polyomavirus is present in common warts and carcinoma in situ of the skin. *Human Pathology*, Vol. 41, No. 10 (October 2010), pp. 1369-1379.

Mertz, K.D.; Junt, T.; Schmid, M.; Pfaltz, M. & Kempf W. (2010b). Inflammatory monocytes are a reservoir for Merkel cell polyomavirus. *Journal of Investigative Dermatology*, Vol. 130, No. 4 (April 2010), pp. 1146-1151, ISSN 0022-202X

Moens, U.; Johansen, T.; Johnsen, J.I.; Seternes, O.M. & Traavik, T. (1995). Noncoding control region of naturally occurring BK virus variants: sequence comparison and functional analysis. *Virus Genes*, Vol. 10, No. 3, pp. 261-275, ISSN 0920-8569

Moens, U.; Seternes, O.M.; Johansen, B. & Rekvig, O.P. (1997) Mechanisms of transcriptional regulation of cellular genes by SV40 large T- and small t-antigens. *Virus Genes*, Vol. 15, No. 2, pp. 135-154, ISSN 0920-8569

Moens, U.; Van Ghelue, M. & Johannessen, M. (2007a). Oncogenic potentials of the human polyomavirus regulatory proteins. *Cellular and Molecular Life Sciences*, Vol. 64, No. 13 (July 2007), pp. 1656-1678, ISSN 1420-682X

Moens, U.; Van Ghelue, M. & Johannessen, M. (2007b). Human polyomaviruses: Molecular mechanisms for transformation and their association with cancers, In: *New Research on Oncogenic Viruses*, Tunely EI, pp. 1-63, Nova Science Publishers, ISBN: 978-1-60021-585-8, New York

Moens, U.; Johannessen, M.; Bárcena-Panero, A.; Gerits, N. & Van Ghelue, M. (2010). Emerging polyomaviruses in the human population. *Reviews in Infection*, Vol. 1, No. 2, (May 2010), pp. 59-93, ISSN 1837-6746

Moens, U.; Ludvigsen, M.; & Van Ghelue, M. (2011). Human polyomaviruses in skin diseases. Pathology Research International, in press.

Mogha, A.; Fautrel, A.; Mouchet, N.; Guo, N.; Corre, N.; Adamski, H.; Watier, E.; Misery, L. & Galibert, M.D. (2010). Merkel cell polyomavirus small T antigen mRNA level is increased following in vivo UV-radiation. *PLoS One*, Vol.5, No. 7 (July 2010), pp. e11423, ISSN.

Moll, I.; Roessler, M.; Brandner, J.M.; Eispert A.C.; Houdek, P. & Moll, R. (2005). Human Merkel cells--aspects of cell biology, distribution and functions. *European Journal of Cell Biology*, Vol. 84, No. 2-3 (March 2005), pp. 259-271, ISSN 0171-9335

Nakajima, H.; Takaishi, M.; Yamamoto, M.; Kamijima, R.; Kodama, H.; Tarutani, M. & Sano, S. (2009). Screening of the specific polyomavirus as diagnostic and prognostic tools for Merkel cell carcinoma. *Journal of Dermatological Science*, Vol. 56, No. 3 (December 2009), pp. 210-212, ISSN 0923-1811

Nakamura, T.; Sato, Y.; Watanabe, D.; Ito, H.; Shimonohara, N.; Tsuji, T.; Nakajima, N.; Suzuki, Y.; Matsuo, K.; Nakagawa, H.; Sata, T. & Katano, H. (2010). Nuclear localization of Merkel cell polyomavirus large T antigen in Merkel cell carcinoma. *Virology*, Vol. 398, No. 2, pp. 273-279, ISSN 0042-6822

Padgett, B.L.; Walker, D.L.; Zu Rhein, G.M.; Eckroade, R.J. & Dessel, B.H. (1971). Cultivation of papova-like virus from human brain with progressive multifocal leukoencephalopathy. *Lancet* Vol.1, No. 7712, (June 1971), pp.1257-1260, ISSN 0140-6736

Paik, J.Y.; Hall, G.; Clarkson, A.; Lee, L.; Toon, C.; Colebatch, A.; Chou, A. & Gill, A.J. (2011). Immunohistochemistry for Merkel cell polyomavirus is highly specific but not sensitive for the diagnosis of Merkel cell carcinoma in the Australian population. *Human Pathology*. (March 2011). [Epub ahead of print] ISSN 1532-8392

Pancaldi, C.; Corazzari, V.; Maniero, S.; Mazzoni, E.; Martini, F. & Tognon, M. (2011). Merkel cell polyomavirus DNA sequenze in the buffy coats of healthy blood donors. *Blood*. Vol. 117, No. 26 (June 2011), pp. 7099-7101, ISSN 0006-4971

Paolini, F.; Donati. P.; Amantea, A.; Bucher, S.; Migliano, E. & Venuti, A. (2011). Merkel cell polyomavirus in Merkel cell carcinoma of Italian patients. *Virology Journal*, Vol. 8, (March 2011), pp. 103-105 , ISSN 1743-422X

Pastrana, D.V.; Tolstov Y.L.; Becker, J.C.; Moore, P.S.; Chang, Y. & Buck, C.B. (2009). Quantitation of human seroresponsiveness to Merkel cell polyomavirus. *PLoS Pathogens*, Vol. 5, No. 9 (September 2009), pp. e1000578, ISSN 1553-7366

Paulson, K.G.; Lemos, B.D.; Feng, B.; Jaimes, N.; Penas, P.F.; Bi, X.; Maher, E.; Cohen, L.; Leonard, J.H.; Granter, S.R.; Chin, L. & Nghiem, P. (2009). Array-CGH reveals recurrent genomic changes in Merkel cell carcinoma including amplification of L-Myc. *Journal of Investigative Dermatology*, Vol. 129, No. 6 (June 2009), pp. 1547-1555, ISSN 0022-202X

Paulson, K.G.; Carter, J.J.; Johnson, L.G.; Cahill, K.W.; Iyer, J.G.; Schrama, D.; Becker, J.C.; Madeleine, M.M.; Nghiem, P. & Galloway, D.A. (2010). Antibodies to Merkel cell polyomavirus T antigen oncoproteins reflect tumor burden in Merkel cell carcinoma carcinoma patients. *Cancer Research*, Vol. 70, No. 21 (November 2010), pp. 8388-8397, ISSN 1538-7445

Paulson, K.G.; Iyer, J.G.; Tegeder, A.R.; Thibodeau, R.; Schelter, J.; Koba, S.; Schrama, D.; Simonson, W.T.; Lemos, B.D.; Byrd, D.R.; Koelle, D.M.; Galloway, D.A.; Leonard,

J.H.; Madeleine, M.M.; Argenyi, Z.B.; Disis, M.L.; Becker, J.C.; Cleary, M.A. & Nghiem, P. (2011). Transcriptome-Wide studies of Merkel cell carcinoma and calidation of intratumoral CD8+ lymphocyte invasion as an independent predictor of survival. *Journal of Clinical Oncology*, Vol. 29, No. 12, (April 2011), pp. 1539-1546, ISSN 1527-7755

Pectasides, D.; Pectasides, M. & Economopoulos, T. (2006). Merkel cell cancer of the skin. *Annals of Oncology*, Vol. 17, No. 10 (October 2006), pp. 1489-1495, ISSN 0923-7534

Pulitzer, M.P.; Amin, B.D. & Busam, K.J. (2009). Merkel cell carcinoma. *Advances in Anatomic Pathology*, Vol. 16, No. 3 (June 2009), pp. 135-144, ISSN 1072-4109

Ramahi, E.; Choi, J.; Fuller, C.D. & Eng, T.Y. (2011). Merkel cell carcinoma. *American Journal of Clinical Oncology*, March 17 [Epub ahead of print].ISSN 0277-3732

Rathi, A.V.; Sáenz Robles, M.T.; Cantalupo, P.G.; Whitehead, R.H. & Pipas, J.M. (2009). Simina virus T-antigen-mediated gene regulation in enterocytes is controlled primarily by the Rb-E2F pathway. *Journal of Virology*, Vol. 83, No. 18 (September 2009), pp. 9521-9531, ISSN 0022 538X

Ricciardiello, L.; Chang, D.K.; Laghi, L.; Goel, A.; Chang, C.L. & Boland, C.R. (2001). Mad-1 is the exclusive JC strain present in the human colon, and its transcriptional control region has a deleted 98-base-pair sequence in colon cancer tissues. *Journal of Virology*, Vol. 75, No. 4 (February 2001), pp. 1996-2001, ISSN 0022-538X

Ridd, K.; Yu, S. & Bastian, B.C. (2009). The presence of polyomavirus in non-melanoma skin cancer in organ transplant recipients is rare. *Journal of Investigative Dermatology*, Vol. 129, No. 1, (January 2009), pp.250-252, ISSN 0022-202X

Sariyer, I.K.; Akan, I.; Palermo, V.; Gordon, J.; Khalili, K. & Safak, M. (2006), Phosphorylation mutants of JC virus agnoprotein are unable to sustain the viral infection cycle. *Journal of Virology*, Vol. 80, No. 8 (April 2006), pp. 3893-3903, ISSN 0022-538X

Sastre-Garau, X.; Peter, M.; Avril, M.F.; Laude, H.; Couturier, J.; Rozenberg, F.; Almeida, A.; Boitier, F.; Carlotti, A.; Couturaud, B. & Dupin, N. (2009). Merkel cell carcinoma of the skin: pathological and molecular evidence for a causative role of MCV in oncogenesis. *Journal of Pathology*, Vol. 218, No. 1 (May 2009), pp. 48-56, ISSN 1096-9896

Schowalter, R.M.; Pastrana, D.V.; Pumphrey, K.A.; Moyer, A.L. & Buck, C.B. (2010). Merkel cell polyomavirus and two previously unknown polyomaviruses are chronically shed from human skin. *Cell Host & Microbe*, Vol.7, No. 6 (June 2010), pp. 509-515, ISSN 1931-3128

Schmitt, M.; Hofler, D.; Koleganova, N. & Pawlita, M. (2011). Human polyomaviruses and other human viruses in neuroendocrine tumors. *Cancer Epidemiology Biomarkers & Prevention*, Vol. 20, No.7 (July 2011), pp. 1558-1561

Schrama, D.; Thiemann, A.; Houben, R. Kähler, K.C.; Becker, J.C. & Hauschild A. (2010). Distinction of 2 different primary Merkel cell carcinomas in 1 patient by Merkel cell polyomavirus genome analysis. *Archives of Dermatology*. Vol. 146, No. 6 (June 2010), pp. 687-689, ISSN 0003-987X

Scuda, N.; Hofmann, J.; Calvignac-Spencer, S.; Ruprecht, K.; Liman, P.; Kühn, J.; Hengel, H. & Ehlers, B. 2011. A novel human polyomavirus closely related to the African green monkey-derived lymphotropic polyomavirus (LPV). *Journal of Virology*, Vol. 85, No. 9 (May 2011), ISSN 0022-538X

Seo, G.J.; Fink, L.H.L.; O'Hara, B.; Atwood, W.J. & Sullivan, C.S. (2008). Evolutionarily conserved function of a viral microRNA. *Journal of Virology*, Vol 82, No. 20 (October 2008), pp. 9823-9828, ISSN 0022-538X

Seo, G.J.; Chen, C.J. & Sullivan, C.S. (2009). Merkel cell polyomavirus encodes a microRNA with the ability to autoregulate viral gene expression," *Virology*, Vol. 382, No. 2 (January 2009), pp. 183-187, ISSN 0042-6822

Sharp, C.P.; Norja, P.; Anthony, I.; Bell, J.E. & Simmonds, P. (2009). Reactivation and mutation of newly discovered WU, KI, and Merkel cell carcinoma polyomaviruses in immunosuppressed individuals. *Journal of Infectious Diseases*, Vol. 199, No. 2 (July 2009), pp. 398-404, ISSN 0022-1899

Shuda, M.; Arora, R.; Kwun, H.J.; Feng, H.; Sarid, R.; Fernandez-Figueras, M.T.; Tolstov, Y.; Gjoerup, O.; Mansukhani, M.M.; Swerdlow, S.H.; Chaudhary, P.M.; Kirkwood, J.M.; Nalesnik, M.A.; Kant, J.A.; Weiss, L.M.; Moore, P.S. & Chang, Y. (2009). Human Merkel cell polyomavirus infection I. MCV T antigen expression in Merkel cell carcinoma, lymphoid tissues and lymphoid tumors. *International Journal of Cancer*, Vol.125, No. 6 (September 2009), pp, 1243-1249, ISSN 1097-0215

Sihto, H.; Kukko, H.; Koljonen, V.; Sankila, R.; Böhling, T. & Joensuu H. (2009). Clinical factors associated with Merkel cell polyomavirus infection in Merkel cell carcinoma. *Journal of the National Cancer Institute*, Vol. 101, No. 13 (July 2009), pp. 938-945, ISSN 0027-8874

Sihto, H.; Kukko, H.; Koljonen, V.; Sankila, R.; Böhling, T. & Joensuu H. (2011). Merkel cell polyomavirus infection, large T antigen, retinoblastoma protein and outcome in Merkel cell carcinoma. *Clinical Cancer Research*, Vol. 17, No. 14 (July 2011), pp. 4806-4813, ISSN 1078-0432

Simmons, D.T.; Gai, D.; Parsons, R.; Debes, A. & Roy, R. (2004). Assembly of the replication initiation complex on SV origin DNA. *Nucleic Acids Research*, Vol. 32, No. 3 (February 2004), pp. 1103-1112, ISSN 0305-1048

Skalsky, R.L. & Cullen, B.R. (2010). Viruses, microRNAs, and host interactions. *Annual Reviews of Microbiology*, Vol. 64, pp. 123-141, ISSN 0066-4227

Southgate, J.; Harnden, P. & Trejdosiewicz, L.K. (1999). Cytokeratin expression patterns in normal and malignant urothelium: a review of the biological and diagnostic implications. *Histology and Histopathology*, Vol. 14 No. 2 (April 1999), pp. 657-664, ISSN 0213-3911

Stoner, G.L. & Hübner, R. (2001). The human polyomaviruses: past, present, and future, In: *Human polyomaviruses. Molecular and clinical perspectives*, Khalili, K.; & Stoner, G.L. pp. 611-663, Wiley-Liss, ISBN 0-471-39009-7, New York.

Sullivan, C.S.; Grundhoff, A.T.; Tevethia, S.; Pipas, J.M. & Ganem, D. (2005). SV40-encoded microRNAs regulate vral gene expression and reduce susceptibility to cytotoxic T cells. *Nature*, Vol. 435, No. 7042 (June 2005), pp. 682-686 ISSN 0028-0836

Suzuki, T.; Orba, Y.; Okada, Y.; Sunden, Y.; Kimura, T.; Tanaka, S.; Nagashima, K.; Hall, W.W. & Sawa, H. (2010). The human polyoma JC virus agnoprotein acts as a viroporin. *PLoS Pathogens*, Vol. 6, No. 3 (March 2010), pp. e1000801, ISSN 1553-7366

Szeder, V.; Grim, M.; Halata, Z. & Sieber-Blum, M. (2003). Neural crest origin of mammalian Merkel cells. *Developmental Biology*, Vol. 253, No. 2 (January 2003), pp. 258-263, ISSN 0012-1606

Tai, P. (2008). Merkel cell cancer: update on biology and treatment. *Current Opinion in Oncology*, Vol. 20, No. 2 (March 2008), pp. 196-200, ISSN 1040-8746

The Rockville Merkel cell carcinoma group (2009). Merkel cell carcinoma: recent progress and current priorities on etiology, pathogenesis, and clinical management. *Journal of Clinical Oncology*, Vol. 27, No. 24 (August 2009), pp. 4021-4026, ISSN 0732-183X

Toker, C. (1972). Trabecular carcinoma of the skin. *Archives of Dermatology*, Vol. 105, No.1 (January 1972), pp. 107-110, ISSN 0003987X

Tolstov, Y.L.; Pastrana, D.V.; Feng, H.; Becker, J.C.; Jenkins, F.J.; Moschos, S.; Chang, Y.; Buck, C.B. & Moore, P.S. (2009). Human Merkel cell polyomavirus infection II. MCV is a common human infection that can be detected by conformational capsid epitope immunoassays. *International Journal of Cancer*, Vol. 125, No. 6 (September 2009) , pp. 1250-1256, ISSN 1097-0215

Toracchio, S.; Foyle, A.; Sroller, V.; Reed, J.A.; Wu, J.; Kozinetz, C.A. & Butel, J.S. (2010). Lymphotropism of Merkel cell polyomavirus infection, Nova Scotia, Canada. *Emerging Infectious Diseases*, Vol. 16, No. 11 (November 2010), pp. 1702-1709, ISSN 1080-0059.

Touzé, A.; Gaitan, J.; Maruani, A.; Le Bidre, E.; Doussinaud, A.; Clavel, C.; Durlach, A.; Aubin, F.; Guyétant, S.; Lorette, G. & Coursaget, P. (2009). Merkel cell polyomavirus strains in patients with merkel cell carcinoma. *Emerging Infectious Diseases*, Vol. 15, No. 6, (June 2009), pp. 960-962, ISSN 1080-6059

Touzé, A.; Le Bidre, E.; Laude, H.; Fleury, M.J.; Cazal, R.; Arnold, F.; Carlotti, A.; Maubec, E.; Aubin, F.; Avril, M.F.; Rozenberg, F.; Tognon, M.; Maruani, A.; Guyetant, S.; Lorette, G. & Coursaget P. (2011). High Levels of Antibodies Against Merkel Cell Polyomavirus Identify a Subset of Patients With Merkel Cell Carcinoma With Better Clinical Outcome. *Journal of Clinical Oncology*, Vol. 29, No. 12 (April 2011), pp. 1612-1619, ISSN 0732-183X

Tsai, W.L. & Chung, R.T. (2010). Viral hepatocarcinogenesis. *Oncogene*, Vol. 29, No. 16 (April 2010), pp. 2309-2324, ISSN 0950-9232

van der Meijden, E.; Janssens, R.W.A.; Lauber, C.; Bavinck, J.N.; Gorbalenya, A.E. & Feltkamp, M.C.W. (2010). Discovery of a new human polyomavirus associated with trichodysplasia spinulosa in an immunocompromized patient. *PLoS Pathogens*, Vol. 6, No. 7 (July 2010), pp. e1001024, ISSN 1553-7366

Van Gele, M.; Leonard, J.H.; Van Roy, N.; Cook, A.L.; De Paepe, A. & Speleman, F. (2001). Frequent allelic loss at 10q23 but low incidence of PTEN mutations in Merkel cell carcinoma. *International Journal of Cancer*, Vol. 92, No. 3 (May 2001), pp. 409-413, ISSN 1097-0215

Van Gele, M.; Boyle, G.M.; Cook, A.L.; Vandesompele, J.; Boonefaes, T.; Rottiers, P.; Van Roy N, De Paepe, A.; Parsons, P.G.; Leonard, J.H. & Speleman, F. (2004). Gene-expression profiling reveals distinct expression patterns of Classic versus variant Merkel cell phenotype and new classifier genes to distinguish Merkel cell from small-cell lung carcinoma. *Oncogene*, Vol. 23, No.15 (April 2004), pp. 2732-2742, ISSN 0950-9232

Van Keymeulen A, Mascre G, Youseff, K.K.; Harel, I.; Michaux, C.; de Geest, N.; Szpalski, C.; Achouri, Y.; Bloch, W.; Hassan, B.A. & Blanpain, C. (2009). Epidermal progenitors give rise to Merkel cells during embryonic development and adult homeostasis. *Journal of Cell Biology*, Vol. 187, No. 1 (October 2009), pp. 91-100, ISSN 1540-8140

Varga, E.; Kiss, M.; Szabó, K. & Kemény, L. (2009) Detection of Merkel cell polyomavirus DNA in Merkel cell carcinomas. *British Journal of Dermatology*, Vol. 16, No. 4 (October 2009), pp. 930-932, ISSN 1365-2133

Vilchez, R.A. & Butel, J.S. (2004). Emergent human pathogen simian virus 40 and its role in cancer. *Clinical Microbiology Reviews* Vol. 17, No. 3 (July 2004), pp. 495-508, ISSN 0893-8512

Vogelstein, B.; Lane, D. & Levine, A.J. (2000). Surfing the p53 network. *Nature*, Vol. 408, No. 6810 (November 2000), pp. 307-310, ISSN 0028-0836

Vousden, K. H. & Prives, C. (2009). Blinded by the light: the growing complexity of p53. Cell, Vol. 137, No. 3 (January 2009), pp. 413–431 ISSN 0092-8674

Waltari, M.; Sihto, H.; Kukko, H.; Koljonen, V.; Sankila, R.; Böhling, T. & Joensuu, H. Association of Merkel cell polyomavirus infection with tumor p53, KIT, stem cell factor, PDGFR-alpha and survival in Merkel cell carcinoma. *International Journal of Cancer*, 2010 Oct 14. DOI: 10.1002/ijc.25720 ISSN (electronic): 1097-0215 PMID: 20949558

Wang, Q.; Li, D.C.; Li, Z.F.; Liu, C.X.; Xiao, Y.M.; Zhang, B.; Li, X.D.; Zhao, J.; Chen, L.P.; Xing, X.M.; Tang, S.F.; Lin, Y.C.; Lai, Y.D.; Yang, P.; Zeng, J.L.; Xiao, Q.; Zeng, X.W.; Lin, Z.N.; Zhuang, S.M. & Chen, W. (2011). Upregulation of miR-27a contributes to the malignant transformation of human bronchial epithelial cells induced by SV40 small T antigen. *Oncogene*, Apr 4 [Epub ahead of print].

Werling, A.M.; Doerflinger, Y.; Brandner, J.M.; Fuchs, F.; Becker, J.C.; Schrama, D.; Kurzen, H.; Goerdt, S. & Peitsch, W.K. (2011). Homo- and heterotypic cell-cell contacts in Merkel cells and Merkel cell carcinomas: heterogeneity and indications for cadherin switching. *Histopathology*, Vol. 58, No. 2, (January 2011), pp. 286-303, ISSN: 1365-2559

Wetzels, C.T.; Hoefnagel, J.G.; Bakkers, J.M.; Dijkman, H.B.; Blokx, W.A. & Melchers, W.J. (2009). Ultrastructural proof of polyomavirus in Merkel cell carcinoma tumour cells and its absence in small cell carcinoma of the lung. *PLoS One*. Vol. 4, No 3 (March 2009) e4958, ISSN 1932-6203

Wieland, U.; Mauch, C.; Kreuter, A.; Krieg, T. & Pfister, H. (2009). Merkel cell polyomavirus DNA in persons without Merkel cell carcinoma. *Emerging Infectious Diseases*, Vol. 15, No. 9 (September 2009), pp. 1496-1498, ISSN 1080-6059

Wieland, U.; Silling, S.; Scola, N.; Potthoff, A.; Gambichler, T.; Brockmeyer, N.H.; Pfister, H. & Kreuter, A. (2011). Merkel cell polyomavirus infection in HIV-positive men. *Archives of Dermatology*, Vol. 147, No. 4 (April 2011), pp. 401-406, ISSN 0003987X

Wong, H.H.; & Wang, J. (2010). Merkel cell carcinoma. *Archives of Pathology & Laboratory Medicine*, Vol. 134, No. 11 (November 2010), pp. 1711-1716, ISSN 0003-9985

Woo, K.J.; Choi, Y.L.; Jung, H.S.; Jung, G.; Shin, Y.K.; Jang, K.T.; Han, J. & Pyon, J.K. (2010). Merkel cell carcinoma: our experience with seven patients in Korea and a literature review. *Journal of Plastic, Reconstructive & Aesthetic Surgery*, Vol. 63, No. 12 (December 2010), pp. 2064-2070, ISSN 1748-6815

Wu, K.N.; McCue, P.A.; Berger, A.; Spiegel, J.R.; Wang, Z.X. & Witkiewicz, A.K. (2010). Detection of Merkel cell carcinoma polyomavirus in mucosal Merkel cell carcinoma. *International Journal of Surgical Pathology*, Vol. 18, No. 5 (October 2010), pp. 342-346, ISSN 1066-8969

Yoshiike, K. & Takemoto, K.K. (1986) Studies with BK virus and monkey lymphotropic papovavirus. In: *The Papovaviridae: The polyomaviruses*. Salzman, N.P. pp. 295-326, Plenum Press, ISBN 0-306-42308-1, New York and London.

zur Hausen, H. (2008a). Novel human polyomaviruses - re-emergence of a well known virus family as possible human carcinogens. *International Journal of Cancer*, Vol. 123, No. 2 (July 2008), pp. 247-250, ISSN 1097-0215

zur Hausen, H. (2008b). A specific signature of Merkel cell polyomavirus persistence in human cancer cells. *Proceedings of the National Academy of Sciences of the United States of America*, Vol. 105, No. 42 (October 2008), pp. 16063-16064, ISSN 0027-8424

zur Hausen, H. (2009). Papillomaviruses in the causation of human cancers - a brief historical account. *Virology*, Vol. 384, No. 2 (February 2009), pp. 260-265, ISSN 0042-6822

6

Macrophage Migration Inhibitory Factor (MIF) Overexpression Accelerates Photocarcinogenesis in the Skin

Tadamichi Shimizu
Department of Dermatology, Graduate School of Medicine and Pharmaceutical Sciences, University of Toyama, Japan

1. Introduction

The effects of sunlight have fascinated researchers for decades because nearly every living organism on earth is exposed to sunlight, including its ultraviolet (UV) fraction. UV radiation is divided into 3 subtypes, UVA (320–400nm), UVB (280–320nm) and UVC (200–280nm), each of which has distinct biological effects. Although UVC is blocked by stratospheric ozone, UVB (1–10%) and UVA (90–99%) reach the surface of the earth and cause skin damage (Matsumura and Ananthaswamy, 2002). An increased risk of skin damage from UV light has recently been linked to the decrease in stratospheric ozone (Ma et al., 2001). The health risks associated with ozone depletion are caused by enhanced UVA irradiation in the environment and increased penetration of the UVB light (Tenkate, 1999, Ma et al., 2001).

The skin is the body's main interface with the environment, and is frequently exposed to UV light. Exposure to UV radiation substantially increases the risk of actinic damage to the skin. UV irradiation leads to various acute deleterious cutaneous effects, including sunburn, as well as long-term consequences such as wrinkling, elastosis, irregular pigmentation, telangiectasia and the potential development of skin cancers (Young, 1990). In recent years, there has been increased interest in the contribution of UVA to skin carcinogenesis (Ridley et al., 2009). However, UVB has been demonstrated to be a causal factor for basal cell carcinoma, squamous cell carcinoma, and lentigo maligna in epidemiological and experimental studies, and UVB exposure has been shown to induce the superficial spread of melanoma in humans and other animals (Kraemer et al., 1997). Chronic UVB-induced inflammatory responses, immunosuppression, and direct DNA damage can be correlated with skin tumor formation (Fischer et al., 1999, Pentland et al., 1999). Furthermore, the inability to adequately repair DNA after UVB irradiation can result in the formation of skin cancers (Cleaver et al., 2002) (Figure 1).

2. Keratinocytes and UV-induced inflammatory cytokines

UV exposure can result in numerous changes in human skin, particularly on the face, neck, and arms. Keratinocytes, melanocytes, fibroblasts, and endothelial cells are all affected by

UV radiation. Epidermal cells are considered to be the major target of UVB radiation, as the vast majority of UVB is absorbed within the epidermis. There is emerging evidence that keratinocytes participate in cutaneous inflammatory reactions and immune responses by producing a variety of cytokines. UV irradiation may trigger cutaneous inflammatory responses by stimulating epidermal keratinocytes to produce biologically potent cytokines such as interleukin (IL)-1 (Ansel et al., 1988, Kupper et al., 1987), IL-6 (Kirnbauer et al., 1991), and tumor necrosis factor (TNF)-α (Köck et al., 1990). Once expressed, TNF-α affects a variety of cell types. It increases MHC class I expression on endothelial cells and dermal fibroblasts, induces the production of IL-1α (Dinarello et al., 1986), increases the expression of adhesion molecules, including ICAM-1, VCAM-1 and E-selectin, and it promotes the formation of sunburn in cells (Schwarz et al., 1995). Furthermore, these cytokines are involved not only in the mediation of local inflammatory reactions but also play discrete roles in tumor promotion (Suganuma et al., 2002).

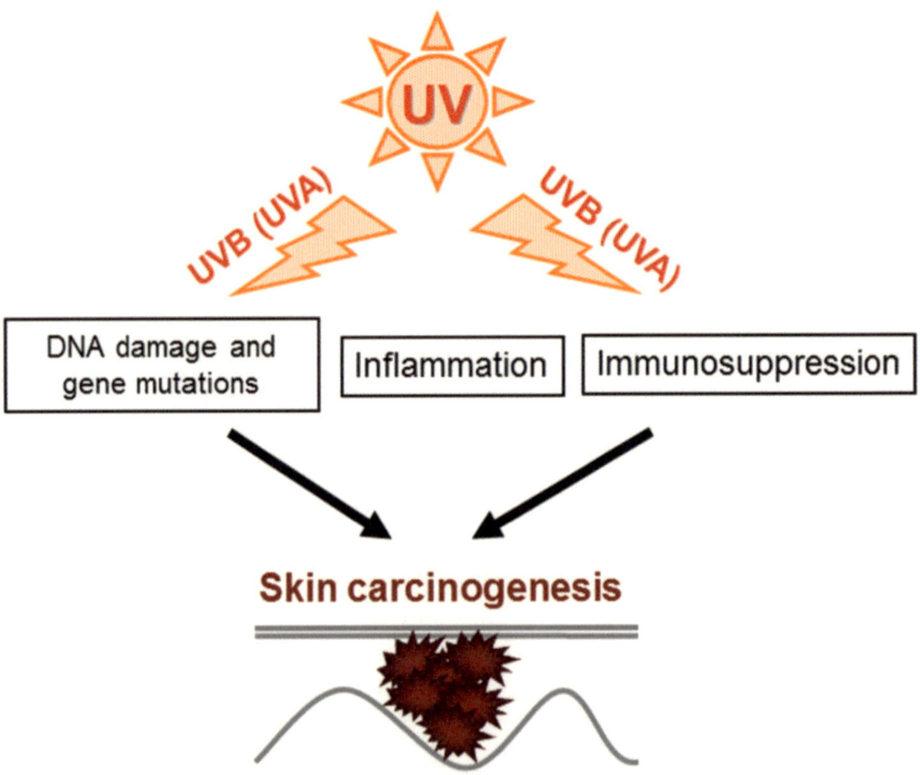

Fig. 1. UV-induced carcinogenesis in the skin.
UV radiation is carcinogenic because it induces DNA damage, gene mutation and chronic inflammation and has immunosuppressive effects on the skin.

UV radiation is also carcinogenic because of its immunosuppressive effect on the skin, and skin cancer patients have greater susceptibility to UV-induced immunosuppression (Streilein et al., 1994). The UV-induced keratinocyte-derived immunosuppressive mediators may enter the circulation and inhibit immune reactions in the skin-draining lymph nodes, or at skin areas not directly exposed to UV radiation, thereby explaining the systemic immunosuppression often observed in skin cancer patients (de Gruijl, 2008). A major soluble factor involved in systemic UV-induced immunosuppression appears to be IL-10. UV-induced DNA damage can result in the release of IL-10, a potent immunosuppressive cytokine, from keratinocytes. It has been hypothesized that the production of IL-10 by keratinocytes or tumor-infiltrating cells may contribute to the immunosuppressive and anti-inflammatory effects, allowing them to escape the immune response (Salazar-Onfray et al., 1999, Weiss et al., 2004).

3. Macrophage Migration Inhibitory Factor (MIF) function in the skin

3.1 Rediscovery of MIF

Macrophage Migration Inhibitory Factor (MIF) was originally identified as a lymphokine that concentrates macrophages at inflammatory loci. MIF is a potent activator of macrophages *in vivo* and is considered to play an important role in cell-mediated immunity (Bloom and Bennett, 1966, David, 1966). Since the molecular cloning of MIF cDNA, MIF has been reevaluated as a proinflammatory cytokine and pituitary-derived hormone that potentiates endotoxemia (Weiser et al., 1989). Subsequent work has shown that T cells and macrophages secrete MIF in response to glucocorticoids, as well as upon activation by various proinflammatory stimuli (Calandra et al., 1994). MIF has been reported to be primarily expressed in T cells and macrophages, however, recent studies have revealed this protein to be ubiquitously expressed by various other cell types, thus indicating that it has more far-reaching non-immunological role(s) in a variety of pathological states (Lanahan et al., 1992, Wistow et al., 1993, Bucala, 1996, Bacher et al., 1997, Nishihira, 2000).

MIF has broad activity on the induction of matrix metalloproteinases (Onodera et al., 2000), glucocorticoid-induced immunomodulation (Calandra et al., 1995), D-dopachrome tautomerase activity (Rosengren et al., 1996), innate immunity relevant to Toll-like receptor 4 (Roger et al., 2001) and is a crucial effector of hypoxia-inducible factor 1α that delays senescence (Welford et al., 2006). It is known that MIF binds to the CD74 extracellular domain, a process that results in the initiation of a signaling pathway in a CD44-dependent manner (Shi et al., 2006, Leng et al., 2003). Recently, it was demonstrated that CD74 forms functional complexes with CXCR4 that mediate MIF-specific signaling (Schwartz et al., 2009). It has also been reported that a small-molecule MIF antagonist increased mesenchymal stem cell (MSC) migration (Barrilleaux et al., 2009). MIF may act on MSCs, at least in part, through CD74 (Barrilleaux et al., 2010). These recent findings suggest that MIF and its antagonists may have therapeutic applications in controlling MSC homing during repair of injury and in other clinically relevant situations.

3.2 The role of MIF in the skin after UV radiation

In the skin, MIF is expressed in the epidermal keratinocytes and fibroblasts (Shimizu et al., 1996, Watanabe et al., 2004). MIF is known to play an important role in the skin with regard to inflammation, the immune response, cutaneous wound healing (Zhao et al., 2005, Dewor et al., 2007) and skin diseases, such as atopic dermatitis (Shimizu et al., 1999a, Hamasaka et al., 2009). In addition, skin melanoma cells express MIF mRNA and produce MIF protein (Shimizu et al., 1999b). The expression of MIF mRNA and the production of MIF protein have been shown to be substantially higher in human melanoma cells than in cultured normal melanocytes. Therefore, MIF functions as a novel growth factor that stimulates the uncontrolled growth and invasion of tumor cells (Shimizu et al., 1999b, Chesney et al., 1999, Shimizu, 2005) (Figure 2).

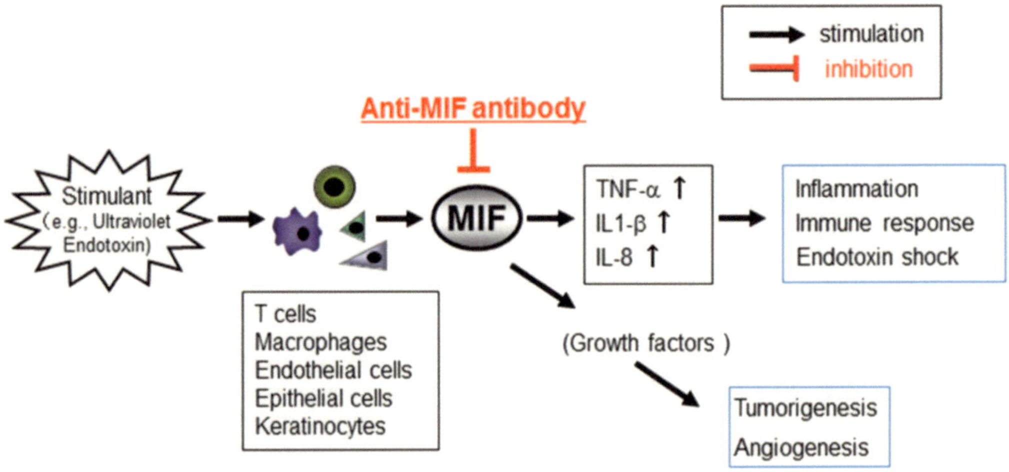

Fig. 2. Biological functions of MIF in the skin.
MIF is readily released into the extracellular space and circulation in response to various stimuli, such as endotoxins and UV irradiation. MIF functions as a multifunctional cytokine, not only during inflammation and immune responses, but also during cell proliferation and angiogenesis. Anti-MIF antibodies effectively suppress these pathophysiological conditions.

Keratinocytes are capable of enhancing MIF production in the skin after UV radiation (Shimizu et al., 1999c). UV radiation indirectly regulates melanogenesis in melanocytes through a paracrine regulatory mechanism involving keratinocytes. Recently, it was demonstrated that the back skin of MIF transgenic (Tg) mice had a higher melanin content than that of wild-type (WT) mice after 12 weeks of UVB exposure. MIF mediated melanogenesis occurs mainly through the activation of protease-activated receptor-2 and stem cell factor expression in keratinocytes after exposure to UVB radiation (Enomoto et al., 2011). It has also been reported that MIF-deficient macrophages suppress the enhanced apoptosis and have restored proinflammatory function. MIF also inhibits p53 activity in macrophages via an autocrine regulatory pathway, thus resulting in a decrease in cellular p53 accumulation and subsequent function (Mitchell et al., 2002). Recent studies have therefore suggested a potentially broader role for MIF in growth regulation because of its ability to antagonize p53-mediated gene activation and apoptosis (Hudson et al., 1999, Nemajerova et al., 2007).

4. MIF and photocarcinogenesis

4.1 MIF and UV-induced gene mutations

Apoptosis and enhanced DNA repair are both mediated by the p53 tumor suppressor (Levine, 1997). The most commonly known UV-induced mutations occur in the p53 gene (TP53), and chronic UV exposure can increase the occurrence of TP53 mutations, leading to dysregulation of apoptosis, and the initiation of skin cancer (Stenback et al., 1998). UV-induced DNA lesions can lead to cell cycle arrest, DNA repair, and apoptosis if the DNA damage is beyond repair. In cells with wild type p53, UV radiation induces p53 expression, which in turn leads to increased p21 synthesis, which arrests the cell cycle in the S1 phase, enabling DNA repair to occur. However, p53 can also participate in the initiation and regulation of the DNA repair process. In response to UV exposure, the protein bax is activated, which induces apoptosis and leads to the safe elimination of damaged cells. Therefore, it is important that apoptosis is induced immediately after UV irradiation. Any dysregulation in p53 signaling, especially with regard to its effects on the transcription of cell cycle regulatory and DNA damage response proteins, can result in cellular transformation.

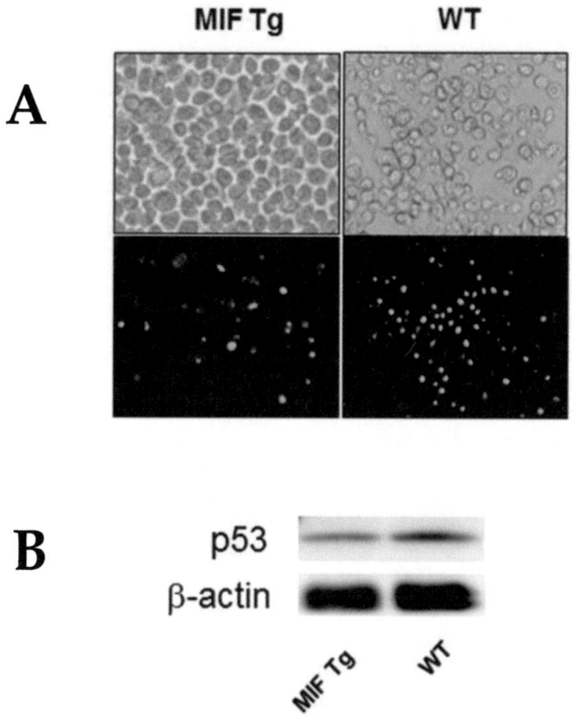

Fig. 3. UVB-induced apoptosis in cultured keratinocytes of MIF Tg and WT mice.
(**A**) Cultured keratinocytes from the MIF Tg or WT mice were irradiated with UVB at 50 mJ/cm^2, and the irradiated cells were analyzed by the TUNEL assay. The upper panels show morphological images. The lower panels show the results of the TUNEL assay. There were significantly fewer apoptotic keratinocytes (TUNEL positive) in MIF Tg mice than in WT mice ($p < 0.005$). (**B**) The p53 protein expression of UVB irradiated keratinocytes was analyzed by a Western blot analysis. The p53 expression in the MIF Tg keratinocytes was lower than that of keratinocytes from WT mice.

MIF is a cytokine that not only plays a critical role in several inflammatory conditions but also inhibits the p53-dependent apoptotic processes (Fingerle-Rowson et al., 2003). Studies indicate that MIF treatment can overcome p53 activity and inhibit its transcriptional activity. Recently, it has been demonstrated that after chronic UVB irradiation, an early onset of carcinogenesis and a higher tumor incidence were observed in MIF Tg mice compared to WT mice (Honda et al., 2009). In addition, the UVB-induced apoptosis of epidermal keratinocytes was inhibited in the MIF Tg mice. Significantly fewer terminal deoxyribonucleotidyl transferase (TDT)-mediated dUTP-digoxigenin nick end labeling (TUNEL)-positive cells were detected in MIF Tg mice than in WT mice. There was also a decrease in the expression of apoptosis regulatory genes (i.e., p53 and bax), in the MIF Tg mice after UVB irradiation (Figure 3). A previous study also demonstrated similar protective effects in the corneas of MIF Tg mice in response to acute UVB light (Kitaichi et al., 2008). MIF is upregulated by UVB irradiation in the mouse cornea, and MIF Tg mice showed fewer apoptotic corneal cells. Similarly, other studies have reported that MIF-deficient mice showed a significant increase in p53 activity and reduced tumor incidence compared to WT mice after acute and chronic exposure to UVB radiation, respectively (Martin et al., 2009). MIF has also been shown to have an inhibitory effect on UVB-induced photo-damage by blocking the expression of apoptosis-regulatory genes (Honda et al., 2009).

Recent evidence suggests that the pathways responsible for the removal of UV-mediated DNA damage can be modulated by several inflammatory cytokines. It has been observed that IL-12, which is an immunomodulatory cytokine, reduces UV-induced apoptosis *in vitro*. This was confirmed *in vivo,* because an injection of IL-12 into the skin of UV exposed mice significantly reduced the number of apoptotic keratinocytes (Schwarz et al., 2002). IL-18 seems to exert similar effects as IL-12. The injection of IL-18 into the UV exposed skin of mice reduced the amount of DNA damage (Schwarz et al., 2006).

4.2 MIF overexpression accelerates photocarcinogenesis

In addition to decreasing protective DNA damage repair, MIF also exhibits direct pro-neoplastic activity. In many tumor cells and pre-tumor states, for example, in prostate (Meyer-Siegler et al., 1998), colon (Legendre et al., 2003), and hepatocellular cancers (Ren et al., 2003), adenocarcinomas of the lung (Kamimura et al., 2000), glioblastomas (Rogge, 2002), and melanomas (Shimizu, 1999b), increased MIF mRNA levels can be detected. The pro-neoplastic role of MIF has been studied by several groups. Fingerle *et al.* reported that embryonic fibroblasts from MIF-deficient mice exhibit p53-dependent growth alterations, increased p53 transcriptional activity, and resistance to ras-mediated transformation (Fingerle-Rowson et al., 2003). The concurrent deletion of the p53 gene *in vivo* reversed the observed phenotype of cells deficient in MIF. *In vivo* studies showed that fibrosarcomas are smaller in size and have a lower mitotic index in MIF-deficient mice relative to their WT counterparts. The authors concluded that there is direct evidence for a functional link between MIF and the p53 tumor suppressor (Fingerle-Rowson et al., 2003).

Using an anti-MIF antibody has also been reported to be effective for reducing tumor growth and neovascularization in lymphoma cells and vascular endothelial cells *in vivo* (Nishihira, 2000). Consistent with this finding, anti-MIF antibodies were found to be effective for reducing tumor angiogenesis in melanoma cells (Shimizu, 1999b) This was demonstrated *in vitro* by using recombinant MIF in fibroblasts, where growth-factor-induced stimulation of these cells resulted in increased MIF concentrations, activation of the extracellular regulated kinase/mitogen-activated protein (ERK-MAP) kinase pathway, and a subsequent increase in cell proliferation (Takahashi et al., 1998). In addition, it has been shown that exposure to TGF-β results in increased MIF expression in a colon cancer cell line (Meyer-Siegler et al., 2006). Furthermore, other investigators observed an increase in the level of cytotoxic T lymphocytes following MIF inhibition achieved by using specific antibodies, and the number of apoptotic tumor cells increased following MIF inhibition (Abe et al., 2001). Tumors arising in the MIF-knockdown cells grew less rapidly and also showed an increased degree of apoptosis (Hagemann et al., 2007). These findings, therefore, suggest that once keratinocytes acquire mutations by UVB-induced DNA damage, they may become malignant, and MIF may thus play a dual role in promoting the growth of these tumor cells and inhibiting their apoptosis.

4.3 MIF and UV-Induced skin inflammatory responses

UVB stimulates the production of several proinflammatory cytokines, including TNF-α, IL-1 and IL-6 in the skin, and these proinflammatory cytokines are considered to be closely related to the progression of skin carcinogenesis (Moore et al., 1999, Murphy et al., 2003, Kim et al., 2010). UVB-induced inflammatory responses, such as the production of cytokines and the infiltration of inflammatory cells, are clearly associated with the development of skin tumors. The inhibition of this inflammatory response via topical application of an anti-inflammatory drug inhibits the acute inflammatory responses after UVB exposure, and decreases tumor formation after chronic exposure (Wilgus et al., 2003).

MIF plays a direct role in both inflammation and tumorigenesis (Bach et al., 2008). UVB exposure in MIF Tg mice resulted in greater leukocyte infiltration than in WT mouse skin (Honda et al., 2009). Moreover, UVB irradiation enhances the expression of MIF in the epidermis, and MIF Tg mice showed higher levels of MIF mRNA expression after UVB exposure (Shimizu, 1999c). Once released, MIF acts as a proinflammatory cytokine to induce the expression of other inflammatory cytokines, including IL-1, IL-6 and TNF-α (Toh et al., 2006, Sanchez-Zamora et al., 2010, Donnelly, 1997). Since the intense inflammation in the skin in response to UVB irradiation was found to correlate with the early onset of carcinogenesis and a higher incidence of tumors after chronic UVB exposure, this finding confirms the likely role of MIF in this process.

5. Conclusions

Chronic exposure to UV irradiation induces early-onset skin carcinogenesis, and many inflammatory cytokines are related to the induction and progression of UV-induced skin cancer (Table 1). Chronic UVB exposure enhances MIF production, which may inhibit the p53-dependent apoptotic processes, thereby inducing photocarcinogenesis in the skin (Figure 4). This newly identified mechanism may positively contribute to our overall understanding of photo-induced skin damage, which ultimately results in carcinogenesis.

Progression of carcinogen	cytokines	References
Modulation of UV-induced apoptosis	MIF	Honda *et al.*, 2009 Martin *et al.*, 2009
	IL-12	Schwarz *et al.*, 2002
	IL-18	Schwarz *et al.*, 2006
Chronic inflammation	TNF-α	Moore *et al.*, 1999
	IL-1	Murphy *et al.*, 2003
	IL-6	Kim *et al.*, 2010
	MIF	Honda *et al.*, 2009
Immunosuppression	IL-10	Salazar-Onfray *et al.*, 1999 Weiss *et al.*, 2004

Table 1. Skin cancer and related inflammatory cytokines

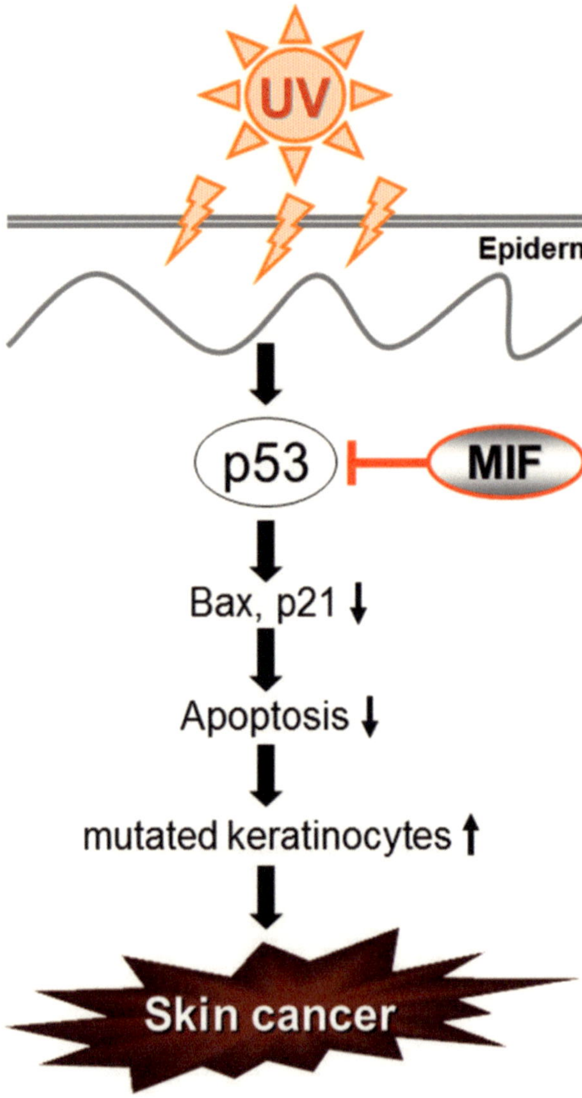

Fig. 4. MIF inhibits p53-dependent apoptotic processes.
UVB exposure enhances MIF production, which may inhibit the p53-dependent apoptotic processes by blocking the relevant expression of apoptosis-regulatory genes, including those encoding p53, p21 and bax, thereby inducing photocarcinogenesis in the skin.

6. References

Abe, R., Peng, T., Sailors, J., Bucala, R. and Metz, C.N. (2001). "Regulation of the CTL response by macrophage migration inhibitory factor." J Immunol 166(2): 747-53.

Ansel, J.C., Luger, T.A., Lowry, D., Perry, P., Roop, D.R. and Mountz, J.D. (1988). "The expression and modulation of IL-1 alpha in murine keratinocytes." J Immunol 140(7): 2274-8.

Bach, J.P., Rinn, B., Meyer, B., Dodel, R. and Bacher, M. (2008). "Role of MIF in inflammation and tumorigenesis." Oncology 75(3-4): 127-33.

Bacher, M., Meinhardt, A., Lan, H.Y., Mu, W., Metz, C.N., Chesney, J.A., Calandra, T., Gemsa, D., Donnelly, T., Atkins, R.C. and Bucala, R. (1997). "Migration inhibitory factor expression in experimentally induced endotoxemia." Am J Pathol 150(1): 235-46.

Barrilleaux, B.L., Phinney, D.G., Fischer-Valuck, B.W., Russell, K.C., Wang, G., Prockop, D.J. and O'Connor, K.C. (2009). "Small-molecule antagonist of macrophage migration inhibitory factor enhances migratory response of mesenchymal stem cells to bronchial epithelial cells." Tissue Eng Part A 15(9): 2335-46.

Barrilleaux, B.L., Fischer-Valuck, B.W., Gilliam, J.K., Phinney, D.G. and O'Connor, K.C. (2010). "Activation of CD74 inhibits migration of human mesenchymal stem cells." In Vitro Cell Dev Biol Anim 46(6): 566-72.

Bloom, B.R. and Bennett, B. (1966). "Mechanism of a reaction in vitro associated with delayed-type hypersensitivity." Science 153(731): 80-2.

Bucala, R. (1996). "MIF re-discovered." pituitary hormone and glucocorticoid-induced regulator of cytokine production." Cytokine Growt Factor Rev 7(1): 19-24.

Calandra, T., Bernhagen, J., Metz, C.N., Spiegel, L.A., Bacher, M., Donnelly, T., Cerami, A. and Bucala, R. (1995). "MIF as a glucocorticoid-induced modulator of cytokine production." Nature 377(6544): 68-71.

Calandra, T., Bernhagen, J., Mitchell, R.A. and Bucala, R. (1994). "The macrophage is an important and previously unrecognized source of macrophage migration inhibitory factor." J Exp Med 179(6): 1895-902.

Chesney, J., Metz, C., Bacher, M., Peng, T., Meinhardt, A. and Bucala, R. (1999). "An essential role for macrophage migration inhibitory factor (MIF) in angiogenesis and the growth of a murine lymphoma." Mol Med 5(3): 181-91.

Cleaver, J.E. and Crowley, E. (2002). "UV damage, DNA repair and skin carcinogenesis." Front Biosci 7: d1024-43.

David, J.R. (1966). "Delayed hypersensitivity in vitro: its mediation by cell-free substances formed by lymphoid cell-antigen interaction." Proc Natl Acad Sci USA 56(1): 72-7.

de Gruijl, F.R. (2008). "UV-induced immunosuppression in the balance." Photochem Photobiol 84(1): 2-9.

Dewor, M., Steffens, G., Krohn, R., Weber, C., Baron, J. and Bernhagen, J. (2007). "Macrophage migration inhibitory factor (MIF) promotes fibroblast migration in scratch-wounded monolayers in vitro." FEBS Lett 581(24): 4734-42.

Dinarello, C.A., Cannon, J.G., Wolff, S.M., Bernheim, H.A., Beutler, B., Cerami, A., Figari, I.S., Palladino, M.A. Jr. and O'Connor, J.V. (1986). "Tumor necrosis factor (cachectin) is an endogenous pyrogen and induces production of interleukin 1." J Exp Med 163(6): 1433-50.

Donnelly, S.C., Haslett, C., Reid, P.T., Grant, I.S., Wallace, W.A., Metz, C.N., Bruce, L.J. and Bucala, R. (1997). "Regulatory role for macrophage migration inhibitory factor in acute respiratory distress syndrome." Nat Med 3(3): 320-3.

Enomoto, A., Yoshihisa, Y., Yamakoshi, T., Ur Rehman, M., Norisugi, O., Hara, H., Matsunaga, K., Makino, T., Nishihira, J. and Shimizu, T. (2011). "UVB radiation induces macrophage migration inhibitory factor-mediated melanogenesis through activation of PAR-2 and SCF in keratinocytes." Am J Pathol 178(2): 679-87.

Fingerle-Rowson, G., Petrenko, O., Metz, C.N., Forsthuber, T.G., Mitchell, R., Huss, R., Moll, U., Muller, W. and Bucala, R. (2003). "The p53-dependent effects of macrophage migration inhibitory factor revealed by gene targeting." Proc Natl Acad Sci USA 100(16): 9354-9.

Fischer, S.M., Lo, H.H., Gordon, G.B., Seibert, K., Kelloff, G., Lubet, R.A. and Conti, C.J. (1999). "Chemopreventive activity of celecoxib, a specific cyclooxygenase-2 inhibitor, and indomethacin against ultraviolet light-induced skin carcinogenesis." Mol Carcinog 25(4): 231-40.

Hagemann, T., Robinson, S.C., Thompson, R.G., Charles, K., Kulbe, H. and Balkwill, F.R. (2007). "Ovarian cancer cell-derived migration inhibitory factor enhances tumor growth, progression, and angiogenesis." Mol Cancer Ther 6(7): 1993-2002.

Hamasaka, A., Abe, R., Koyama, Y., Yoshioka, N., Fujita, Y., Hoshina, D., Sasaki, M., Hirasawa, T., Onodera, S., Ohshima, S., Leng, L., Bucala, R., Nishihira, J., Shimizu, T. and Shimizu, H. (2009). "DNA-vaccination against macrophage migration inhibitory factor improves atopic dermatitis in murine models." J Allergy Clin Immunol 124(1): 90-9.

Honda, A., Abe, R., Yoshihisa, Y., Makino, T., Matsunaga, K., Nishihira, J., Shimizu, H. and Shimizu, T. (2009). "Deficient deletion of apoptotic cells by macrophage migration inhibitory factor (MIF) overexpression accelerates photocarcinogenesis." Carcinogenesis 30(9): 1597-605.

Hudson, J.D., Shoaibi, M.A., Maestro, R., Carnero, A., Hannon, G.J. and Beach, D.H. (1999). "A proinflammatory cytokine inhibits p53 tumor suppressor activity." J Exp Med 190(10): 1375-82.

Kamimura, A., Kamachi, M., Nishihira, J., Ogura, S., Isobe, H., Dosaka-Akita, H., Ogata, A., Shindoh, M., Ohbuchi, T. and Kawakami, Y. (2000). "Intracellular distribution of macrophage migration inhibitory factor predicts the prognosis of patients with adenocarcinoma of the lung." Cancer 89(2): 334-41.

Kim, E.J., Park, H., Kim, J. and Park, J.H. (2010). "3,3'-diindolylmethane suppresses 12-O-tetradecanoylphorbol-13-acetate-induced inflammation and tumor promotion in mouse skin via the downregulation of inflammatory mediators." Mol Carcinog 49(7): 672-83.

Kirnbauer, R., Kock, A., Neuner, P., Forster, E., Krutmann, J., Urbanski, A., Schauer, E., Ansel, J.C., Schwarz, T. and Luger, T.A. (1991). "Regulation of epidermal cell interleukin-6 production by UV light and corticosteroids." J Invest Dermatol 96(4): 484-9.

Kitaichi, N., Shimizu, T., Yoshida, K., Honda, A., Yoshihisa, Y., Kase, S., Ohgami, K., Norisugi, O., Makino, T., Nishihira, J., Yamagishi, S. and Ohno, S. (2008). "Macrophage migration inhibitory factor ameliorates UV-induced photokeratitis in mice." Exp Eye Res 86(6): 929-35.

Köck, A., Schwarz, T., Kirnbauer, R., Urbanski, A., Perry, P., Ansel, J.C. and Luger, T.A. (1990). " Human keratinocytes are a source for tumor necrosis factor alpha : evidence for synthesis and release upon stimulation with endotoxin or ultraviolet light." J Exp Med 172(6): 1609-14.

Kraemer, K.H. (1997). "Sunlight and skin cancer : another link revealed." Proc Natl Acad Sci USA 94(1): 11-4.

Kupper, T.S., Chua, A.O., Flood, P., McGuire, J. and Gubler, U. (1987). " Interleukin 1 gene expression in cultured human keratinocytes is augmented by ultraviolet irradiation." J Clin Invest 80(2): 430-6.

Lanahan, A., Williams, J.B., Sanders, L.K. and Nathans, D. (1992). "Growth factor-induced delayed early response genes." Mol Cell Biol 12(9): 3919-29.

Legendre, H., Decaestecker, C., Nagy, N., Hendlisz, A., Schuring, M.P., Salmon, I., Gabius, H.J., Pector, J.C. and Kiss, R. (2003). "Prognostic values of galectin-3 and the macrophage migration inhibitory factor (MIF) in human colorectal cancers." Mod Pathol 16(5): 491-504.

Leng, L., Metz, C.N, Fang, Y., Xu, J., Donnelly, S., Baugh, J., Delohery, T., Chen, Y., Mitchell, R.A. and Bucala, R. (2003). "MIF signal transduction initiated by binding to CD74." J Exp Med 197(11): 1467-76.

Levine, A.J. (1997). "p53, the cellular gatekeeper for growth and division." Cell 88(3): 323-31.

Ma, W., Wlaschek, M., Tantcheva-Poór, I., Schneider, L.A., Naderi, L., Razi-Wolf, Z., Schüller, J. and Scharffetter-Kochanek, K. (2001). "Chronological ageing and photoageing of the fibroblasts and the dermal connective tissue." Clin Exp Dermatol 26(7): 592-9.

Martin, J., Duncan, F.J., Keiser, T., Shin, S., Kusewitt, D.F., Oberyszyn, T., Satoska,r A.R. and VanBuskirk, A.M. (2009). "Macrophage migration inhibitory factor (MIF) plays a critical role in pathogenesis of ultraviolet-B (UVB)-induced nonmelanoma skin cancer (NMSC)." FASEB J 23(3): 720-30.

Matsumura, Y. and Ananthaswamy, H.N. (2002). "Short-term and long-term cellular and molecular events following UV irradiation of skin: implications for molecular medicine." Expert Rev Mol Med 4(26): 1-22.

Meyer-Siegler, K., Fattor, R.A. and Hudson, P.B. (1998). "Expression of macrophage migration inhibitory factor in the human prostate." Diagn Mol Pathol 7(1): 44-50.

Meyer-Siegler, K.L., Iczkowski, K.A., Leng, L., Bucala, R. and Vera, P.L. (2006). "Inhibition of macrophage migration inhibitory factor or its receptor (CD74) attenuates growth and invasion of DU-145 prostate cancer cells." J Immunol 177(12) 8730-9.

Mitchell, R.A., Liao, H., Chesney, J., Fingerle-Rowson, G., Baugh, J., David, J. and Bucala, R. (2002). "Macrophage migration inhibitory factor (MIF) sustains macrophage proinflammatory function by inhibiting p53: regulatory role in the innate immune response." Proc Natl Acad Sci USA 99(1): 345-50.

Moore, R.J., Owens, D.M., Stamp, G., Arnott, C., Burke, F., East, N., Holdsworth, H., Turner, L., Rollins, B., Pasparakis, M., Kollias, G. and Balkwill, F. (1999). "Mice deficient in tumor necrosis factor-alpha are resistant to skin carcinogenesis." Nat Med 5(7): 828-31.

Murphy, J.E., Morales, R.E., Scott, J. and Kupper, T.S. (2003). "IL-1 alpha, innate immunity, and skin carcinogenesis: the effect of constitutive expression of IL-1 alpha in epidermis on chemical carcinogenesis." J Immunol 170(11): 5697-703.

Nemajerova, A., Mena, P., Fingerle-Rowson, G., Moll, U.M. and Petrenko, O. (2007). "Impaired DNA damage checkpoint response in MIF-deficient mice." EMBO J 26(4): 987-97.

Nishihira, J. (2000). "Macrophage migration inhibitory factor (MIF): its essential role in the immune system and cell growth." J Interferon Cytokine Res 20(9): 751-62.

Onodera, S., Kaneda, K., Mizue, Y., Koyama, Y., Fujinaga, M. and Nishihira, J. (2000). "Macrophage migration inhibitory factor up-regulates expression of matrix metalloproteinases in synovial fibroblasts of rheumatoid arthritis." J Biol Chem 275(1): 444-50.

Pentland, A.P., Schoggins, J.W., Scott, G.A., Khan, K.N. and Han, R. (1999). "Reduction of UV-induced skin tumors in hairless mice by selective COX-2 inhibition." Carcinogenesis 20(10): 1939-44.

Ren, Y., Tsui, H.T., Poon, R.T., Ng, I.O., Li, Z., Chen, Y., Jiang, G., Lau, C., Yu, W.C., Bacher, M. and Fan, S.T. (2003). "Macrophage migration inhibitory factor: roles in regulating tumor cell migration and expression of angiogenic factors in hepatocellular carcinoma." Int J Cancer 107(1): 22-9.

Ridley, A.J., Whiteside, J.R., McMillan, T.J. and Allinson, S.L. (2009). " Cellular and sub-cellular responses to UVA in relation to carcinogenesis." Int J Radiat Biol 85(3): 177-95.

Roger, T., David, J., Glauser, M.P. and Calandra, T. (2001). "MIF regulates innate immune responses through modulation of Toll-like receptor 4." Nature 414(6866): 920-4.

Rogge, L. (2002). "A genomic view of helper T cell subsets." Ann N Y Acad Sci 975: 57-67.

Rosengren, E., Bucala, R., Aman, P., Jacobsson, L., Odh, G., Metz, C.N. and Rorsman, H. (1996). "The immunoregulatory mediator macrophage migration inhibitory factor (MIF) catalyzes a tautomerization reaction." Mol Med 2(1): 143-9.

Salazar-Onfray, F. (1999). "Interleukin 10: A cytokine used by tumors to escape immunosurveillance." Med Oncol 16(2): 86-94.

Sanchez-Zamora, Y., Terrazas, L.I., Vilches-Flores, A., Leal, E., Juárez, I., Whitacre, C., Kithcart, A., Pruitt, J., Sielecki, T., Satoskar, A.R. and Rodriguez-Sosa, M. (2010). "Macrophage migration inhibitory factor is a therapeutic target in treatment of non-insulin-dependent diabetes mellitus." FASEB J 24(7): 2583-90.

Schwartz, V., Lue, H., Kraemer, S, Korbiel, J., Krohn, R., Ohl, K., Bucala, R., Weber, C. and Bernhagen, J. (2009). "A functional heteromeric MIF receptor formed by CD74 and CXCR4." FEBS Lett 583(17): 2749-57.

Schwarz, A., Bhardwaj, R, Aragane, Y., Mahnke, K., Riemann, H., Metze, D., Luger, T.A. and Schwarz, T. (1995). "Ultraviolet-B-induced apoptosis of keratinocytes: evidence for partial involvement of tumor necrosis factor-alpha in the formation of sunburn cells." J Invest Dermatol 104(6): 922-7.

Schwarz, A., Maeda, A., Ständer, S., van Steeg, H. and Schwarz, T. (2006). "IL-18 reduces ultraviolet radiation-induced DNA damage and thereby affects photoimmunosuppression." J Immunol 176(5): 2896-901.

Schwarz, A., Ständer, S., Berneburg, M., Böhm, M., Kulms, D., van Steeg, H., Grosse-Heitmeyer, 38 K., Krutmann, J. and Schwarz, T. (2002). "Interleukin-12 suppresses ultraviolet radiation-induced apoptosis by inducing DNA repair." Nat Cell Biol 4(1): 26-31.

Shi, X., Leng, L., Wang, T., Wang, W., Du, X., Li, J., McDonald, C., Chen, Z., Murphy, J.W., Lolis, E., Noble, P., Knudson, W. and Bucala, R. (2006). "CD44 is the signaling component of the macrophage migration inhibitory factor-CD74 receptor complex." Immunity 25(4): 595-606.

Shimizu, T. (2005). "Role of macrophage migration inhibitory factor (MIF) in the skin." J Dermatol Sci 37(2): 65-73.

Shimizu, T., Ohkawara, A., Nishihira, J. and Sakamoto, W. (1996). "Identification of macrophage migration inhibitory factor (MIF) in human skin and its immunohistochemical localization." FEBS Lett 381(3): 199-202.

Shimizu, T., Abe, R., Ohkawara, A. and Nishihira, J. (1999a). "Increased production of macrophage migration inhibitory factor by PBMCs of atopic dermatitis." J Allergy Clin Immunol 104(3): 659-64.

Shimizu, T., Abe, R., Nakamura, H., Ohkawara, A., Suzuki, M. and Nishihira, J. (1999b). "High expression of macrophage migration inhibitory factor in human melanoma cells and its role in tumor cell growth and angiogenesis." Biochem Biophys Res Commun 264(3): 751-8.

Shimizu, T., Abe, R., Ohkawara, A. and Nishihira, J. (1999c). "Ultraviolet B radiation upregulates the production of macrophage migration inhibitory factor (MIF) in human epidermal keratinocytes." J Invest Dermatol 112(2): 210-5.

Stenback, F., Makinen, M. and Jussila, T. (1998). "p53 expression in skin carcinogenesis and its relationship to cell proliferation and tumour growth." Eur J Cancer 34(9): 1415-24.

Streilein, J.W., Taylor, J.R., Vincek, V., Kurimoto, I., Shimizu, T., Tie, C. and Golomb, C. (1994). "Immune surveillance and sunlight-induced skin cancer." Immunol Today 15(4): 174-9.

Suganuma, M., Okabe, S., Kurusu, M., Iida, N., Ohshima, S., Saeki, Y., Kishimoto, T. and Fujiki, H. (2002). "Discrete roles of cytokines, TNF-alpha, IL-1, IL-6 in tumor promotion and cell transformation." Int J Oncol 20(1): 131-6.

Takahashi, N., Nishihira, J., Sato, Y., Kondo, M., Ogawa, H., Ohshima, T., Une, Y. and Todo, S. (1998). "Involvement of macrophage migration inhibitory factor (MIF) in the mechanism of tumor cell growth." Mol Med 4(11): 707-14.

Tenkate, T.D. (1999). "Occupational exposure to ultraviolet radiation : a health risk assessment." Rev Environ Health 14(4): 187-209.

Toh, M.L., Aeberli, D., Lacey, D., Yang, Y., Santos, L.L., Clarkson, M., Sharma, L., Clyne, C. and Morand, E.F. (2006). "Regulation of IL-1 and TNF receptor expression and function by endogenous macrophage migration inhibitory factor." J Immunol 177(7): 4818-25.

Watanabe, H., Shimizu, T., Nishihira, J., Abe, R., Nakayama, T., Taniguchi, M., Sabe, H., Ishibashi, T. and Shimizu, H. (2004). "Ultraviolet A-induced production of matrix metalloproteinase-1 is mediated by macrophage migration inhibitory factor (MIF) in human dermal fibroblasts." J Biol Chem 279(3): 1676-83.

Weiser, W.Y., Temple, P.A., Witek-Giannotti, J.S., Remold, H.G., Clark, S.C. and David, J.R. (1989). "Molecular cloning of a cDNA encoding a human macrophage migration inhibitory factor." Proc Natl Acad Sci USA 86(19): 7522-6.

Weiss, E., Mamelak, AJ., La Morgia, S., Wang, B., Feliciani, C., Tulli, A. and Sauder, DN. (2004). "The role of interleukin 10 in the pathogenesis and potential treatment of skin diseases." J Am Acad Dermatol 50(5): 657-75.

Welford, S.M., Bedogni, B., Gradin, K., Poellinger, L., Broome Powell, M. and Giaccia, A.J. (2006). "HIF1alpha delays premature senescence through the activation of MIF." Genes Dev 20(24): 3366-71.

Wilgus, T.A., Koki, A.T., Zweifel, B.S., Kusewitt, D.F., Rubal, P.A. and Oberyszyn, T.M. (2003). "Inhibition of cutaneous ultraviolet light B-mediated inflammation and tumor formation with topical celecoxib treatment." Mol Carcinog. 38(2): 49-58.

Wistow, G.J., Shaughnessy, M.P., Lee, D.C., Hodin, J. and Zelenka, P.S. (1993). "A macrophage migration inhibitory factor is expressed in the differentiating cells of the eye lens." Proc Natl Acad Sci USA 90(4): 1272-5.

Young, A.R. (1990). "Cumulative effects of ultraviolet radiation on the skin : cancer and photoaging." Semin Dermatol 9(1): 25-31.

Zhao, Y., Shimizu, T., Nishihira, J., Koyama, Y., Kushibiki, T., Honda, A., Watanabe, H., Abe, R., Tabata, Y. and Shimizu, H. (2005). "Tissue regeneration using macrophage migration inhibitory factor (MIF)-impregnated gelatin microbeads in cutaneous wounds." Am J Pathol 167(6): 1519-29.

Part 2

Skin Cancer Diagnosis

7

Optical Imaging as Auxiliary Tool in Skin Cancer Diagnosis

S. Pratavieira, C. T. Andrade, A. G. Salvio, V.S. Bagnato and C. Kurachi
Instituto de Física de São Carlos - Universidade de São Paulo, São Carlos, SP, Brasil

1. Introduction

Clinical detection of early malignant and premalignant skin lesions is not simple due to their similar features with the more common benign lesions. The traditional skin cancer screening is based on careful whole body visual inspection, and if a suspected lesion is noticed, further examination with biopsy is required. Visual examination relies heavily on the experience and skills of the physician to identify and delineate the initial changes related to carcinogenesis and cancer progression. White light dermatoscope is the most used conventional tool for skin cancer screening, used by dermatologists for a magnified visualization of the skin. Optical imaging at widefield and microscopic levels has been presented as clinical tools for aiding lesion detection and discrimination. Optical techniques are non-invasive, with fast response through an *in situ* interrogation, and are potentially sensitive to biochemical and structural changes presented in skin cancer development. For skin cancer diagnostics the main used techniques are: widefield imaging, optical spectroscopy and microscopy imaging. Widefield imaging allows the examination of large areas and has the potential of improving detection of occult lesions, margin delimitation, and of guiding biopsy site determination. Optical spectroscopy presents more detailed information on tissue composition, through the light intensity for each collected emission wavelength, which might be later correlated to specific biomolecules. Microscopy imaging has a main advantage of the evaluation of the tissue characteristics at cellular level, but only a small fraction of the lesion volume is interrogated. Distinct optical techniques offer different tissue/cellular information that is complimentary, even though for cancer screening, widefield optical imaging may represent the first best option, when compared to point spectroscopy or optical microscopy. The combination of information from different imaging modalities has the potential of revealing tissue features resulting in an improved diagnostic performance, due to their distinct provided tissue information. In this chapter an overview of the optical clinical methods and the instruments developed for skin cancer detection of published studies will be discussed.

2. Interaction visible light – skin

The electromagnetic radiation extends, in order of increasing energy, from radio waves with low energy (long wavelengths), to high-energy radiation (X-ray and gamma radiation). Include regions of radiation with intermediate energies between the ultraviolet and microwave, passing by the visible light. Each of these regions has distinct ways to be produced and detected, and each interacts with matter differently, which may reveal certain characteristics of the system investigated. Due to the distinct energy characteristics, different light/biological tissue interaction occurs. This is the reason, for instance, why the x-rays may induce DNA damage (Karagas, et al. 1996, McLaren, et al. 1975), and the violet light is used for jaundice treatment of new-borns (Bauer, et al. 2004). Optical diagnostic systems are the system that uses the visible light for diagnostics. The visible light or white light is composing by all colors, with the range of wavelength of 400 - 700 nanometers (when the light is understood as a wave). All optical diagnostic systems are based on the one or more types of light-tissue interactions to provide biochemical and/or structural tissue information. This idea relies on the fact that tissue changes alters light-tissue interaction, and if the re-emitted light exiting the tissue is collected and analyzed, a correlation may be obtained. Each specific light wavelength (or color) has a particular interaction with the tissue.

When the light is incident in a biological tissue, the main following events occur:

a. Specular scattering: the light is reflected at the tissue surface with the same incident angle relative to the normal orientation.
b. Diffuse scattering: the light is diffusely scattered inside the tissue. Due to the different refractive indexes of biological components, the photon (when the light can be understood as constitute by photons) travelling within the tissue suffers multiple direction changes.
c. Transmission: the light is transmitted through the tissue and may exit without changing its incident direction.
d. Absorption: the light is absorbed by biological chromophores and this energy may result in molecular vibration (heat), and luminescent emission. The most important biological absorbers are hemoglobin and melanin.
e. Luminescence: after light absorption, some excited biological chromophores may lose this excess of energy through light emission (fluorescence and phosphorescence). The prevalent optical luminescent event in biological tissues is the fluorescence.

These are the most important events of the light-tissue interaction (figure 1), but there are many others phenomena that can be explored by an optical technique. Light polarization, Raman scattering, lifetime fluorescence, phase coherence, non-linear effects, are some examples. All these effects can be used to form an optical image. Biological tissues, especially the skin, are considered turbid media, where the diffuse scattering is the most important optical event in the visible range, i.e., the incident photons have multiple scattering before they are absorbed. Biological fluorophores will emit fluorescence in several directions, and these fluorescent photons will scattered and can also be absorbed by other chromophores. Tissue native fluorescence will result from the contribution of all fluorophores present in the interrogated tissue. This detected tissue fluorescence is also influenced by the presence and concentration of absorbers and scatterers. The influence of absorbance and structural tissue properties is even more relevant whereas the collected fluorescence is obtained at the tissue surface result from the exiting photons.

The main endogenous fluorophores are tryptophan, nicotinamide adenine dinucleotide (NADH), flavin adenine dinucleotide (FAD), collagen, elastin, and keratin. Main absorbers non-fluorescent are hemoglobin and melanin; and the scatterers are the cell membrane, organelles, and collagen fibers, that indirectly modifies the intensity and shape of the fluorescence collected spectrum. For the imaging widefield devices, the most important light-tissue interactions are the fluorescence and diffuse reflectance (de Veld, et al. 2005).

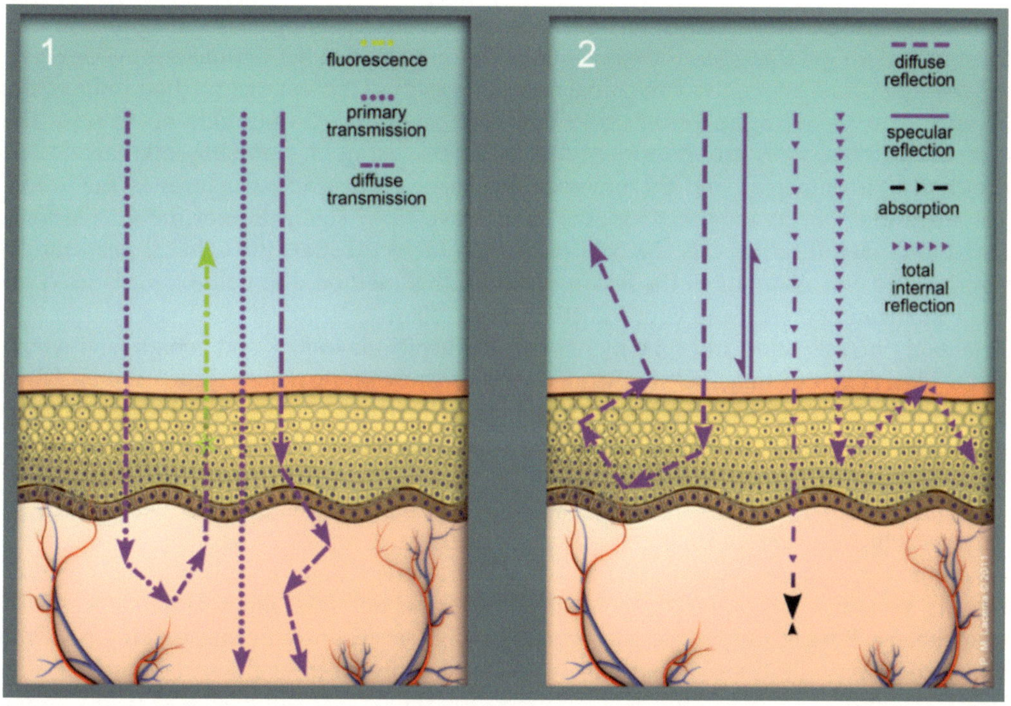

Fig. 1. Main optical events that occur when a light beam is incident to the skin surface. These schematic diagrams are illustrative for single photo pathways.

During neoplastic progression, the optical properties of both superficial epithelium and underlying stroma are altered. Optical effects like reflectance and fluorescence are considerably modified during the time evolution of the lesion. The perceived loss of fluorescence in dysplatic and malignant tissues compared to normal tissues has been mainly attributed to decreasing collagen signal from the stroma, due to fiber crosslink breakdown. Reflectance analysis, that is the analysis of the diffuse scattering, can detect local tissue changes in scattering and absorption properties. Absorption is affected by changes in some endogenous cromophores, blood content and tissue oxygenation, which are related to altered tissue metabolism and neovascularization presented at carcinomas (Gillenwater, et al. 2008, Kwasniak and Garcia-Zuazaga 2011).

Optical imaging can be performed at cellular level (microscopy) or tissue level (widefield). The advantage of the microscopy imaging is the evaluation of cellular characteristics, but in a small fraction of the lesion volume. Widefield imaging allows the examination of large areas and has the potential of improving detection of occult lesions, margin delimitation, and of guiding biopsy site determination. Distinct optical techniques offer different tissue/cellular information that is complimentary, but widefield optical imaging may represent the best option for cancer screening due to the possibility of analysis of large areas with fast response and less inter-operator variance (Laine, et al. 2008).

3. Clinical procedures

Nowadays, conventional examination for skin cancer screening is based on the visualization provided by a dermatoscope, a well-established modality in Dermatology.

Dermatoscopy (or dermoscopy or epiluminescence microscopy) uses a magnifying lens through an oil/gel interface, the conventional immersion contact dermatoscopy, or cross-polarizing optical filters, the non-contact dermatoscopy. This last one method reduces the amount of reflected light, resulting in the visualization of deeper skin structures. The clinical features that are important for analysis using a dermatoscope are color, dimensions (symmetry), and the presence or absence of certain structures in the lesion. The main idea of this diagnostic tool is to improve the visualization of the skin lesions, based on magnification, so the physician can detect better the clinical features to discriminate and distinguish the lesion types. In this method, the white light is used for this visualization (Ferris and Divito 2010, Tanaka 2006).

Total body investigation and time monitoring of suspicious lesions and benign nevi would be the ideal skin screening, but this is unpractical because of the required clinical time. Some studies have showed improved early detection of melanoma when the dermatoscopy is associated with time series photography. The disadvantage of this method, concerning health policies, is the high cost that is around thousands US$ per person. Incidence of new and changed nevi and melanomas detected using baseline images and dermoscopy in patients at high risk for melanoma (Banky, et al. 2003).

When the clinician detects a lesion, its visual characteristics as color, architecture, texture, and its palpation are carefully evaluated under white light illumination, the ABCD (Asymmetry, Border, Color, Diameter) rule. If malignant features are suspected, a biopsy is indicated to provide tissue sample for histological analysis, the golden standard for skin cancer diagnostics. In the cases of punch biopsies, the biopsy site is chosen based on the individual clinician criteria to determine the more representative area of the lesion. This procedure is highly subjective and variable comparing dermatologists with distinct experience and training (Kittler, et al. 2011, Bono, et al. 1999). The biopsy is indicated when the clinician recognizes clinical features that are potential indicatives of a malignant condition. At non-homogenous and extent lesions, the biopsy site determination may not be simple. It is not unusual that a lesion shows distinct histological patterns, as different dysplasia degrees, carcinoma *in situ*, and even invasive carcinoma. As a result, the chosen lesion sample may not be representative, and initial carcinoma can be missed. On the other hand, multiple biopsies at once are not well accepted by the patient, since it is an invasive procedure. After tissue removal, the material is sent to a laboratory for processing and analysis by a pathologist. This method takes time and cannot be performed *in situ*, and besides the fresh frozen tissue protocol for resected specimens, the pathology result is usually obtained only after a few days (Patel, et al. 2008).

4. Optical systems for aid in skin cancer diagnostics

Visual examination and the methods of the last section relies heavily on the experience and skills of the physician to identify and delineate premalignant and early cancer changes, which is not simple due to the similar clinical characteristics compared to the more common benign lesions. Gold standard diagnostics is obtained only after a tissue sample removal and processing for microscopic evaluation and its classification based on morphological characteristics at cellular level.

Enhancing the visual contrast between normal and altered skin has the potential to contribute for biopsy site determination, as well as for lesion margin delimitation before surgical resection. Optical widefield imaging has been presented as an attractive technique for this purpose (Marcon, et al. 2007, Ramanujam 2000, Marghoob, et al. 2003). Main advantages are a non-invasive and objective in situ procedure with real time response and a potential technique to the identification of occult lesions under the conventional with light examination (Carli, et al. 2001, Bono, et al. 2002, Braun, et al. 2002, MacKie, et al. 2002, McGovern 2003).

There are several optical imaging systems with direct visualization (naked eye) or visualization through electronic devices. Both methodologies allow the visualization of fluorescence and/or reflectance. When a set of images of the same skin location is taken at different spectral bands (reflectance and/or fluorescence); the result can be a multispectral or hiperspectral image. The difference between a multispectral or hiperspectral image is the number of images acquired. A multispectral imaging is a technique with a promising potential for *in vivo* skin diagnostics. Fluorescence usually has as tissue targets the NADH/FAD from the epithelial cells, and the collagen at the stroma. Reflectance using different excitation wavelength will focused on the absorption by specific chromospheres mainly hemoglobin and melanin.

There are some multispectral systems, acquiring reflectance images (RL) with several excitation wavelengths, or fluorescence images (FL) with several excitation/emission wavelengths (Dhawan, et al. 2009, Carrara, et al. 2005, Kapsokalyvas, et al. 2009). More recently, a few systems with combination of both modalities have been used and proposed for the diagnostics of skin cancer (Pratavieira, et al. 2009) and other cancer types as oral (Roblyer, et al. 2009), and cervical (Benavides, et al. 2003, Agrawal, et al. 2001). Individual analysis of fluorescence, narrowband reflectance or white light image may not be sufficient for the final discrimination, characterization, and classification of the lesion. Combining information from different imaging modalities has the potential of revealing tissue features resulting in an improved diagnostic performance, due to their distinct provided information. In table 1 we present the most important tissue information provided by each imaging modality.

Several commercial systems are available: Dermlite (3Gen, LLC, Dana Point, CA, U.S.A.), Dyaderm (Biocam GmbH, Regensburg, Germany), Dermascope (AMD Telemedicine, Elizabeth, NJ, U.S.A.), MelaFind (Electro-Optical Sciences, Irvington, NY, U.S.A.), Molemax (Derma Medical Systems, Vienna, Austria), Microderm (Visiomed Comp.,Bochum, Germany), Multiderm (Light4tech, Scandicci, Fi, Italy), Nevoscope (Translite LLC, Sugar Land, TX, U.S.A.), Siascopy (Astron Clinica, Cambridge, UK), SolarScan (Polartechnics Ltd, Sydney, Australia), and many others. All have been specifically designed for the detection/interpretation of skin lesions. Some of those commercial imaging systems are multispectral.

Image Modality:	*Tissue information by optical detection:*
FL, ME=400nm	Fluorescence of Collagen, Elastin, NADH, and Flavins.
RL ME=400nm	Absorption of Collagen, Elastin, NADH, and Flavins.
RL ME=530nm	Absorption of hemoglobin, morphology and identification of blood vessels.
RL ME=630nm	Observation of scatter structures and surface texture.
RL ME=470nm	Absorption of keratin and melanin.
RL White Light	Global analysis.

Table 1. Most relevant tissue information for cancer diagnostics provided by some optical modalities.

The image, in general, can be obtained placing the instrument in contact with the skin, where the surface reflection of light is reduced by either an oil-glass interface at the skin or through cross-polarization setup to remove the specular reflectance before forming the image. Other systems do not have any contact with the interrogated skin. Some limitations of the widefield fluorescence image are very limited interrogation depth, photobleaching of biomolecules, and high signal background. The main advantages are lower instrumentation cost, when compared to others optical techniques, and with potential portable and friendly-use systems.

In figure 2 an example of this instrumentation is presented. This system was assembled by our group, this is based on light emitting diodes (LED) illumination for reflectance modality at red, green and blue (RGB) spectrum and white light, and for fluorescence modality at 400 nm excitation (Pratavieira, et al. 2009). The main optical components a widefield fluorescence system are presented at figure 2, the light source, some lens and filters to remove the backscattering light at the excitation wavelength and the detection mode. For the detection, the visualization can be performed directly with the naked eye, or it can be digitalized and saved as an image by a conventional digital camera or a CCD. Besides the LED illumination other sources can be also chose as a lamp or laser.

When the image is digitalized, a mathematical processing, using computational algorithm, can be performed for image segmentation. The segmentation performed may be helpful for enhancing lesion discrimination, in choosing the biopsy site and in the delimitation of lesion margins, aiding in surgical resection. Also this technique provides a quantitative and less subjective analysis of the image, compared to only its visualization. The computational algorithm may vary from simple image addition or/and subtraction, the widely accepted ABCD (Asymmetry, Border, Color, Diameter) rule when comparing skin lesions against the database, until advanced texture analysis using fractal geometry (Schaefer, et al. 2011, Tasoulis, et al. 2010, Ogorzalek, et al. 2009).

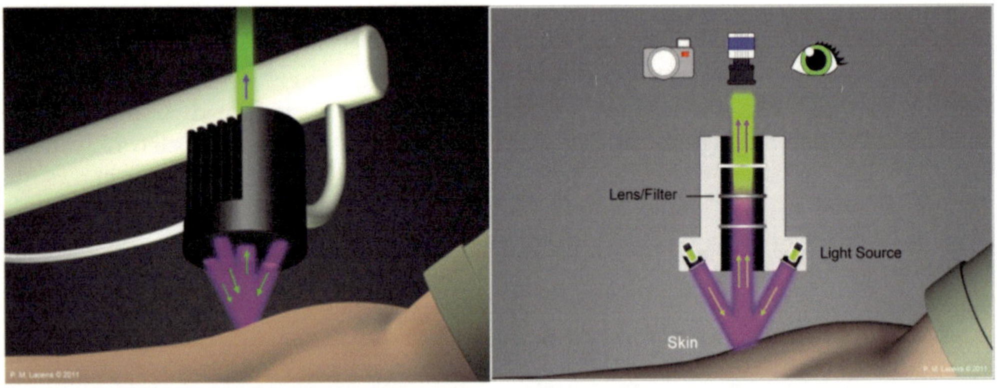

Fig. 2. Possible configuration of an image system. The light interacts with the skin and is re-emitted. The emission can be magnified by lens and the colors selected by optical filters. The visualization can be performed by a camera or naked eye.

Fluorescence imaging can also be performed using an exogenous component for increasing contrast between lesion and normal skin. In this case, the fluorescence analysis is not based on the contribution of the endogenous biomolecules present in the lesion, but on the presence of a fluorescent marker with enhanced concentration at the malignant cells. The most common technique is the previous topical application of a 15-20% aminolevulinic acid (ALA) or metil-ALA cream, a pro-drug for photodynamic therapy. ALA or Me-ALA enhances the cellular production of protoporphyrin IX (PpIX), a fluorescent biomolecule. When the pretreated tissue with ALA or Me-ALA is visualized with widefield fluorescence imaging, a strong red fluorescence, originated from the produced PpIX, lesions discrimination is improved. This technique is known as photodynamic detection (Hewett, et al. 2000, Orenstein, et al. 1998, Hewett, et al. 2001).

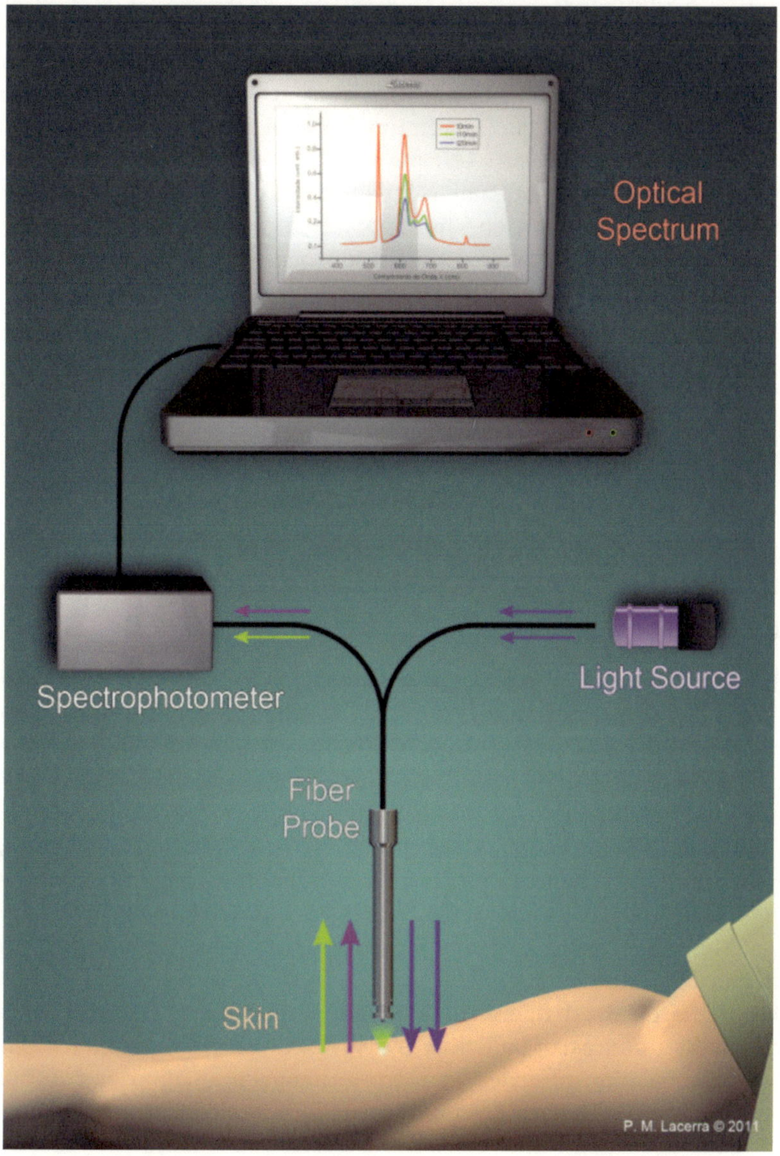

Fig. 3. Typical configuration of a spectroscopy system, the light is emitted by a lamp, laser or a LED. The light is guided by the optical fiber to the skin. The re-emmited light is analyzed at a spectrometer, which shows the intensity light emitted at each wavelength.

Another commonly investigated technique is the point spectroscopy by fluorescence (FL) and/or reflectance (RL), with single or multiple wavelengths. In this case, the result is not an image, but a graph showing the spectral information present at the re-emitted light. The spectroscopy methods show good specificity and sensitivity on cancer discrimination however, the obtained information is punctual, which makes the analysis difficult for large areas and the diagnostics is dependent on and specific for the interrogated site. Point spectroscopy uses optical fibers that deliver the excitation light to the tissue surface and collect the re-emitted light. Depending on the spectrometer and optical design, fluorescence or reflectance is investigated. The result showed after this optical measurement is a graph with the emitted light intensity as a function of the wavelength (Sterenborg, et al. 1994, Utz, et al. 1994, Kollias, et al. 2000, Ramanujam 2000, Panjehpour, et al. 2002, Panjehpour, et al. 2002). In figure 3 a typical configuration of this setup is presented.

Microscopy imaging is another punctual technique. For skin investigation, common systems are confocal scanning microscopy, and multiphoton tomography, where a laser is used to excite the skin fluorophores, or scatterers components. For one or two photon excitation some commercial system are available such as Lucid's VivaScope (Rochester, NY, U.S.A.), and DermaInspect (JenLab GmbH, Jena, Germany). This technique has a great advantage in comparison with the others (widefield, spectroscopy) because in this method, the image resolution is at cellular level. For some instrumentation, the cellular and tissue features may be similar to what is visualized by histological slides. Characteristics used for conventional diagnostics as cellular shape, nuclei structure and tissue organization may be also obtained. The microscopy images has the advantage of very high resolution, very low out-of-focus signal, but the main limitation is still the high cost (Roberts, et al. 2011, Koehler, et al. 2011, Garbe, et al. 2011, Breunig, et al. 2010).

5. Widefield fluorescence image in skin cancer diagnostics

In this section, we are going to present a widefield fluorescence device assembled by our group and some of the images taken at patients with skin lesions. The illumination device is based on an array of two LEDs composing an UV-blue range light. This spectral region was chosen for its already well-known use to excite endogenous fluorophores at skin. Light intensity is around 50 mW/cm^2. A handheld device enclose the illumination part and also the optical components to provide fluorescence imaging: a dichroic mirror, a longpass filter to remove the light at excitation wavelengths, and another filter to remove the yellow spectral range. This set of filters allows the fluorescence viewing in the green and red range (Costa, et al. 2010). A schematic diagram of the configuration of the widefield fluorescence image is presented at figure 4.

An example of the obtained fluorescence image is showed at figure 5. A basocellular carcinoma lesion at a Caucasian patient was visualized using the system. The comparison between the discrimination provided at a white light illumination and the fluorescence imaging can be observed. The cancer lesion is usually visualized at the fluorescence image as a darker region, correlated with the less tissue fluorescence, mainly due to the changes on collagen structure induced by the carcinoma progression. The tumor margins can be better discriminate using the fluorescence, the contrast between lesion and normal tissue is enhanced.

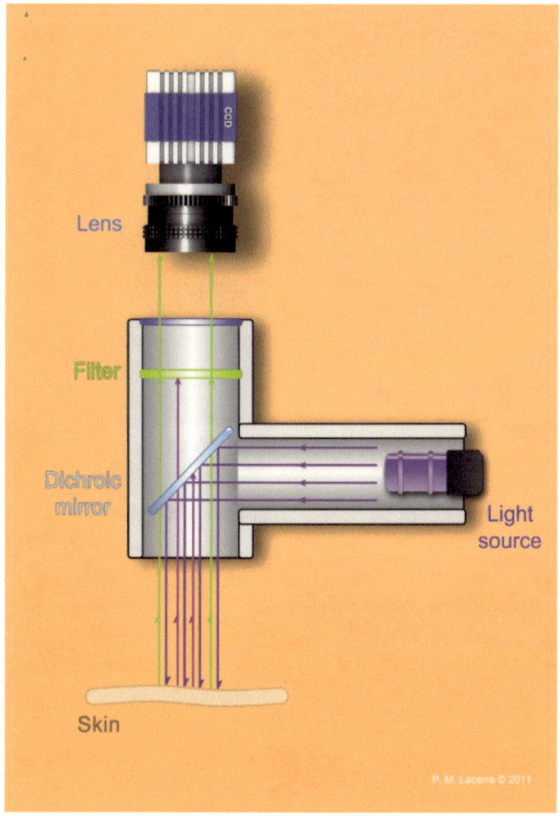

Fig. 4. Configuration of the fluorescence imaging device used.

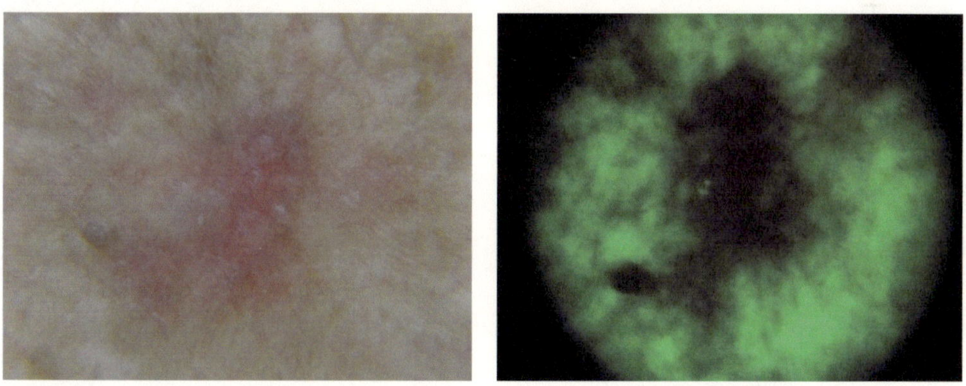

Fig. 5. Basocellular carcinoma under white light illumination (left hand picture) and visualized using the widefield fluorescence modality (right hand picture).

Another important issue in skin diagnostics is the lesion discrimination between melanoma and seborrheic keratosis. At conventional white light illumination, without magnification, both lesions may appear similar. The fluorescence widefield imaging has the potential to overcome this problem. In figure 6 and 7, we present the examination of two patients, one with a seborrheic keratosis (fig.6) and another with melanoma. At white light illumination the clinical features may appear similar for a not well trained physician, but at the fluorescence image the discrimination is evident due to the presence of the corneal pseudocists. All pigmented lesions show low fluorescence compared to the normal skin, and at seborrheic keratosis, the corneal pseudocists are evident due to its high fluorescence emission.

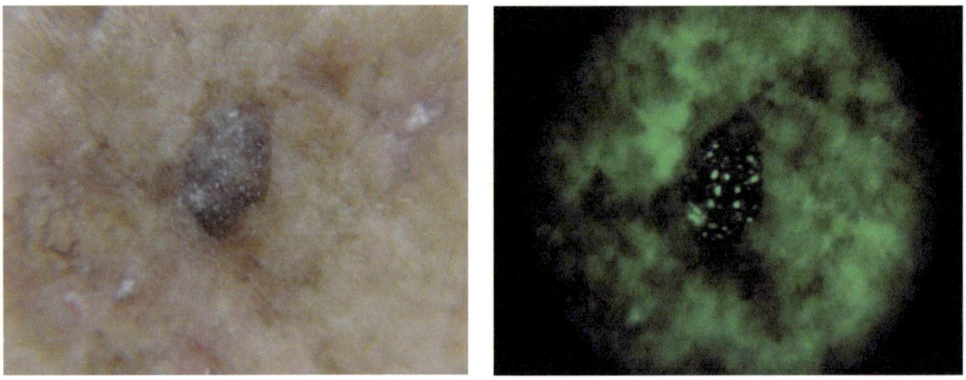

Fig. 6. Seborrheic keratosis under white light illumination (left hand picture) and at fluorescence imaging visualization (right hand picture).

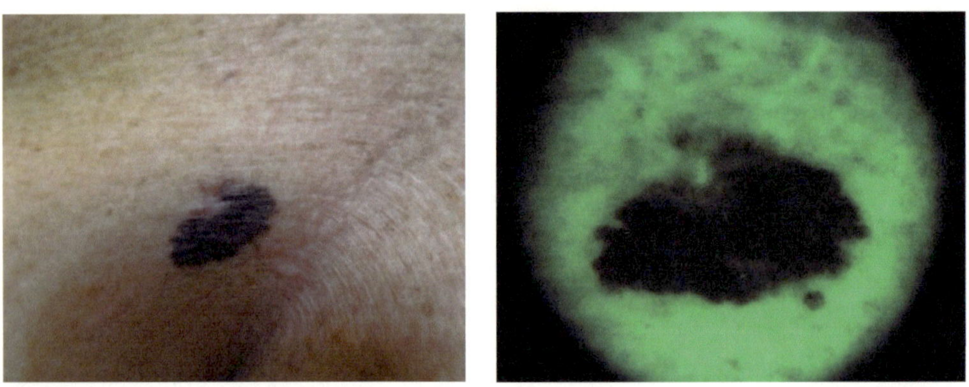

Fig. 7. Melanoma under white light illumination (left hand picture) and at fluorescence imaging visualization (right hand picture).

To improve the contrast visualization of tumor imaging using fluorescence, a biomarker can be used, such as protoporphyrin IX (PpIX), which is a photosensitizer that occurs in cells, but at low levels. In the example showed at figure 8, the basocellular carcinoma lesion was pre-treated with a topical application of a 10% ALA solution. Sixty minutes after, a high concentration of PpIX production is observed at the lesion and not at the surrounding normal cells. This photodynamic optical diagnostics may be useful for the detection of occult lesions, but the efficacy of this indication needs still to be defined.

To show the potential use of the photodynamic diagnostics to aid in the differentiation of benign and malignant lesions, the same protocol was used for the investigation of a nevi. As it is showed at figure 9, no PpIX production is observed.

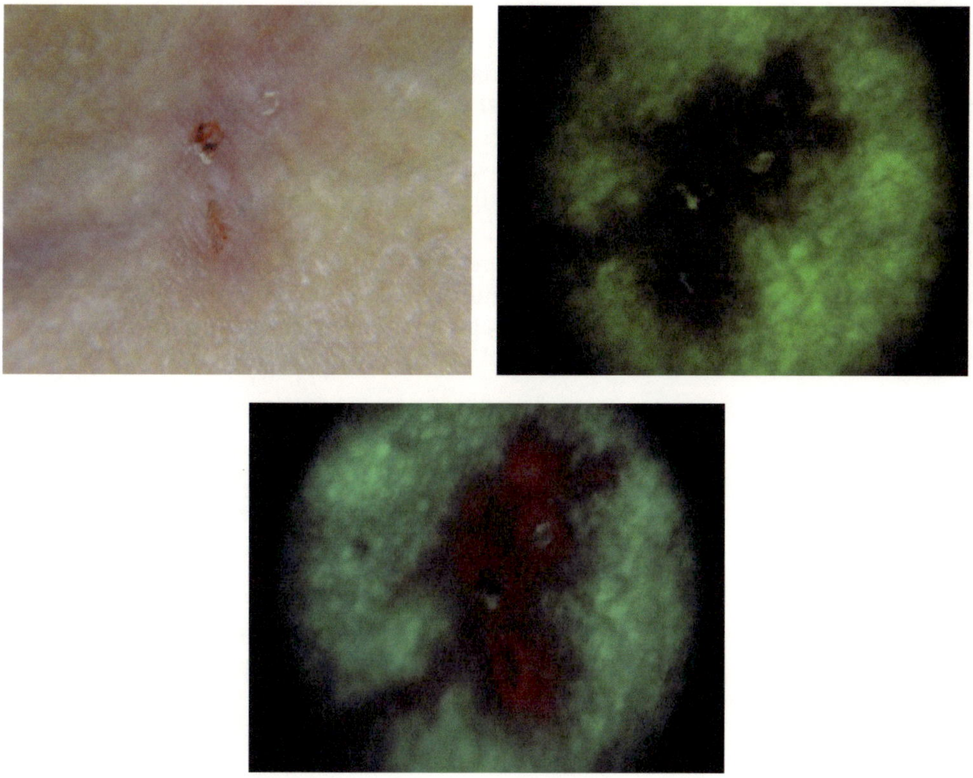

Fig. 8. Basocellular carcinoma under white light illumination (upper left hand picture), visualized using the widefield fluorescence modality (upper right hand picture), and under photodynamic diagnostic image using ALA (lower picture).

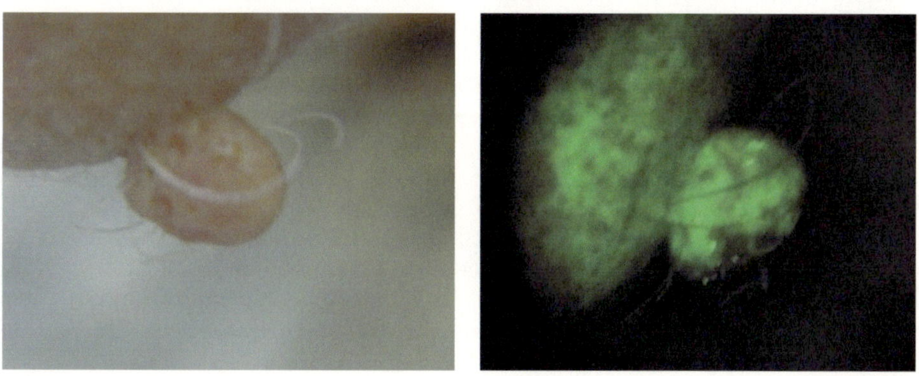

Fig. 9. Nevi under white light (right hand picture) and the photodynamic diagnostic image using ALA (left hand picture).

Photodynamic diagnostics does not show satisfactory results for hyperkeratinized lesions, since the keratin layer is a physical barrier for ALA penetration, and so the induction of PpIX production does occur properly. For these lesions, it is recommended a superficial lesion curettage before ALA solution application.

6. Conclusion

Several optical modalities, including spectroscopy and imaging techniques, have been presented as potential tools to improve cancer diagnostics. Widefield fluorescence imaging is the most attractive technique for skin cancer screening. Tissue fluorescence has correlated information of biochemical and structural features, which can be used for discrimination of normal and tumor tissues. Some examples of fluorescence images obtained by a homemade device were presented, showing a better discrimination of basocellular carcinoma and melanoma lesions based on tissue autofluorescence. Clinical studies must be performed to determine the efficacy of the optical techniques for the skin cancer diagnostics, based on specificity and sensitivity rates. We believe that the optical technologies have great potential to become important auxiliary tools for clinical examination of skin.

7. Acknowledgments

The authors acknowledge the support provided by CNPq (INOF - INCT Program), FAPESP (CEPOF - CEPID Program and S.P. scholarship) and CAPES scholarship.

8. References

Agrawal, A., T. Harrell, S. Bambot, M. Faupel, and D. Ferris. Multimodal Multispectral Imaging of the Cervix in Vivo for the Detection of Neoplasia. *Biomarkers and Biological Spectral Imaging,* 2, no. 16 (2001): 68-74.

Banky, J. P., D. English, J. W. Yeatman, J. P. Dowling, and J. W. Kelly. Incidence of New and Changed Melanocytic Naevi and Melanoma Detected Using Baseline Images in a Population at Increased Risk for Melanoma. *British Journal of Dermatology,* 149 (Jul 2003): 105-05.

Bauer, J., P. Buttner, H. Luther, T. S. Wiecker, M. Mohrle, and C. Garbe. Blue Light Phototherapy of Neonatal Jaundice Does Not Increase the Risk for Melanocytic Nevus Development. *Arch Dermatol,* 140, no. 4 (Apr 2004): 493-4.

Benavides, J. M., S. Chang, S. Y. Park, R. Richards-Kortum, N. Mackinnon, C. MacAulay, A. Milbourne, A. Malpica, and M. Follen. Multispectral Digital Colposcopy for in Vivo Detection of Cervical Cancer. *Optics Express,* 11, no. 10 (May 19 2003): 1223-36.

Bono, A., C. Bartoli, N. Cascinelli, M. Lualdi, A. Maurichi, D. Moglia, G. Tragni, S. Tomatis, and R. Marchesini. Melanoma Detection - a Prospective Study Comparing Diagnosis with the Naked Eye, Dermatoscopy and Telespectrophotometry. *Dermatology,* 205, no. 4 (2002): 362-66.

Bono, A., S. Tomatis, C. Bartoli, G. Tragni, G. Radaelli, A. Maurichi, and R. Marchesini. The Abcd System of Melanoma Detection - a Spectrophotometric Analysis of the Asymmetry, Border, Color, and Dimension. *Cancer,* 85, no. 1 (Jan 1 1999): 72-77.

Braun, R. P., H. Rabinovitz, M. Oliviero, A. W. Kopf, J. H. Saurat, and L. Thomas. Dermatoscopy of Pigmented Lesions. *Annales De Dermatologie Et De Venereologie,* 129, no. 2 (Feb 2002): 187-202.

Breunig, H. G., H. Studier, and K. Konig. Multiphoton Excitation Characteristics of Cellular Fluorophores of Human Skin in Vivo. *Optics Express,* 18, no. 8 (Apr 12 2010): 7857-71.

Carli, P., V. De Giorgi, and B. Giannotti. Dermoscopy and Early Diagnosis of Melanoma - the Light and the Dark. *Archives of Dermatology,* 137, no. 12 (Dec 2001): 1641-44.

Carrara, M., S. Tomatis, A. Bono, C. Bartoli, D. Moglia, M. Lualdi, A. Colombo, M. Santinami, and R. Marchesini. Automated Segmentation of Pigmented Skin Lesions in Multispectral Imaging. *Phys Med Biol,* 50, no. 22 (Nov 21 2005): N345-57.

Costa, M. M. ;, C. ; Kurachi, V. S. ; Bagnato, and L. Ventura. "Development of an Optical Fluorescence Imaging System for Medical Use." Paper presented at the 19th International Laser Physics Workshop, 2010, Foz do Iguaçu. BOOK OF ABSTRACTS, 2010. p. 123-123., 2010.

de Veld, D. C. G., M. Skurichina, M. J. H. Wities, R. P. W. Duin, H. J. C. M. Sterenborg, and J. L. N. Roodenburg. Autofluorescence and Diffuse Reflectance Spectroscopy for Oral Oncology. *Lasers Surg Med,* 36, no. 5 (Jun 2005): 356-64.

Dhawan, A. P., B. D'Alessandro, S. Patwardhan, and N. Mullani. Multispectral Optical Imaging of Skin-Lesions for Detection of Malignant Melanomas. *Conf Proc IEEE Eng Med Biol Soc,* 2009 (2009): 5352-5.

Ferris, L. K., and S. J. Divito. Advances and Short Comings in the Early Diagnosis of Melanoma. *Melanoma Research,* 20, no. 6 (Dec 2010): 450-58.

Garbe, C., D. Leupold, M. Scholz, G. Stankovic, J. Reda, S. Buder, R. Eichhorn, *et al.* The Stepwise Two-Photon Excited Melanin Fluorescence Is a Unique Diagnostic Tool for the Detection of Malignant Transformation in Melanocytes. *Pigment Cell & Melanoma Research,* 24, no. 3 (Jun 2011): 438-45.

Gillenwater, A., I. Pavlova, M. Williams, A. El-Naggar, and R. Richards-Kortum. Understanding the Biological Basis of Autofluorescence Imaging for Oral Cancer Detection: High-Resolution Fluorescence Microscopy in Viable Tissue. *Clinical Cancer Research,* 14, no. 8 (Apr 15 2008): 2396-404.

Hewett, J., T. McKechnie, and W. Sibbett. Fluorescence Detection of Superficial Skin Cancers. *Journal of Modern Optics,* 47, no. 11 (Sep 2000): 2021-27.

Hewett, J., V. Nadeau, J. Ferguson, H. Moseley, S. Ibbotson, L. Brancaleon, D. Birkin, W. Sibbett, and M. Padgett. Multispectral Monitoring of Fluorescence During Ala-Pdt of Superficial Skin Cancers. *Optical Methods for Tumor Treatment and Detection: Mechanisms and Techniques in Photodynamic Therapy X,* 2, no. 5 (2001): 68-75.

Kapsokalyvas, D., N. Bruscino, G. Cannarozzo, V. de Giorgi, T. Lotti, and F. S. Pavone. Multispectral Dermoscope. *Clinical and Biomedical Spectroscopy,* 7368 (2009).

Karagas, M. R., J. A. McDonald, E. R. Greenberg, T. A. Stukel, J. E. Weiss, J. A. Baron, and M. M. Stevens. Risk of Basal Cell and Squamous Cell Skin Cancers after Ionizing Radiation Therapy. For the Skin Cancer Prevention Study Group. *J Natl Cancer Inst,* 88, no. 24 (Dec 18 1996): 1848-53.

Kittler, H., C. Rosendahl, P. Tschandl, C. Med, and A. Cameron. Diagnostic Accuracy of Dermatoscopy for Melanocytic and Nonmelanocytic Pigmented Lesions. *Journal of the American Academy of Dermatology,* 64, no. 6 (Jun 2011): 1068-73.

Koehler, M. J., M. Speicher, S. Lange-Asschenfeldt, E. Stockfleth, S. Metz, P. Elsner, M. Kaatz, and K. Konig. Clinical Application of Multiphoton Tomography in Combination with Confocal Laser Scanning Microscopy for in Vivo Evaluation of Skin Diseases. *Experimental Dermatology,* 20, no. 7 (Jul 2011): 589-94.

Kollias, N., R. Gillies, G. Zonios, and R. R. Anderson. Fluorescence Excitation Spectroscopy Provides Information About Human Skin in Vivo. *Journal of Investigative Dermatology,* 115, no. 4 (Oct 2000): 704-07.

Kwasniak, L. A., and J. Garcia-Zuazaga. Basal Cell Carcinoma: Evidence-Based Medicine and Review of Treatment Modalities. *International Journal of Dermatology,* 50, no. 6 (Jun 2011): 645-58.

Laine, A. F., A. R. Kherlopian, T. Song, Q. Duan, M. A. Neimark, M. J. Po, and J. K. Gohagan. A Review of Imaging Techniques for Systems Biology. *Bmc Systems Biology,* 2 (Aug 12 2008).

MacKie, R. M., C. Fleming, A. D. McMahon, and P. Jarrett. The Use of the Dermatoscope to Identify Early Melanoma Using the Three-Colour Test. *British Journal of Dermatology,* 146, no. 3 (Mar 2002): 481-84.

Marcon, N. E., R. S. DaCosta, and B. C. Wilson. Fluorescence and Spectral Imaging. *Thescientificworldjournal,* 7 (2007): 2046-71.

Marghoob, A. A., L. D. Swindle, C. Z. Moricz, F. A. Sanchez Negron, B. Slue, A. C. Halpern, and A. W. Kopf. Instruments and New Technologies for the in Vivo Diagnosis of Melanoma. *J Am Acad Dermatol,* 49, no. 5 (Nov 2003): 777-97; quiz 98-9.

McGovern, V. Digital Diagnosis: New Tool for Detecting Skin Cancer. *Environ Health Perspect,* 111, no. 14 (Nov 2003): A770-3.

McLaren, J. R., A. J. Maruszczak, and Z. L. Olkowski. Short Term Effects of Ionizing Radiation on the Recurrent or Metastatic Skin Cancer--a Quantitative DNA Study. *Strahlentherapie,* 149, no. 2 (Feb 1975): 166-72.

Orenstein, A., G. Kostenich, C. Rothmann, Barshack I, and Z. Malik. Imaging of Human Skin Lesions Using Multipixel Fourier Transform Spectroscopy. *Lasers in Medical Science,* 13, no. 2 (1998): 112-18.

Panjehpour, M., C. E. Julius, M. N. Phan, T. Vo-Dinh, and S. Overholt. Laser-Induced Fluorescence Spectroscopy for in Vivo Diagnosis of Non-Melanoma Skin Cancers. *Lasers in Surgery and Medicine,* 31, no. 5 (2002): 367-73.

Panjehpour, M., C. Julius, M. N. Phan, T. Vo-Dinh, and S. Overholt. In Vivo Fluorescence Spectroscopy for Diagnosis of Skin Cancer. *Biomedical Diagnostic, Guidance, and Surgical-Assist Systems Iv,* 4615 (2002): 20-31.

Patel, J. K., S. Konda, O. A. Perez, S. Amini, G. Elgart, and B. Berman. Newer Technologies/Techniques and Tools in the Diagnosis of Melanoma. *European Journal of Dermatology,* 18, no. 6 (Nov-Dec 2008): 617-31.

Pratavieira, S., P. L. A. Santos, V. S. Bagnato, and C. Kurachi. "Development of a Widefield Reflectance and Fluorescence Imaging Device for the Detection of Skin and Oral Cancer." In *Photodynamic Therapy: Back to the Future.* Seattle: edited by David H. Kessel, Proceedings of SPIE Vol. 7380 (SPIE, Bellingham, WA 2009) 73805G, 2009.

Ramanujam, N. Fluorescence Spectroscopy of Neoplastic and Non-Neoplastic Tissues. *Neoplasia,* 2, no. 1-2 (Jan-Apr 2000): 89-117.

Roberts, MS Roberts, M. S., Y. Dancik, T. W. Prow, C. A. Thorling, L. L. Lin, J. E. Grice, T. A. Robertson, K. Konig, and W. Becker. Non-Invasive Imaging of Skin Physiology and Percutaneous Penetration Using Fluorescence Spectral and Lifetime Imaging with Multiphoton and Confocal Microscopy. *European Journal of Pharmaceutics and Biopharmaceutics,* 77, no. 3 (Apr 2011): 469-88.

Roblyer, D., C. Kurachi, A. M. Gillenwater, and R. Richards-Kortum. In Vivo Fluorescence Hyperspectral Imaging of Oral Neoplasia. *Advanced Biomedical and Clinical Diagnostic Systems Vii,* 7169 (2009).

Sterenborg, H. J. C. M., M. Motamedi, R. F. Wagner, M. Duvic, S. Thomsen, and S. L. Jacques. In-Vivo Fluorescence Spectroscopy and Imaging of Human Skin Tumors. *Lasers in Medical Science,* 9, no. 3 (Sep 1994): 191-201.

Tanaka, M. Dermoscopy. *Journal of Dermatology,* 33, no. 8 (Aug 2006): 513-17.

Utz, S. R., Y. P. Sinichkin, I. V. Meglinski, and H. A. Pilipenko. Fluorescence Spectroscopy in Combine with Reflectance Measurements in Human Skin Examination - What for and How. *Optical Biopsy and Fluorescence Spectroscopy and Imaging, Proceedings Of,* (1994): 125-36.

Part 3

Prevention and Therapy for Skin Cancer

8

Cyclooxygenase-2 Overexpression in Non-Melanoma Skin Cancer: Molecular Pathways Involved as Targets for Prevention and Treatment

Daniel H. González Maglio, Mariela L. Paz,
Eliana M. Cela and Juliana Leoni
University of Buenos Aires, Pharmacy and Biochemistry School
Argentina

1. Introduction

Non melanoma skin cancers (NMSCs) are the most frequent malignancies in humans (Geller & Annas, 2003). It comprises many different types of tumors, such as Squamous Cell Carcinoma (SCC) and Basal Cell Carcinoma (BCC), which are the main ones among the NMSCs. There are 100.000 new cases of these neoplasms per year in the UK (Aitken *et al.*, 2007) and about a millon in the US (Kuchide, 2003). NMSC incidence is estimated to increase in a 10% by 2060 -taking into account the Copenhagen Amendments scenario for protection of ozone layer- (Slaper *et al.*, 1996).

The development of both SCC and BCC implies a malignant transformation of keratinocytes, the most abundant cells in the epidermis. In addition to genetic factors, there are a variety of stimulus that can induce this transformation, like viral or bacterial infections and chemical agents (such as 7,12-dimethyl benzanthracene -DMBA- or Benzo[a]pyrene-7,8-diol-9,10-epoxide -B[a]PDE-), (Aubin *et al.*, 2003; Bouwes Bavinck *et al.*, 2001; Madan *et al.*, 2006). However, the most important carcinogen of the skin is the solar ultraviolet radiation (UVr), mainly the UVB component (280-310 nm), which is able to reach the earth surface (Armstrong & Kricker, 2001).

All of those carcinogens promote molecular and cellular changes, modifying different functions like cell cycle control or apoptotic cell death. In this way, the affected cells lose their capacity to regulate their proliferation properly and have the potential to generate an uncontrolled linage of cells, which may ultimately lead to tumor formation and growth.

There are many gene products that have been found to be involved in skin cancer development. Some of them are related to cell cycle -like cyclin D1- (Liang *et al.*, 2000), apoptosis -like Bax, Bcl-2, and others- or in both processes -like p53 and p21- (Coultas & Strasser, 2003; Murphy *et al.*, 2002). Additionally, skin UVB irradiation has been proven to induce an increment in the levels of a significant number of immune system mediators, such as tumor necrosis factor-α (TNF-α), interleukins 6 (IL-6), 10 (IL-10), 8 (IL-8), 4 (IL-4), prostaglandins (PGs), nitric oxide (NO) and vascular endothelial growth factor (VEGF), among others (Paz *et al.*, 2008; Trompezinski *et al.*, 2001). Some of these molecules are known to mediate an important outcome of UVB irradiation: immunosuppression. It has been vastly proved since Margaret Kripke's first description (Fisher & Kripke, 1977) that UVr-induced DNA damage is not sufficient to lead to skin cancer development; there must be a concomitant decrease in normal immunosurvillance (Aubin, 2003; Ullrich & Kripke, 1984). This immunosuppression is mainly mediated by IL-4, IL-10 and prostaglandin-E_2 (PGE_2) (Shreedhar *et al.*, 1998).

PGs -including PGE_2- and thromboxanes (TXs), are subproducts of key enzymes in the inflammatory response: cyclooxygenases (COXs). There are two isoforms described for COX: COX-1, which is constitutively expressed in many tissues and the inducible isoform COX-2, which is up-regulated under physiological and pathophysiological conditions.

The relationship between COX-2 over-expression and non-melanoma skin cancer development and progression has been very well documented and described. Along this chapter we will discuss different aspects concerning this relationship, including molecular pathways involved in COX-2 expression, cellular effects of COX-2 products and experimental treatments for non-melanoma skin cancer, which comprises the modulation of the COX-2 pathway.

2. Molecular pathways involved in COX-2 expression

COX-2 is a single copy gene, whose location was identified in chromosome 1 by a fluorescence in situ hybridization technique (locus 1q25.2-25.3) (Tay *et al.*, 1994). Its gene size is about 8 kb and it includes 10 exons with 9 introns, resulting in a primary mRNA of 4.5 kb. The expression of this gene, as it was mentioned before, is inducible. There are many factors which can contribute to the induction of COX-2 expression, including cytokines, growth factors, hormones and bacterial components.

2.1 COX-2 gene structure

COX-2 was first described in 1991 by Kujubu et al. (Kujubu *et al.*, 1991) as a primary response gene, which encodes an amino acid sequence sharing 61% of identity with the COX-1 gene, described in 1988 by Merlie et al. (Merlie *et al.*, 1988).

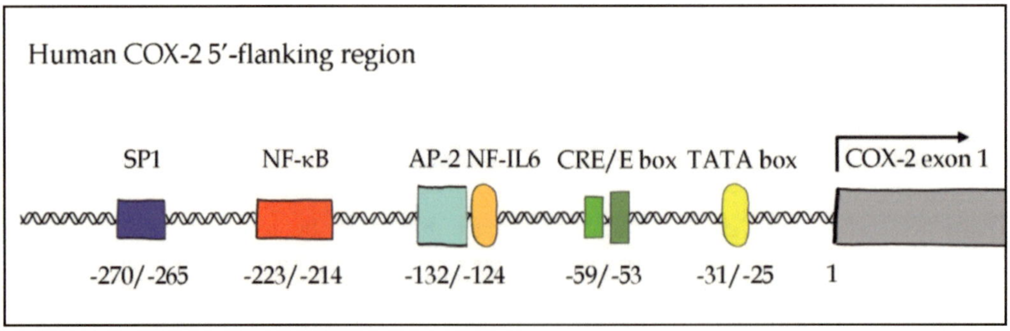

Fig. 1. Estructure of COX-2 gene regulatory region. Transcription regulatory elements are shown, their names (above) and upstream position (below with numbers) are indicated.

In 1995 Inoue et al. analyzed the sequence of the human COX-2 5'-flanking region, describing several transcription regulatory elements (Figure 1), which include a TATA box, a CRE motif, an E-box, a NF-IL6 motif, three Sp1 sites, two AP-2 sites and two NF-κB sites (Inoue *et al.*, 1995). Many animal COX-2 5'-flanking sequences have been characterized, exhibiting similar structures in mouse, horse, cow and rat.
All of these sequence elements have a potential role in the induction of the expression of COX-2. Some inducers and the molecular pathways involved in the activation of transcription factors, which finally lead to COX-2 expression, are described in the next section.

2.2 Stimulus and mechanisms involved in COX-2 expression

Prostaglandins and thromboxanes production are intimately related to inflammation, besides the fact that they produce a regulation of the overall inflammatory response (Ricciotti & FitzGerald, 2011). In this way, it is reasonable that many cytokines and molecules involved in the inflammatory process may play some role in the production of PGs and TXs. Certainly, TNF-α, IL-1 and Toll-like receptors agonists (like bacterial lipopolysaccharide -LPS-) can highly induce the expression of COX-2 gene in many cell types.
Besides the three mentioned molecules, there are other stimuli which are capable of inducing COX-2 expression. Other cytokines and different growth factors -like IL-6, EGF, FGF and PDGF- may lead to its expression (Tanabe & Tohnai, 2002). Keratinocytes, the most abundant cells in the skin, are a cell type that is particularly exposed to natural UVr. This stimulus is sufficient to induce the production of many inflammation-related molecules by the keratinocytes -such as TNF-α, IL-6 and COX-2 itself- among others (Paz *et al.*, 2008). Finally, there are many chemical agents used as tumor promoters (Lim *et al.*, 2011; Rundhaug *et al.*, 2007), which are able to induce the expression of COX-2.
There are two main molecular pathways involved in COX-2 expression (Figures 2 and 3). The first one includes the activation of a transcription factor (NF-κB, nuclear factor kappa B) and the second one involves the mitogen-activated protein kinases (MAPKs) cascade -with three subgroups: p38 MAPK, ERKs and JNK-.
NF-κB is normally inhibited by IκB binding; this inhibitor can be phosphorylated and degraded in the proteasome, releasing the nuclear factor to translocate to the nucleus and to start its transcriptional effects. In this pathway the trigger stimuli is related to the interaction of membrane receptors with their corresponding agonists, like TNF-α receptor (TNFR), IL-1 receptor (IL-1R) and Toll-like receptor 4 (TLR-4). As it is shown in Figure 2 there are several molecules involved in the pathway, relating the membrane receptors with the phosphorylation of IκB. TNFR recruits TRADD (TNFR-associated death domain protein), which recruits TRAF-2 (TNFR-associated factor 2), leading to the final common path: phosphorylation of NIK (NF-κB-inducing kinase), IKK (IκB kinase complex) and the final phosphorylation (and consequent inactivation) of IκB. The other side of this pathway comprises IL-1R and TLR-4. Both molecules use MyD88 (Myeloid differentiation factor 88) as a linker for the recruitment of IRAK (IL-1R-activated kinase) and the consequent phosphorylation of TRAF-6 (TNFR-associated factor 6), which leads to the same final common path above mentioned. Once released, NF-κB translocates to the nucleus activating the transcription of target genes, like COX-2.

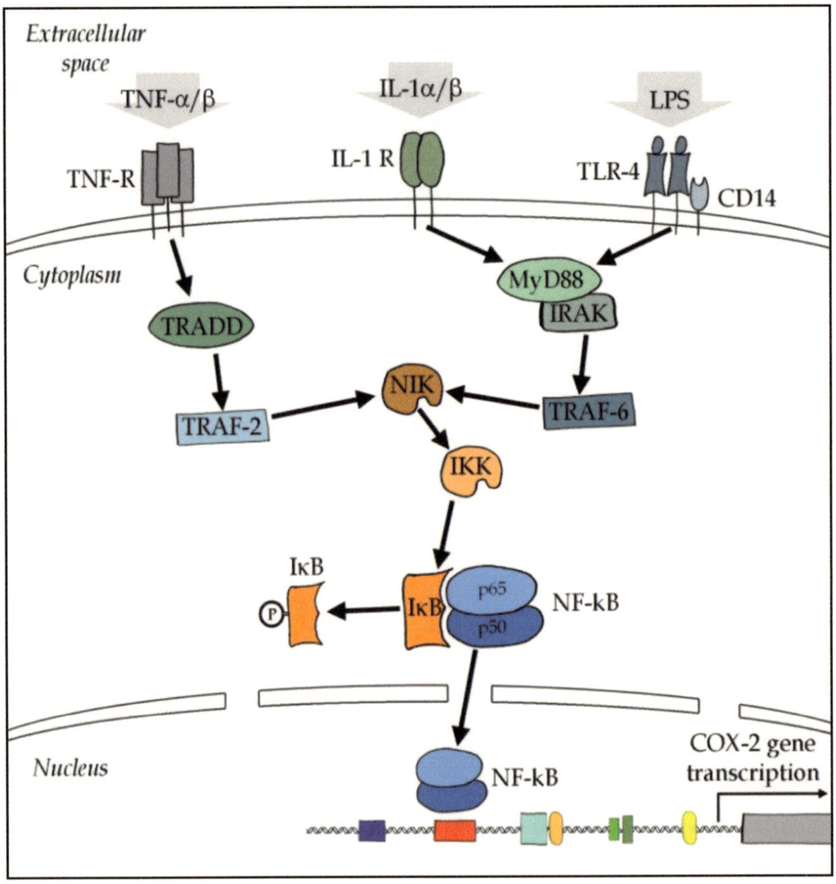

Fig. 2. Nuclear factor kappa B -NF-κB- molecular pathway. Membrane receptors with their corresponding agonists as trigger stimuli (grey arrows) are shown, also the different downstream molecules involved. The common final path, that leads to NF-κB activation and subsequent COX-2 expression, can also be seen. P: phosphorylated molecule.

MAPKs pathway includes a cascade of kinases with specific activity, each of them phosphorylates (and activates) the next kinase in the path, ultimately leading to the activation of transcription factors which promote the transcription of target genes. This pathway is one of the most significant in the activation of COX-2 expression and prostaglandins biosynthesis. JNK (c-Jun N-terminal kinase) and p38 MAPK share some of the activation stimuli -like proinflammatory cytokines and bacterial endotoxins- also environmental stressors, such as heat shock, oxidative stress and ultraviolet light (highly relevant in the development of skin cancer). On the other hand, ERKs (extracellular-regulated kinases) are mainly activated by growth factors and oncogenes, like Ras. As it is shown in Figure 3, the three MAPKs have individual upstream kinases involved in their activation (MAPK kinase). MKK-4/7 activate JNK, while MEK-1/2 activate ERKs and MKK-3/6 activate p38. MKKs and MEKs are known as MAPK kinases, and all of them are under the control of an upstream kinase (generally named as MAPKK kinase). MAPKK kinases are not specific, and in this step the pathways begin to crosslink. We describe only a few examples of these MAPKK kinases: the phosphorylation of MKK-4/7 by MEKK 1,

MEK-1/2 by Raf-1 (which in turn is activated by Ras oncogene) and MKK-3/6 by RIP. Besides these kinases, a family of proteins named SFKs -Src family kinases, including Fyn kinase- can directly activate MAPK kinases. Considering the beginning of the pathway, MAPKK kinases are activated by STE20 kinases or by GTP-binding proteins (Chang & Karin, 2001). Finally, at the end of the pathway MAPK activates transcription factors such as AP-1 (homodimers or heterodimers conformed by Jun, Fos, JDP and ATF families) leading to an increment in COX-2 expression. Another activated transcription factors can be C/EBPs, which play different roles in COX-2 expression, according to the cell type involved (Chun & Surh, 2004).

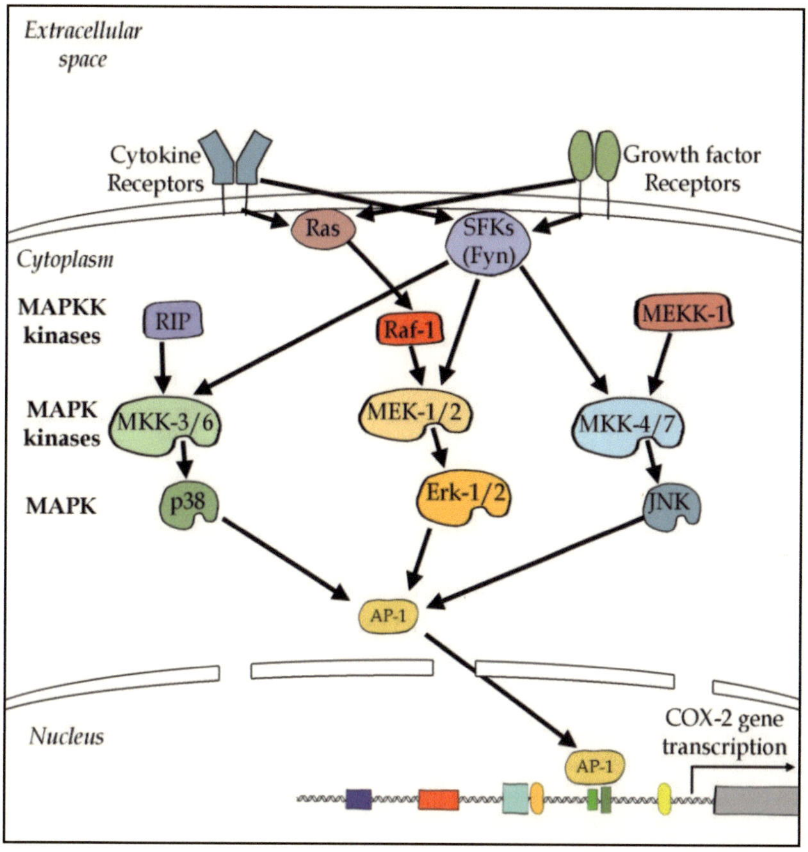

Fig. 3. Mitogen-activated protein kinases -MAPKs- molecular pathway. Membrane receptors which receive the trigger stimuli are shown, also the different downstream molecules involved and their crosslinks. This cascade includes kinases which phosphorylate and activate the next kinase. The common final path through the activation of the transcription factor AP-1, that finally leads to COX-2 expression, can also be seen.

In addition to the described mechanisms, there is an intense crosstalk between NF-κB and MAPKs pathways (Figure 4). For example, MEKK 1 and RIP are activated by TRAF-2 (Wu & Zhou, 2010) and MEKK 1 and JNK can be activated in LPS-treated macrophages through and adapter protein, named ECSIT (Kopp *et al.*, 1999). Besides, MEKK 1 is capable of phosphorylating IκB, releasing in this way an active NF-κB (Chun & Surh, 2004).

Finally, it is worth to notice that there are other pathways involved in the activation of NF-κB or MAPKs (Figure 4). For example, Phosphoinositol triphosphate (PIP_3, produced by active PI3K) activates Akt protein, which is able to phosphorilate IκB, therefore releasing active NF-κB (Ouyang *et al.*, 2006).

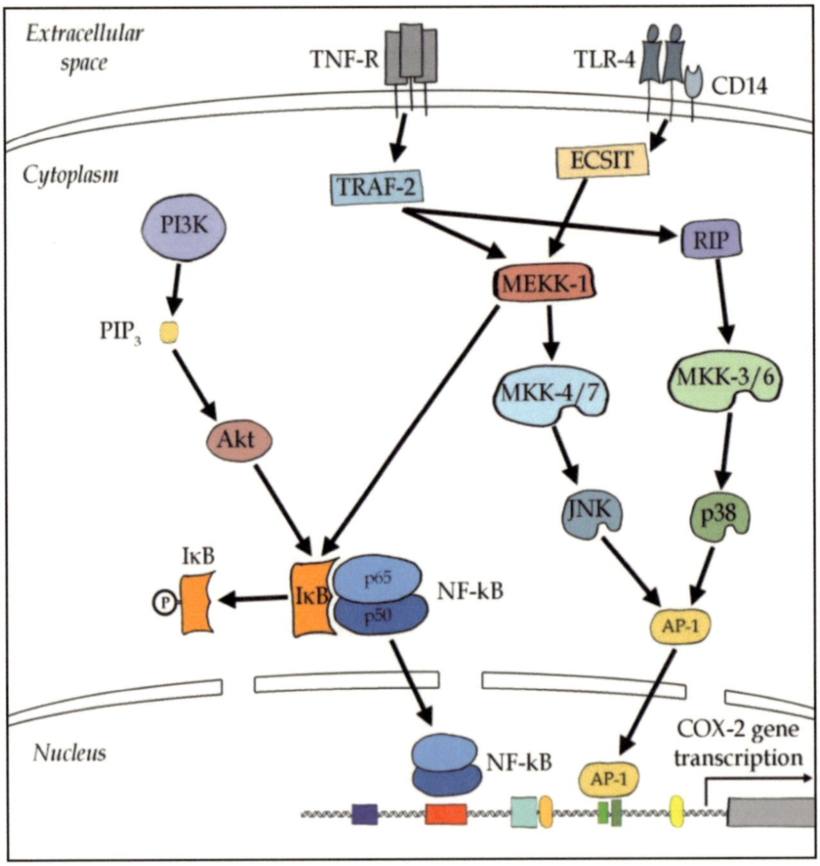

Fig. 4. Crosstalk between MAPKs, PIP_3 and NF-κB pathways. Membrane receptors, the different downstream molecules involved and their crosslinks are shown. The final path, which leads to COX-2 transcription and expression, can also be seen. P: phosphorylated molecule.

3. Molecular and cellular effects of COX-2 products

COXs -also known as PGH synthases- are the enzymes responsible for the conversion of arachidonic acid (AA) into PGH_2. AA is released from the cell membrane phospholipids by Phospholipase-A_2. AA conversion chemical reaction is catalyzed by the two enzymatic activities of COXs: cyclooxigenase (or bis-dioxygenase) activity generates a cyclopentane hydroperoxy endoperoxide (PGG_2) from AA. Peroxidase activity reduces the hydroperoxy group yielding the final product PGH_2 (Figure 5.a). PGH_2 by turns can be transform to different products (PGI_2 or prostacyclin, PGD_2, PGF_{2a}, PGE_2 and TXA_2) by specific synthases (Figure 5.b).

All of these AA-derived molecules, which play different roles in many physiological and pathophysiological mechanisms, have a short half-life *in vivo* (from seconds to minutes), performing its actions in an autocrine and paracrine fashion, rather than in an endocrine way (Ricciotti & FitzGerald, 2011).

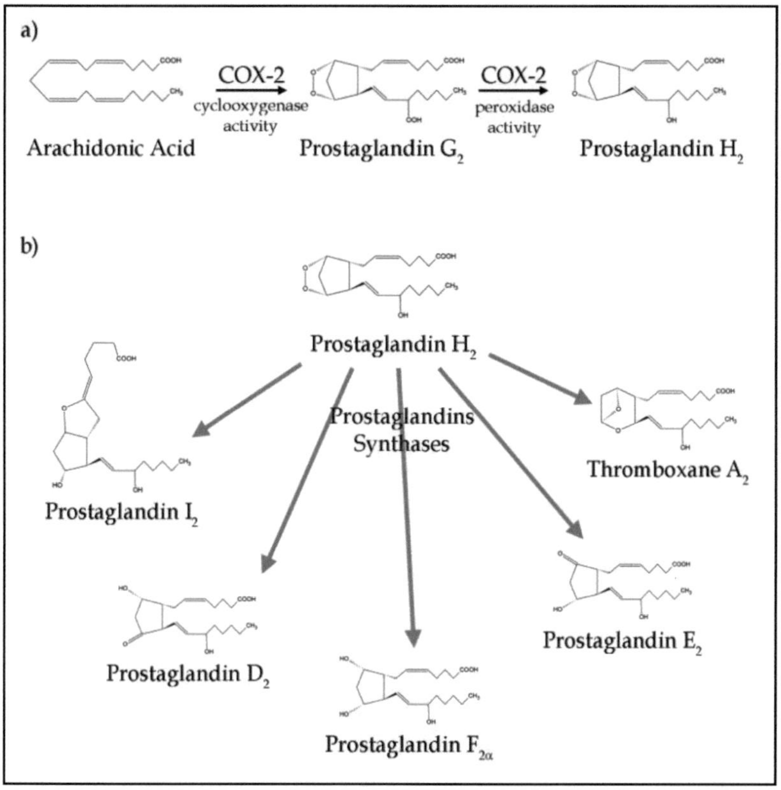

Fig. 5. Prostaglandins synthesis. a) Conversion of arachidonic acid -AA- into prostaglandin H_2 -PGH_2-, by the two enzymatic activities of COX-2. b) Conversion of PGH_2 into different final products, by specific synthases. The chemical structures and names of each product are shown.

3.1 Effects of PGE_2 on cell cycle and proliferation

Prostaglandins, particularly PGE_2, have been related to cell growth in some cell types. The role of PGE_2 has been widely described in keratinocytes, as a cell proliferation inducer. Indeed, it was described at the end of the 1970 decade, that there was an increase in the production of PGE_2 in a mouse model of epidermal hyperproliferation -induced by 12-O-tetradecanoylphorbol-13-acetate (TPA)- (Ashendel & Boutwell, 1979). In this TPA-induced proliferation model, keratinocyte growth was effectively blocked using the Non-Steroidal Anti-Inflammatory Drug indomethacin and successfully restored with an external supplementation of PGE_2 (Furstenberger *et al.*, 1979; Furstenberger & Marks, 1978). A few years later, Pentland described not only the capacity of keratinocytes to produce their own PGs from an external source of AA, but also the autocrine effects of these PGs on the cellular growth rate (Pentland & Needleman, 1986).

Interestingly, the final effect of PGE_2 in a specific cell type depends on the kind of receptor expressed in the target cell. There are four types of PGE_2 receptors, identified as E Prostanoid receptors 1 to 4 (EP_1-EP_4) (Narumiya *et al.*, 1999; Negishi *et al.*, 1993). These receptors are G-protein-coupled receptors which can activate different molecular pathways. EP_1 acts through the activation of Phospholipase C-β leading to an increase of intracellular calcium, while the other three receptors regulate adenylate cyclase activity. Meanwhile EP3 is able to down-regulate its activity, EP_2 and EP_4 can up-regulate it (Negishi *et al.*, 1995). Other PGs also exert their effects through G-protein-coupled receptor, according to Table 1.

Prostaglandin	Prostanoid Receptor Subtype	G-protein coupled	Molecular Effects
PGE_2	EP_1	G_q	↑IP_3
	EP_2	G_s	↑ cAMP
	EP_3	G_i, G_{12}, G_{Rho}	↓ cAMP, ↑ Ca^{2+}
	EP_4	G_s	↑ cAMP
PGD_2	DP	G_s	↑ cAMP
	CRTH2	G_i	↓ cAMP, ↑ Ca^{2+}
$PGF_{2\alpha}$	FP_A, FP_B	G_q, G_{Rho}	↑IP_3
PGI_2	IP-IP	G_s, G_q, G_i	↑ ↓ cAMP, ↑IP_3
	IP-TP_α	G_s	↑ cAMP
TxA_2	TP_α, TP_β	G_q, G_s, G_i, G_h, $G_{12/13}$	↑ Ca^{2+}, ↑ ↓ cAMP, ↑IP_3

Table 1. Molecular effects of prostaglandins –PGs-. The type of PG, subtype of prostanoid receptor involved, G-protein-coupled receptor activated and final molecular effect are shown. ↑: increase, ↓: decrease, ↑ ↓: both effects are possible.

Recently, in a study performed using primary mouse keratinocytes, Ansari et al. demonstrated that PGE_2 is capable of inducing an indirect phosphorilation of epidermal growth factor receptor (EGFR), leading to the activation of Ras/MEK/ERK/AP-1 and PI3-K/Akt/NF-κB pathways; besides the direct activation of Adenylate cyclase/PKA/CREB through EP receptor. Transcription factors CREB, AP-1 and NF-κB lead to its proliferative effects through the activation of the expression of cyclin D1 and VEGF (Ansari *et al.*, 2008).

3.2 Prostaglandins effects on inflammation and immune system

The involvement of PGs in the inflammatory response has been largely known. The typical signs of inflammation -heat, redness, swelling and pain- result from PGs direct effects. Indeed, redness and edema are a consequence of an increased vasodilatation and vascular endothelium permeability, mediated by the interaction of PGI_2 and PGE_2 with vascular smooth muscle cells, respectively (Funk, 2001; Yamamoto *et al.*, 1999). Besides vascular modifications, inflammation-related pain depends on PGE_2 stimulation of peripheral sensory neurons (Ricciotti & FitzGerald, 2011). Additionally, fever caused in many inflammatory processes is also due to the interaction of PGE_2 with the nervous system, in this case with neurons of the organum vasculosa lamina terminalis at the midline of the preoptic area (Funk, 2001). In order to relieve one or all of these effects, inhibitors of PGs synthesis have been used as anti-inflammatory drugs for more than a century (acetylsalicylic acid was released in 1899 by Bayer), even when their molecular target was unknown. Nowadays, all of the Non-Steroidal Anti-Inflammatory Drugs (NSAIDs) are well-known inhibitors of COXs enzymes. There are different groups of NSAIDs each of them with diverse mechanisms of action and also selectivity for the two isoforms of the enzyme.

As it was stated before, PGs and COXs implication in the inflammatory response have been described many decades ago. However, the positive feedback loop that involves these molecules (Figure 6) should be highlighted, since PGE_2 (a sub-product of the enzyme) is able to regulate both COX isoforms expression, as it has been proved in keratinocytes. Amazingly, not only COX-2 expression was increased but also was COX-1 (Maldve *et al.*, 2000). The mechanism underlying this feedback involves EP_2 receptor and the activation of cAMP/CREB pathway (Ansari *et al.*, 2007).

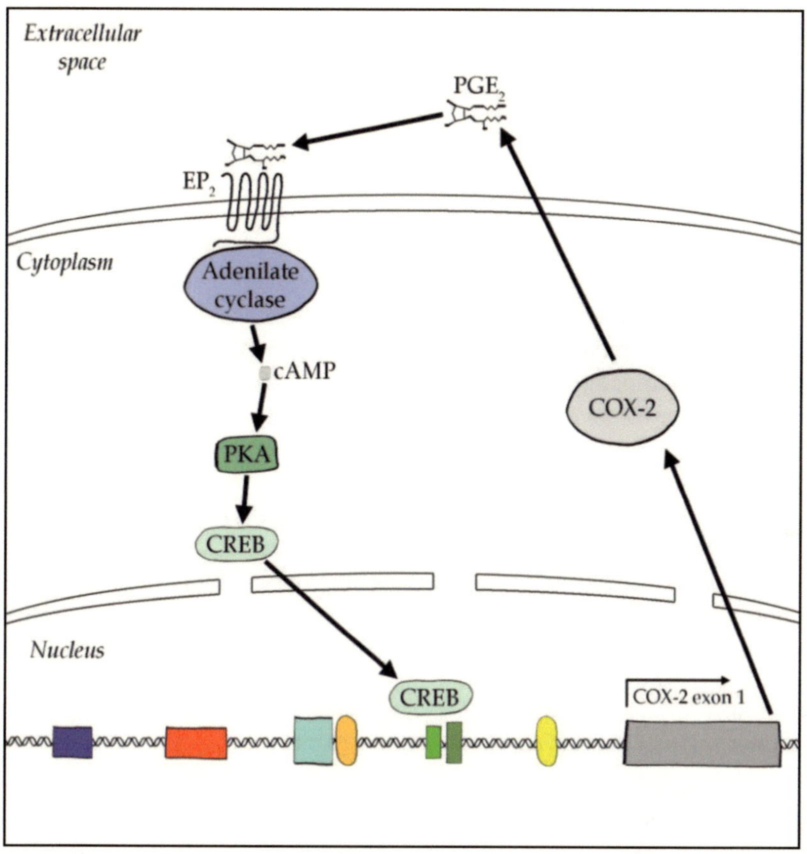

Fig. 6. COX-2 expression positive feedback loop. PGE_2, through its binding to EP_2 receptor, activates the cAMP/CREB pathway that finally leads to COX-2 expression, which synthesizes more PGE_2.

Besides their direct effects on inflammation, PGs play key roles in the development of the immune response, being capable of modifying dendritic cells and T helper (T_h) cells responses. During the activation of naive T_h cells by dendritic cells, or other antigen presenting cells, they can differentiate into different phenotypes: T_h1 cells (characterized by IFN-γ production), T_h2 cells (characterized by IL-4 production), T_h17 cells (characterized by IL-17 production) or T_{reg} cells (characterized by IL-10 production). PGE_2

plays an important role during this phenotypic differentiation of T_h cells. As it has been recently reported, PGE_2 -through its interaction with both EP_2 and EP_4- facilitates T_h1 cells differentiation, by the activation of the PI3K signalling pathway. Moreover, even when it was observed that T_h17 differentiation was not affected directly by PGE_2, an important role in IL-23-mediated T_h17 cells expansion was proved for PGE_2. IL-23 is the cytokine involved in the differentiation of naive T_h cells into T_h17 subset and is produced by dendritic cells, which generate endogenous PGE_2 that acts in an autocrine way through EP_4, activating the cAMP-Epac pathway. PGE_2 did not substantially affect T_h2, while it did inhibit T_{reg} differentiation (Yao *et al.*, 2009). Finally, Langerhans cells (the skin-homing dendritic cells) require the PGE_2-EP_4 signalling to mature and migrate from the epidermis to the draining lymph nodes, in order to perform an appropriate T cells activation (Kabashima *et al.*, 2003).

4. Skin cancer development and COX-2 over-expression

Under physiological conditions a balance exists between cell growth and death, resulting in a "homeostatic regulation". In this way, cells are normally under the control of their environment. Basically, cancer consists of a group of cells -probably originated from only one cell- that presents an "out of control" growth and functional characteristics. Cancer cells exhibit six basic acquired capabilities : i) self-sufficiency in growth signals, ii) insensitivity to anti-growth signals, iii) evading apoptosis, iv) sustained angiogenesis, v) tissue invasion and metastasis and vi) limitless replicative potential (Hanahan & Weinberg, 2000). Different signalling pathways can be affected by environmental stimuli, affecting normal cell growth. UVB radiation, as it was mentioned before in this chapter, is the main environmental carcinogen, affecting in a severe way cell growth control (de Gruijl *et al.*, 2001). As it has been vastly proved, specific mutations in the p53 gene and over-expression of the p53 protein are present in different types of skin cancer (Bolshakov *et al.*, 2003; Brash *et al.*, 1991). However, it is not the only affected gene, as it was demonstrated by Kim et al., among others, who evaluated the expression of p53 and COX-2 in human skin cancers: SCC, BCC, Bowen's disease and actinic keratosis. In this study it was found that both proteins are over-expressed in skin cancer, but there is not a direct correlation between them (Kim *et al.*, 2006). COX-2 over-expression could be a consequence of UVB radiation exposure and the subsequent activation of different signaling pathways, like the ones which include MAPK, PI3K and NF-κB.

4.1 Epidemiological data

It was described that up-regulation of COX-2 expression, which is normally undetected in most human tissues, is related to cancer promotion and development. Indeed, COX-2 has been evaluated in different human and animal malignancies, and it was stated as a probable target for cancer prevention (Hull, 2005; Subbaramaiah & Dannenberg, 2003).

COX-2 over-expression in different types of non-melanoma skin cancers have been assessed by different research groups, mainly by immunohistochemical techniques on human biopsy samples. In this way, human samples of SCC, BCC, Bowen's disease (BD, essentially SCC *in situ*), actinic keratosis (AK, pretumoral lesions that may evolve to SCC) and benign papillomas were studied. Sample positive reaction for COX-2 expression (in many cases with a highly positive result) ranged between 50 and 91% in SCC, 56 and 80% in BCC, 40 and 88% in BD, 50 and 83% in AK and it was of 25% in benign papillomas (An *et al.*, 2002; Kagoura *et al.*, 2001; Kim *et al.*, 2006). COX-2 over-expression has also been determined in mice models of skin abnormalities, such as hyperplasia of the skin, benign papillomas and SCC –resulting from UV chronic irradiation-. In these animal models COX-2 expression was also found increased in all cases, in accordance with the results obtained in human biopsy samples abovementioned (An *et al.*, 2002; Athar *et al.*, 2001).

4.2 Relationships between COX-2 expression, UV radiation and skin cancer development

UV radiation, as the main inducer of skin cancer, activates many molecular pathways in skin cells. There is a vast bibliography about all of these processes, which we described briefly, and it has also been reviewed elsewhere by other authors (Rundhaug & Fischer, 2008).
COX-2 expression can be induced in humans, proved both in cultured skin cells and in whole tissues, after a single or multiple exposures to UVr (Buckman *et al.*, 1998; Tripp *et al.*, 2003). This molecular response to UVr plays a pivotal role in the development of skin malignancies. UVr is able to increase reactive oxygen species (ROS) production, due to an excitation of molecules which act as chromophores and that can finally transfer the absorbed-energy to molecular oxygen, generating ROS. These molecules produce the oxidation of a phosphatase (receptor-type protein tyrosin phosphatase-κ), whose function is to keep the epidermal growth factor receptor (EGFR) unphosphorilated and inactive. Once the phosphatase is inactivated, EGFR becomes active and can transduce the signal through the downstream pathway, which includes Ras/Rac1/p38, leading ultimately to COX-2 transcription (Xu *et al.*, 2006a; Xu *et al.*, 2006b). Besides this mechanism, UVr may transfer its energy to generate a photoproduct of tryptophan, named 6-formylindolo[2,3-b]carbazole (FICZ). This molecule is a ligand for arylhydrocarbon receptor (AhR), which activates Src kinase and finally leads to the over-expression of COX-2 (Fritsche *et al.*, 2007). Another described mechanism underlying UVr-induced COX-2 over-expression is mediated by genotoxic damage. UVr directly affects cells by the generation of thymine dimers in the DNA; this genotoxic damage activates p53 protein, which arrests cell cycle and regulates the activation of apoptotic cell death. p53 also leads to the induction of heparin-binding EGF, which activates Ras/Raf/ERK pathway finally mediating the over-expression of COX-2 (Han *et al.*, 2002).
COX-2 over-expression leads to the many molecular events described before in this chapter. There are some more evidences of the involvement of those molecules and pathways in the development of skin cancer. Transgenic mice that express COX-2 constitutively in the skin-under the regulation of keratin 5 promoter- were studied in terms of alterations of growth or differentiation of the keratinocytes. It was found that constitutive expression of COX-2 in keratinocytes generates epidermal hyperplasia, mainly due to a lack of differentiation instead of an increased growth rate, and other pathological signs-like epidermal invaginations, loss of cell polarity and formation of horn pearls- (Neufang *et al.*, 2001). Moreover, studies performed in knock-out mice for both COX isoforms demonstrated that the absence of any of these enzymes reduces the incidence of skin cancer development, in DMBA-TPA model (Tiano *et al.*, 2002a). Finally, the carcinogenic effect of COX-2-derived PGE_2 is: i) dependent on the expression of EP_2, but not of the expression of EP_3; since knock-out mice lacking these two receptor type respond in different ways to the carcinogenic stimuli of DMBA/TPA treatment (Sung *et al.*, 2005) and ii) dependent on EP_1;

since its specific blockade reduced the number of tumor per mice in a UVB-induced skin cancer model (Tober *et al.*, 2006). However, the four prostanoid receptors EP_1-EP_4 are expressed differentially throughout the skin, and developed different staining patterns after UVB irradiation, suggesting that each receptor might play dissimilar roles in carcinogenesis (Tober *et al.*, 2007).

5. Chemoprovention and treatment of skin cancer

Classical treatment for NMSC consists mainly in surgical excision. Particularly, for the case of BCC, there is no need to perform a follow-up of the patients, since this type of cancer does not have the capacity to metastasize (MacKie, 2006). However, there are enormous efforts being made in order to evaluate alternative non-surgical therapies for NMSC. Many of them are being studied in animal models, and many others in human patients. We make here a brief summary of treatments, highlighting the molecular pathways involved, both for some pharmacological and natural compounds.

5.1 Pharmacological compounds in the skin cancer treatment

As it was mentioned before, most of the knowledge about the role of COX in the development of skin cancer was achieved by studies performed with NSAIDs. In this way, the oldest report on the topic was first published, as far as we know, in 1995 (Reeve *et al.*, 1995). In this study indomethacin (a non-specific NSAID) was administrated in a mouse model of UV-induced skin cancer. Many studies were performed since then, facing the issue in different ways. Non-specific NSAIDs orally administered have the great disadvantage of gastric side-effects, in prolonged treatments. Considering this aspect, the pioneering work of Reeve et al. was discussed by Pentland et al., whose work was performed using celecoxib -a specific COX-2 inhibitor- in the same model: SKH:1 mice chronically exposed to UV radiation (Pentland *et al.*, 1999), results which were further confirmed (Orengo *et al.*, 2002). Pentland demonstrated that, beyond the absence of side-effects, there were much better anti-tumor results using celecoxib instead of indomethacin. Moreover, these conclusions were also achieved by other research group, which directly compared the anti-tumor effects of both celecoxib and indomethacin in parallel experiments (Fischer *et al.*, 1999). Oral celecoxib treatment was recently evaluated in a randomized, double blind, placebo-controlled trial, showing that it would be helpful in the prevention of SCC and BCC in patients who have an extensive actinic damage (Elmets *et al.*, 2010).

In addition to these studies, the idea of skin cancer oral treatments was challenged by another way for drugs application: topical treatment. The present book includes a full chapter related to the topical administration of drugs and skin cancer, written by Taveira & Lopez, which could be of interest. Celecoxib topically applied demonstrated to be useful in the suppression of UVB-induced cutaneous inflammation (Wilgus *et al.*, 2000). Besides, topically applied naproxen -a non-selective NSAID- was useful in the reduction of skin tumors after chronic irradiation of SKH:1 mice, with a marked decrease in the levels of PGE_2 and a surprising increment in the epidermal production of TNF-α (González Maglio *et al.*, 2010). Accordingly, long ago it has been reported that TNF-α production increases after the inhibition of COX (Hart *et al.*, 1989). PGE_2, as it was stated before in this chapter, may act both increasing and decreasing the levels of cAMP (a well-known repressor of TNF-α expression). The NSAID-mediated decrease in PGE_2

production might avoid the inhibition of TNF-α transcription, increasing in this way the level of this cytokine in the treated cells (Grandjean-Laquerriere, 2003). Increases in TNF-α production may explain, at least in part, another important effect of NSAIDs treatment: the induction of apoptosis in the target cells (Fecker *et al.*, 2007). This induction could be mediated by TNF-receptor triggered cell death pathway. Moreover, it is worth to notice that topical treatment could dramatically reduce the gastric side-effects of non-specific NSAIDs prolonged treatment. If this kind of drug application was performed, there would be better results in the anti-tumor effects, since both isoforms of COX mediates skin cancer development (Tiano *et al.*, 2002b). However, in neither of the commented studies the incidence of tumors in treated mice was null, showing that there are cellular alterations remaining that cannot be faced with this kind of drugs.

Aspirin or acetylsalicylic acid -the oldest NSAIDs in use- may capture some special attention, since it has been demonstrated that this drug is not only capable of inhibiting COX enzymatic activity, but also of inhibiting the activity of IκB kinase-β, inhibiting in this way the NF-κB pathway (Yin *et al.*, 1998).

It is of great interest to analyze another drug, imiquimod, recently approved by the US Food and Drug Administration (FDA) to be used topically in the treatment of human SCC and BCC (Love *et al.*, 2009). This drug activates directly TLR-7 and TLR-8 and leads to the activation of NF-κB and AP-1 nuclear factors, resulting in the expression of pro-inflammatory cytokines, and probably -but not proven up to date- COX-2. Another mechanism of action includes a decrease in the cellular levels of cAMP which, as it was explained before, inhibits the transcription of inflammatory cytokines, like TNF-α. Finally, imiquimod can induce directly apoptotic cell death of tumoral cells through the activation of death receptors (Schon & Schon, 2007; Schon *et al.*, 2006).

Drug treatment of skin cancer might affect the COX-2 pathway, but a reduction in this enzyme expression or activity does not necessarily ensure an anti-tumor effect. Besides, by only blocking COX activity, the incidence of cancer can be reduced, but not entirely abolished.

5.2 Natural compounds in the skin cancer treatment

Historically, different human malignancies and pathologies have been treated with medicinal plants and different natural extracts. Nowadays, a great number of natural compounds with anti-tumor effects have been identified and isolated. Many of them have anti-oxidant effects, which are responsible for their protective effects against malignancies. A whole chapter of the present book, written by Filip and Clichici, is completely dedicated to analyze the use of natural compounds in the treatment of skin cancer. Hereafter, we comment the use of some compounds in this field, with some mention to the corresponding molecular pathway involved.

Many natural compounds have the ability of down-regulate *in vitro* or *in vivo* the UV-induced over-expression of COX-2 or the production of PGE_2. Some very well documented examples are curcumin (Cho *et al.*, 2005), apigenin (Tong *et al.*, 2007), nobiletin (Tanaka *et al.*, 2004), cyanidin (Kim *et al.*, 2010), cyaniding-3-glucoside (Lim *et al.*, 2011) and α-linoleic acid (Takemura *et al.*, 2002). This capacity of inhibiting COX-2 expression or function is promising for the use of these compounds in skin cancer treatment. However, not all of the above-mentioned compounds have been properly assayed in animal tumor models.

As an example, cyanidin-3-glucoside (C3G) has been proven to effectively reduce the number of papillomas in TPA-treated mice (Ding *et al.*, 2006). C3G was also demonstrated to attenuate activation of transcription factors AP-1 and NF-κB, and the kinases MEK, MKK4, Akt and MAPKs. However, it does not affect the phosphorylation of the upstream kinase Fyn. Molecular docking analysis has demonstrated the capacity of C3G to directly fit in the pocket responsible for enzymatic activity of Fyn (Lim *et al.*, 2011).
Resveratrol was shown to be useful in the treatment of UV-induced skin cancer in mice (Aziz *et al.*, 2005). Moreover, it has exhibited an interesting decrease in the activation of NF-κB pathway in UVB-exposed cultured keratinocytes (Adhami *et al.*, 2003).
Pathways which are activated by peroxisome proliferator-activated receptors (PPARs) are also of interest. These pathways may be activated by a great number of ligands, including pharmacological compounds, fatty acids and fatty acid-derived molecules. PPAR-α can modulate the expression of COX-2 and VEGF by antagonizing NF-κB and AP-1, inducing the expression of IκB and interfering with the MAPKs pathway (Grau *et al.*, 2008). Indeed, PPAR-α expression is down-regulated in human SCC and AK biopsies (Nijsten *et al.*, 2005) and its activation has shown a partial inhibition in the development of skin tumors in a mice model (Thuillier *et al.*, 2000). Finally, α-linoleic acid (ligand of PPAR-α) can mediate a decrease in the UV-induced PGE_2 production in SKH:1 mice (Takemura *et al.*, 2002).
It is worth to notice that all of these compounds, although promising, are not being used in humans yet. Many of them remain to be thoroughly tested in animal models, before they can be approved for human treatment. Additionally, for natural compounds it is also vacant the analysis of the topical administration, since the majority of the studies have been performed using the classical oral administration. Topical administration can offer the advantages of direct treatment of the lesion and reduction of unwanted side-effects, which have not been well-described and reported yet, for the doses of the natural compounds needed to exhibit anti-tumor effects.

6. Conclusion

COX-2 over-expression is highly related to human NMSC development and progression. Many very well known carcinogens can activate different molecular pathways leading to COX-2 gene transcription. Over-expression of COX-2 enzyme was determined in human NMSC biopsies as well as in animal tissues by different techniques. *In vitro* studies have demonstrated its expression in keratinocytes after carcinogenic stimuli.
The sub-products of COX-2 enzyme activity, mainly PGE_2, lead to many cellular and molecular events related with carcinogenesis. These events include apoptosis resistance, growth signalling, angiogenesis and selective immunosuppression. Many of these events are regulated by the expression of specific receptors expressed in the target cell.
A great number of studies have been performed in order to obtain alternative or adjuvant treatments for NMSC, different from surgical excision. Treatments which regulate COX-2 expression pathways or its own enzymatic activity, altered the whole inflammatory response, as well as the cellular and molecular events mentioned before. All anti-tumor therapies must be analyzed taking into account that malignant-transformed cells can be directly eliminated -by avoiding growth stimuli or inducing cytotoxicity- or indirectly -by the proper activation of the immune response-. In this way, some of the above-mentioned treatments induce preferentially cytotoxic effects, while others increase the immune response. For some others, even when the overall anti-tumor effects were effectively proven,

the exact mechanism was not. Finally, it is important to highlight that opposite effects on the same pathway may result in an equally effective anti-tumor response, i.e. imiquimod activates NF-κB pathway while PPAR-α ligands inhibit it, and both are useful treatments for NMSC.

7. Acknowledgment

Publication of this work was supported by Universidad de Buenos Aires.
The authors would like to thank Dr. Alejandro Ferrari for critical review of the manuscript.

8. References

Adhami VM, Afaq F, Ahmad N (2003) Suppression of ultraviolet B exposure-mediated activation of NF-kappaB in normal human keratinocytes by resveratrol. *Neoplasia* 5:74-82. 1522-8002 (Print) 1476-5586 (Linking).

Aitken GR, Henderson JR, Chang S-C, McNeil CJ, Birch-Machin Ma (2007) Direct monitoring of UV-induced free radical generation in HaCaT keratinocytes. *Clinical and experimental dermatology* 32:722-7.

An KP, Athar M, Tang X, Katiyar SK, Russo J, Beech J, *et al.* (2002) Cyclooxygenase-2 expression in murine and human nonmelanoma skin cancers: implications for therapeutic approaches. *Photochem Photobiol* 76:73-80. 0031-8655 (Print) 0031-8655 (Linking).

Ansari KM, Rundhaug JE, Fischer SM (2008) Multiple signaling pathways are responsible for prostaglandin E2-induced murine keratinocyte proliferation. *Mol Cancer Res* 6:1003-16. 1541-7786 (Print) 1541-7786 (Linking).

Ansari KM, Sung YM, He G, Fischer SM (2007) Prostaglandin receptor EP2 is responsible for cyclooxygenase-2 induction by prostaglandin E2 in mouse skin. *Carcinogenesis* 28:2063-8. 1460-2180 (Electronic) 0143-3334 (Linking).

Armstrong BK, Kricker A (2001) The epidemiology of UV induced skin cancer. *Journal of Photochemistry and Photobiology* 63:8-18.

Ashendel CL, Boutwell RK (1979) Prostaglandin E and F levels in mouse epidermis are increased by tumor-promoting phorbol esters. *Biochem Biophys Res Commun* 90:623-7. 0006-291X (Print) 0006-291X (Linking).

Athar M, An KP, Morel KD, Kim AL, Aszterbaum M, Longley J, *et al.* (2001) Ultraviolet B(UVB)-induced cox-2 expression in murine skin: an immunohistochemical study. *Biochem Biophys Res Commun* 280:1042-7. 0006-291X (Print) 0006-291X (Linking).

Aubin F (2003) Mechanisms involved in ultraviolet light-induced immunosuppression. *European journal of dermatology : EJD* 13:515-23.

Aubin F, Humbey O, Guerrini JS, Mougin C, Laurent R (2003) [Non-melanoma skin cancers and human papillomavirus]. *Ann Dermatol Venereol* 130:1131-8. 0151-9638 (Print) 0151-9638 (Linking).

Aziz MH, Reagan-Shaw S, Wu J, Longley BJ, Ahmad N (2005) Chemoprevention of skin cancer by grape constituent resveratrol: relevance to human disease? *FASEB J* 19:1193-5. 1530-6860 (Electronic) 0892-6638 (Linking).

Bolshakov S, Walker CM, Strom SS, Selvan MS, Clayman GL, El-Naggar A, *et al.* (2003) P53 Mutations in Human Aggressive and Nonaggressive Basal and Squamous Cell Carcinomas. *Clinical cancer research : an official journal of the American Association for Cancer Research* 9:228-34.

Bouwes Bavinck JN, Feltkamp M, Struijk L, ter Schegget J (2001) Human papillomavirus infection and skin cancer risk in organ transplant recipients. *J Investig Dermatol Symp Proc* 6:207-11. 1087-0024 (Print) 1087-0024 (Linking).

Brash DE, Rudolph JA, Simon JA, Lin A, McKenna GJ, Baden HP, *et al.* (1991) A role for sunlight in skin cancer: UV-induced p53 mutations in squamous cell carcinoma. *Proc Natl Acad Sci U S A* 88:10124-8. 0027-8424 (Print) 0027-8424 (Linking).

Buckman SY, Gresham a, Hale P, Hruza G, Anast J, Masferrer J, *et al.* (1998) COX-2 expression is induced by UVB exposure in human skin: implications for the development of skin cancer. *Carcinogenesis* 19:723-9.

Coultas L, Strasser A (2003) The role of the Bcl-2 protein family in cancer. *Seminars in Cancer Biology* 13:115-23.

Chang L, Karin M (2001) Mammalian MAP kinase signalling cascades. *Nature* 410:37-40. 0028-0836 (Print) 0028-0836 (Linking).

Cho J-W, Park K, Kweon GR, Jang B-C, Baek W-K, Suh M-H, *et al.* (2005) Curcumin inhibits the expression of COX-2 in UVB-irradiated human keratinocytes (HaCaT) by inhibiting activation of AP-1: p38 MAP kinase and JNK as potential upstream targets. *Experimental & molecular medicine* 37:186-92.

Chun KS, Surh YJ (2004) Signal transduction pathways regulating cyclooxygenase-2 expression: potential molecular targets for chemoprevention. *Biochem Pharmacol* 68:1089-100. 0006-2952 (Print) 0006-2952 (Linking).

de Gruijl FR, van Kranen HJ, Mullenders LHF (2001) UV-induced DNA damage , repair , mutations and oncogenic pathways in skin cancer. *Journal of Photochemistry and Photobiology B: Biology* 63:19-27.

Ding M, Feng R, Wang SY, Bowman L, Lu Y, Qian Y, *et al.* (2006) Cyanidin-3-glucoside, a natural product derived from blackberry, exhibits chemopreventive and chemotherapeutic activity. *J Biol Chem* 281:17359-68. 0021-9258 (Print) 0021-9258 (Linking).

Elmets CA, Viner JL, Pentland AP, Cantrell W, Lin HY, Bailey H, *et al.* (2010) Chemoprevention of nonmelanoma skin cancer with celecoxib: a randomized, double-blind, placebo-controlled trial. *J Natl Cancer Inst* 102:1835-44. 1460-2105 (Electronic) 0027-8874 (Linking).

Fecker LF, Stockfleth E, Nindl I, Ulrich C, Forschner T, Eberle J (2007) The role of apoptosis in therapy and prophylaxis of epithelial tumours by nonsteroidal anti-inflammatory drugs (NSAIDs). *The British journal of dermatology* 156 Suppl 25-33.

Fischer SM, Lo HH, Gordon GB, Seibert K, Kelloff G, Lubet RA, *et al.* (1999) Chemopreventive activity of celecoxib, a specific cyclooxygenase-2 inhibitor, and indomethacin against ultraviolet light-induced skin carcinogenesis. *Mol Carcinog* 25:231-40. 0899-1987 (Print) 0899-1987 (Linking).

Fisher MS, Kripke ML (1977) Systemic alteration induced in mice by ultraviolet light irradiation and its relationship to ultraviolet carcinogenesis. *Proceedings of the National Academy of Sciences* 74:1688-92.

Fritsche E, Schafer C, Calles C, Bernsmann T, Bernshausen T, Wurm M, *et al.* (2007) Lightening up the UV response by identification of the arylhydrocarbon receptor as a cytoplasmatic target for ultraviolet B radiation. *Proc Natl Acad Sci U S A* 104:8851-6. 0027-8424 (Print) 0027-8424 (Linking).

Funk CD (2001) Prostaglandins and leukotrienes: advances in eicosanoid biology. *Science* 294:1871-5. 0036-8075 (Print) 0036-8075 (Linking).

Furstenberger G, de Bravo M, Bertsch S, Marks F (1979) The effect of indomethacin on cell proliferation induced by chemical and mechanical means in mouse epidermis in vivo. *Res Commun Chem Pathol Pharmacol* 24:533-41. 0034-5164 (Print) 0034-5164 (Linking).

Furstenberger G, Marks F (1978) Indomethacin inhibition of cell proliferation induced by the phorbolester TPA is reversed by prostaglandin E2 in mouse epidermis in vivo. *Biochem Biophys Res Commun* 84:1103-11. 0006-291X (Print) 0006-291X (Linking).

Geller AC, Annas GD (2003) Epidemiology of melanoma and nonmelanoma skin cancer. *Semin Oncol Nurs* 19:2-11. 0749-2081 (Print) 0749-2081 (Linking).

González Maglio DH, Paz ML, Ferrari A, Weill FS, Nieto J, Leoni J (2010) Alterations in Skin Immune Response Throughout Chronic UVB Irradiation—Skin Cancer Development and Prevention by Naproxen. *Photochemistry and Photobiology* 86:146-52.

Grandjean-Laquerriere a (2003) Differential regulation of TNF-α, IL-6 and IL-10 in UVB-irradiated human keratinocytes via cyclic AMP/protein kinase A pathway. *Cytokine* 23:138-49.

Grau R, Diaz-Munoz MD, Cacheiro-Llaguno C, Fresno M, Iniguez MA (2008) Role of peroxisome proliferator-activated receptor alpha in the control of cyclooxygenase 2 and vascular endothelial growth factor: involvement in tumor growth. *PPAR Res* 2008:352437. 1687-4757 (Print).

Han JA, Kim JI, Ongusaha PP, Hwang DH, Ballou LR, Mahale A, *et al.* (2002) P53-mediated induction of Cox-2 counteracts p53- or genotoxic stress-induced apoptosis. *EMBO J* 21:5635-44. 0261-4189 (Print) 0261-4189 (Linking).

Hanahan D, Weinberg RA (2000) The hallmarks of cancer. *Cell* 100:57-70. 0092-8674 (Print) 0092-8674 (Linking).

Hart PH, Whitty GA, Piccoli DS, Hamilton JA (1989) Control by IFN-gamma and PGE2 of TNF alpha and IL-1 production by human monocytes. *Immunology* 66:376-83. 0019-2805 (Print) 0019-2805 (Linking).

Hull MA (2005) Cyclooxygenase-2: how good is it as a target for cancer chemoprevention? *Eur J Cancer* 41:1854-63. 0959-8049 (Print) 0959-8049 (Linking).

Inoue H, Yokoyama C, Hara S, Tone Y, Tanabe T (1995) Transcriptional regulation of human prostaglandin-endoperoxide synthase-2 gene by lipopolysaccharide and phorbol ester in vascular endothelial cells. Involvement of both nuclear factor for interleukin-6 expression site and cAMP response element. *J Biol Chem* 270:24965-71. 0021-9258 (Print) 0021-9258 (Linking).

Kabashima K, Sakata D, Nagamachi M, Miyachi Y, Inaba K, Narumiya S (2003) Prostaglandin E2-EP4 signaling initiates skin immune responses by promoting migration and maturation of Langerhans cells. *Nat Med* 9:744-9. 1078-8956 (Print) 1078-8956 (Linking).

Kagoura M, Toyoda M, Matsui C, Morohashi M (2001) Immunohistochemical expression of cyclooxygenase-2 in skin cancers. *J Cutan Pathol* 28:298-302. 0303-6987 (Print) 0303-6987 (Linking).

Kim JE, Kwon JY, Seo SK, Son JE, Jung SK, Min SY, *et al.* (2010) Cyanidin suppresses ultraviolet B-induced COX-2 expression in epidermal cells by targeting MKK4, MEK1, and Raf-1. *Biochem Pharmacol* 79:1473-82. 1873-2968 (Electronic) 0006-2952 (Linking).

Kim KH, Park EJ, Seo YJ, Cho HS, Kim CW, Kim KJ, *et al.* (2006) Immunohistochemical study of cyclooxygenase-2 and p53 expression in skin tumors. *J Dermatol* 33:319-25. 0385-2407 (Print) 0385-2407 (Linking).

Kopp E, Medzhitov R, Carothers J, Xiao C, Douglas I, Janeway CA, *et al.* (1999) ECSIT is an evolutionarily conserved intermediate in the Toll/IL-1 signal transduction pathway. *Genes Dev* 13:2059-71. 0890-9369 (Print) 0890-9369 (Linking).

Kuchide M (2003) Cancer chemopreventive effects of oral feeding α-tocopherol on ultraviolet light B induced photocarcinogenesis of hairless mouse. *Cancer Letters* 196:169-77.

Kujubu DA, Fletcher BS, Varnum BC, Lim RW, Herschman HR (1991) TIS10, a phorbol ester tumor promoter-inducible mRNA from Swiss 3T3 cells, encodes a novel prostaglandin synthase/cyclooxygenase homologue. *J Biol Chem* 266:12866-72. 0021-9258 (Print) 0021-9258 (Linking).

Liang SB, Furihata M, Takeuchi T, Iwata J, Chen BK, Sonobe H, *et al.* (2000) Overexpression of cyclin D1 in nonmelanocytic skin cancer. *Virchows Arch* 436:370-6. 0945-6317 (Print) 0945-6317 (Linking).

Lim TG, Kwon JY, Kim J, Song NR, Lee KM, Heo YS, *et al.* (2011) Cyanidin-3-glucoside suppresses B[a]PDE-induced cyclooxygenase-2 expression by directly inhibiting Fyn kinase activity. *Biochem Pharmacol* 82:167-74. 1873-2968 (Electronic) 0006-2952 (Linking).

Love WE, Bernhard JD, Bordeaux JS (2009) Topical imiquimod or fluorouracil therapy for basal and squamous cell carcinoma: a systematic review. *Arch Dermatol* 145:1431-8. 1538-3652 (Electronic) 0003-987X (Linking).

MacKie RM (2006) Long-term health risk to the skin of ultraviolet radiation. *Progress in Biophysics and Molecular Biology* 92:92-6.

Madan V, Hoban P, Strange RC, Fryer AA, Lear JT (2006) Genetics and risk factors for basal cell carcinoma. *Br J Dermatol* 154 Suppl 1:5-7. 0007-0963 (Print) 0007-0963 (Linking).

Maldve RE, Kim Y, Muga SJ, Fischer SM (2000) Prostaglandin E(2) regulation of cyclooxygenase expression in keratinocytes is mediated via cyclic nucleotide-linked prostaglandin receptors. *J Lipid Res* 41:873-81. 0022-2275 (Print) 0022-2275 (Linking).

Merlie JP, Fagan D, Mudd J, Needleman P (1988) Isolation and characterization of the complementary DNA for sheep seminal vesicle prostaglandin endoperoxide synthase (cyclooxygenase). *J Biol Chem* 263:3550-3. 0021-9258 (Print) 0021-9258 (Linking).

Murphy M, Mabruk MJEMF, Lenane P, Liew a, McCann P, Buckley a, *et al.* (2002) Comparison of the expression of p53, p21, Bax and the induction of apoptosis between patients with basal cell carcinoma and normal controls in response to ultraviolet irradiation. *Journal of clinical pathology* 55:829-33.

Narumiya S, Sugimoto Y, Ushikubi F (1999) Prostanoid receptors: structures, properties, and functions. *Physiol Rev* 79:1193-226. 0031-9333 (Print) 0031-9333 (Linking).

Negishi M, Sugimoto Y, Ichikawa A (1993) Prostanoid receptors and their biological actions. *Prog Lipid Res* 32:417-34. 0163-7827 (Print) 0163-7827 (Linking).

Negishi M, Sugimoto Y, Ichikawa A (1995) Prostaglandin E receptors. *J Lipid Mediat Cell Signal* 12:379-91. 0929-7855 (Print) 0929-7855 (Linking).

Neufang G, Furstenberger G, Heidt M, Marks F, Muller-Decker K (2001) Abnormal differentiation of epidermis in transgenic mice constitutively expressing cyclooxygenase-2 in skin. *Proc Natl Acad Sci U S A* 98:7629-34. 0027-8424 (Print) 0027-8424 (Linking).

Nijsten T, Geluyckens E, Colpaert C, Lambert J (2005) Peroxisome proliferator-activated receptors in squamous cell carcinoma and its precursors. *J Cutan Pathol* 32:340-7. 0303-6987 (Print) 0303-6987 (Linking).

Orengo IF, Gerguis J, Phillips R, Guevara A, Lewis AT, Black HS (2002) Celecoxib, a cyclooxygenase 2 inhibitor as a potential chemopreventive to UV-induced skin cancer: a study in the hairless mouse model. *Arch Dermatol* 138:751-5. 0003-987X (Print) 0003-987X (Linking).

Ouyang W, Li J, Ma Q, Huang C (2006) Essential roles of PI-3K/Akt/IKKbeta/NFkappaB pathway in cyclin D1 induction by arsenite in JB6 Cl41 cells. *Carcinogenesis* 27:864-73. 0143-3334 (Print) 0143-3334 (Linking).

Paz ML, Ferrari A, Weill FS, Leoni J, Maglio DHG (2008) Time-course evaluation and treatment of skin inflammatory immune response after ultraviolet B irradiation. *Cytokine* 44:70-7.

Pentland AP, Needleman P (1986) Modulation of keratinocyte proliferation in vitro by endogenous prostaglandin synthesis. *J Clin Invest* 77:246-51. 0021-9738 (Print) 0021-9738 (Linking).

Pentland aP, Schoggins JW, Scott Ga, Khan KN, Han R (1999) Reduction of UV-induced skin tumors in hairless mice by selective COX-2 inhibition. *Carcinogenesis* 20:1939-44.

Reeve VE, Matheson MJ, Bosnic M, Boehm-Wilcox C (1995) The protective effect of indomethacin on photocarcinogenesis in hairless mice. *Cancer Lett* 95:213-9. 0304-3835 (Print) 0304-3835 (Linking).

Ricciotti E, FitzGerald GA (2011) Prostaglandins and inflammation. *Arterioscler Thromb Vasc Biol* 31:986-1000. 1524-4636 (Electronic) 1079-5642 (Linking).

Rundhaug JE, Fischer SM (2008) Cyclo-oxygenase-2 plays a critical role in UV-induced skin carcinogenesis. *Photochem Photobiol* 84:322-9. 0031-8655 (Print) 0031-8655 (Linking).

Rundhaug JE, Pavone A, Kim E, Fischer SM (2007) The effect of cyclooxygenase-2 overexpression on skin carcinogenesis is context dependent. *Mol Carcinog* 46:981-92. 1098-2744 (Electronic) 0899-1987 (Linking).

Schon MP, Schon M (2007) Imiquimod: mode of action. *Br J Dermatol* 157 Suppl 2:8-13. 0007-0963 (Print) 0007-0963 (Linking).

Schon MP, Schon M, Klotz KN (2006) The small antitumoral immune response modifier imiquimod interacts with adenosine receptor signaling in a TLR7- and TLR8-independent fashion. *J Invest Dermatol* 126:1338-47. 0022-202X (Print) 0022-202X (Linking).

Shreedhar V, Giese T, Sung VW, Ullrich SE (1998) A cytokine cascade including prostaglandin E2, IL-4, and IL-10 is responsible for UV-induced systemic immune suppression. *Journal of immunology (Baltimore, Md : 1950)* 160:3783-9.

Slaper H, Velders GJ, Daniel JS, de Gruijl FR, van der Leun JC (1996) Estimates of ozone depletion and skin cancer incidence to examine the Vienna Convention achievements. *Nature* 384:256-8. 0028-0836 (Print) 0028-0836 (Linking).

Subbaramaiah K, Dannenberg AJ (2003) Cyclooxygenase 2: a molecular target for cancer prevention and treatment. *Trends Pharmacol Sci* 24:96-102. 0165-6147 (Print) 0165-6147 (Linking).

Sung YM, He G, Fischer SM (2005) Lack of expression of the EP2 but not EP3 receptor for prostaglandin E2 results in suppression of skin tumor development. *Cancer Res* 65:9304-11. 0008-5472 (Print) 0008-5472 (Linking).

Takemura N, Takahashi K, Tanaka H, Ihara Y, Ikemoto A, Fujii Y, *et al.* (2002) Dietary, but not Topical , Alpha-linolenic Acid Suppresses UVB-induced Skin Injury in Hairless Mice when Compared with Linoleic Acid {. *Photochemistry and Photobiology* 76:657-63.

Tanabe T, Tohnai N (2002) Cyclooxygenase isozymes and their gene structures and expression. *Prostaglandins Other Lipid Mediat* 68-69:95-114. 1098-8823 (Print) 1098-8823 (Linking).

Tanaka S, Sato T, Akimoto N, Yano M, Ito A (2004) Prevention of UVB-induced photoinflammation and photoaging by a polymethoxy flavonoid, nobiletin, in human keratinocytes in vivo and in vitro. *Biochemical pharmacology* 68:433-9.

Tay A, Squire JA, Goldberg H, Skorecki K (1994) Assignment of the human prostaglandin-endoperoxide synthase 2 (PTGS2) gene to 1q25 by fluorescence in situ hybridization. *Genomics* 23:718-9. 0888-7543 (Print) 0888-7543 (Linking).

Thuillier P, Anchiraico GJ, Nickel KP, Maldve RE, Gimenez-Conti I, Muga SJ, *et al.* (2000) Activators of peroxisome proliferator-activated receptor-alpha partially inhibit mouse skin tumor promotion. *Mol Carcinog* 29:134-42. 0899-1987 (Print) 0899-1987 (Linking).

Tiano HF, Loftin CD, Akunda J, Lee CA, Spalding J, Sessoms A, *et al.* (2002a) Deficiency of either cyclooxygenase (COX)-1 or COX-2 alters epidermal differentiation and reduces mouse skin tumorigenesis. *Cancer Res* 62:3395-401. 0008-5472 (Print) 0008-5472 (Linking).

Tiano HF, Loftin CD, Akunda J, Lee Ca, Spalding J, Sessoms A, *et al.* (2002b) Deficiency of either cyclooxygenase (COX)-1 or COX-2 alters epidermal differentiation and reduces mouse skin tumorigenesis. *Cancer research* 62:3395-401.

Tober KL, Thomas-Ahner JM, Kusewitt DF, Oberyszyn TM (2007) Effects of UVB on E prostanoid receptor expression in murine skin. *J Invest Dermatol* 127:214-21. 1523-1747 (Electronic) 0022-202X (Linking).

Tober KL, Wilgus TA, Kusewitt DF, Thomas-ahner JM, Maruyama T, Oberyszyn TM (2006) Importance of the EP1 Receptor in Cutaneous UVB-Induced Inflammation and Tumor Development. *Journal of Investigative Dermatology* 126:205-11.

Tong X, Van Dross RT, Abu-Yousif A, Morrison AR, Pelling JC (2007) Apigenin prevents UVB-induced cyclooxygenase 2 expression: coupled mRNA stabilization and translational inhibition. *Mol Cell Biol* 27:283-96. 0270-7306 (Print) 0270-7306 (Linking).

Tripp CS, Blomme EAG, Chinn KS, Hardy MM, LaCelle P, Pentland AP (2003) Epidermal COX-2 Induction Following Ultraviolet Irradiation: Suggested Mechanism for the Role of COX-2 Inhibition in Photoprotection. *Journal of Investigative Dermatology* 121:853-61.

Trompezinski S, Pernet I, Schmitt D, Viac J (2001) UV radiation and prostaglandin E2 up-regulate vascular endothelial growth factor (VEGF) in cultured human fibroblasts. *Inflammation research : official journal of the European Histamine Research Society [et al]* 50:422-7.

Ullrich SE, Kripke ML (1984) Mechanisms in the suppression of tumor rejection produced in mice by repeated UV irradiation. *Journal of immunology (Baltimore, Md : 1950)* 133:2786-90.

Wilgus TA, Ross MS, Parrett ML, Oberyszyn TM (2000) Topical application of a selective cyclooxygenase inhibitor suppresses UVB mediated cutaneous inflammation *Prostaglandins & other Lipid Mediators* 62:367-84.

Wu Y, Zhou BP (2010) TNF-alpha/NF-kappaB/Snail pathway in cancer cell migration and invasion. *Br J Cancer* 102:639-44. 1532-1827 (Electronic) 0007-0920 (Linking).

Xu Y, Shao Y, Voorhees JJ, Fisher GJ (2006a) Oxidative inhibition of receptor-type protein-tyrosine phosphatase kappa by ultraviolet irradiation activates epidermal growth factor receptor in human keratinocytes. *J Biol Chem* 281:27389-97. 0021-9258 (Print) 0021-9258 (Linking).

Xu Y, Voorhees JJ, Fisher GJ (2006b) Epidermal growth factor receptor is a critical mediator of ultraviolet B irradiation-induced signal transduction in immortalized human keratinocyte HaCaT cells. *Am J Pathol* 169:823-30. 0002-9440 (Print) 0002-9440 (Linking).

Yamamoto M, Aoyagi M, Fukai N, Matsushima Y, Yamamoto K (1999) Increase in prostaglandin E(2) production by interleukin-1beta in arterial smooth muscle cells derived from patients with moyamoya disease. *Circ Res* 85:912-8. 1524-4571 (Electronic) 0009-7330 (Linking).

Yao C, Sakata D, Esaki Y, Li Y, Matsuoka T, Kuroiwa K, *et al.* (2009) Prostaglandin E2-EP4 signaling promotes immune inflammation through Th1 cell differentiation and Th17 cell expansion. *Nat Med* 15:633-40. 1546-170X (Electronic) 1078-8956 (Linking).

Yin MJ, Yamamoto Y, Gaynor RB (1998) The anti-inflammatory agents aspirin and salicylate inhibit the activity of I(kappa)B kinase-beta. *Nature* 396:77-80. 0028-0836 (Print) 0028-0836 (Linking).

9

Chemoprevention of Skin Cancer by Natural Compounds

Gabriela Adriana Filip and Simona Clichici
Department of Physiology, University of Medicine and Pharmacy, Cluj-Napoca Romania

1. Introduction

Skin tumors in humans represent about 30% of all new cancers reported annually (Yusuf et al, 2007); their incidence is expected to increase substantially because of increased recreational exposure to sunlight and depletion of the ozone layer. The main factor incriminated in skin cancer is represented by the ultraviolet radiation, especially type B (UVB), which accounts for 90% of the skin cancer cases (Azis, 2005). Currently, between 2 and 3 million non-melanoma skin cancers and 132.000 melanoma skin cancers occur each year and one in every three cancers diagnosed is a skin cancer according to World Health Organization (WHO, 2004). Further more so, it is estimated that one in five persons will develop a basal cell or squamous cell carcinoma in its life time (Robinson, 2005). The identification of the critical molecular targets and signaling pathways involved in the development of premalign and malign lesions UV-induced and the development of agents that modulate these targets are important steps in the management of skin cancer. In 1894 Paul Gerson Unna established that there was a direct causal relationship between exposure to sunlight and the development of the skin carcinomas (Unna, 1894). The acute exposure to UV radiation leads to erythema, edema, burns, pain, thickening and pigmentation of the skin (Afaq & Mukhtar, 2001) while chronic exposure induces immunosuppression (Aziz, 2005), premature aging (Jurkiewicz et al, 1995; Lopez-Torres et al, 1998) and skin cancers (Katiyar & Mukhtar, 2001; Katiyar, 2008; Taylor et al, 1990). The sunlight UV spectrum can be separated into three wavelengths: UVA (320-400 nm), UVB (280-320 nm) and UVC (200-280 nm). Primarily UVA and UVB reach the earth's surface as UVC is filtered out by the ozone layer (Shae & Parrish, 1991). Though the UVB radiations is a small part of UV emissions (4 - 5%), they are extremely aggresive being 1000 times more carcinogenic than UVA (Bowden, 2004; Mukhtar & Elmets, 1996). UVB directly or through the reactive oxygen species (ROS) affects the genetic material of exposed cells forming photoproducts such as DNA cyclobutane pyrimidine dimers (CPDs) and pyrimidine (6-4) pyrimidone (Afaq et al, 2007) respective 8-oxo-7, 8-dihydroguanine (8-oxo-dG) and 8-hydroxy-20-deoxyguanosine (8-OHdG) (Kawachi et al, 2008). Multistage carcinogenesis is a widely accepted hypothesis for the development of skin cancer. Skin carcinogenesis is divided into three stages namely: initiation, promotion and progression. Both UVA and UVB radiation have been shown to be complete carcinogens, capable of initiation, promotion and progression of carcinogenetic process (Aziz et al, 2005; Brash et al, 1996; Elmets et al, 2001). Actually, UV has dual actions in the development of skin cancers, it damages DNA and induces mutations of cellular genes crucial for oncogenesis; it induces immunosuppresion, which prevents tumor rejection by the host. To exert its biological effects, UV must be first absorbed by cellular chromophore, which transforms the energy into a biochemical signal. Nucleic acids and proteins, especially tryptophan and tyrosine, are the major cellular chromophores in skin. In the DNA molecule, after the absorption of UVB radiation, dimeric photoproducts between adjacent pyrimidine bases are formed (Afaq et al, 2007). Usually the photoproducts formed are repaired effectively, but if the solar exposure is chronic and excessive, the process of repair is exceeded, the photoproducts persist and replicate, which may lead to transcriptional errors and, finally, to cancer (Kane & Kumar, 1999). The most frequent DNA mutations irradiation include the substitution of cytosine base by thymine (Mitchell et al, 1999). It was noticed that the methylation of the cytosine residues in the 5′-CCG and 5′-TCG sequences increased the formation of CPDs over 10 times, preferentially in *p53* gene (Lou et al, 2001). Disregulated sunburn apoptosis together with loss of normal function of the product of the *p53* gene may lead to transcriptional errors and, finally, to cancer. In addition, UVB radiation produces reactive oxygen species that can also damage DNA molecules and generate mainly 8-hydroxy-2′-deoxyguanosine (8-OHdG) (Ahmed et al, 1999). Formation of 8-OHdG induces G-C→T-A transversions during DNA replication especially in *ras* and *p53* genes initiating the carcinogenetic process (Basset-Seguin et al, 1994). Changes in the gene expression after UV irradiation are grouped as follows: initial changes (from 0.5 to 2 h), intermediate changes (from 4 to 8 h), and late ones (from 16 to 24 h). Firstly, UV activates several transcription factors - junB, junD, c-fos, ETR101, EGR1, and URY, up-regulates several mitochondrial proteins involved in the removal of reactive oxygen species - and suppresses c-Myc (Mlakar & Glava, 2007). The intermediate phase shows expression of genes of chemokines, cytokines, and growth factors (IL-8, Gro-α, Gro-β, MDNCF, and MIP2-β). In the late phase, the strongest induced genes are: keratinocyte differential markers, p53 and p21WAF1, ERK3, growth arrest and DNA-damage-induced protein (GADD45) (Murakami et al, 2001). The DNA damage response culminates in activation of cell cycle checkpoints and the appropriate DNA repair pathways or, in certain contexts, initiation of apoptotic programs. Progression of normal cell division depends on cyclin interaction with cyclin dependent kinase (CDKs) and the degradation of cyclins before chromosomal segregation. Deregulation of CDK-cyclin complexes or CDKs regulators result in continued proliferation or unscheduled re-entry into the cell cycle. There is ample evidence that UVB induces reactive oxygen species which have been involved in the pathogenesis of skin cancer (Bartsch & Nair, 2004; Halliday, 2005; Trouba et al, 2002). UVB exposure induces generation of reactive oxygen species in keratinocytes and fibroblasts: superoxide anion radical (O_2 ·), hydrogen peroxide (H_2O_2), the hydroxyl radical (HO·) and singlet oxygen ($1O_2$ ·). An imbalance between the generation of ROS and cellular antioxidant capacity leads to a state of oxidative stress that contributes to various pathological conditions including cancer (Katiyar & Elmets, 2001). Beside ROS, reactive nitrogen species (RNS), including nitric oxide (NO·), play a role in oxidative damage of proteins *via* nitrosylation reactions. More importantly, NO· can react with superoxide and produce peroxynitrite anion ($ONOO^-$), a toxic product involved in the apoptosis process and DNA cleavage (Katiyar et al, 2001). Defence mechanisms to remove the ROS include enzymes such as: superoxide dismutase (SOD), catalase (CAT), glutathione peroxidase (GPx), heme oxygenase-1 (HO-1), metallothionein - 2 (MT-2), glutathione S-transferases (GSTs), and small molecules with antioxidant activity such as: glutathione reduced (GSH), vitamin C, E, ubiquinona, β-carotene, etc., (Droge, 2002). Superoxide dismutase belongs to major antioxidant enzymes that contribute to the homeostasis of oxygen radicals in the skin. The dismutation of superoxide by SOD results in the production of hydrogen peroxide, which is subsequently converted to water and oxygen through a reaction catalyzed by CAT. An imbalance in the ratio of antioxidant enzymes may thus contribute to an excessive accumulation of ROS, increasing oxidative stress and skin damage (Sharma et al, 2004). GPx is a selenoprotein that catalyses the conversion of UV-induced hydrogen peroxide into water and molecular oxygen using GSH as unique hydrogen donor. Besides the regulatory effect of GSH on the activity of redox sensitive cysteine-containing enzymes (Klatt & Lamas, 2000), it modulates the activation and binding of transcription factors. The cellular concentration of the GSH is up to 100 fold higher than glutathione oxidized (GSSG) so, minor increase in GSH oxidation can significantly affect the GSH:GSSG ratio and consequently influences signal transduction and cell cycle progression (Klaunig & Kamendulis, 2004). The balance can be restored by NADPH-dependent glutathione reductase or the thioredoxin/glutaredoxin systems that catalyze the reduction of GSSG to GSH or by elimination of the GSSG from the cell (Schafer & Buettner, 2001). In addition, GSH contributes to the regeneration of ascorbate and α-tocopherol and detoxifies reactive species via its ability to conjugate pro-oxidants (Heck et al, 2003). Nrf2 (Nuclear factor-erythroid 2-related factor) and Keap1 (Kelch-like-ECH-associated protein 1) are key proteins in the coordinated transcriptional induction of various antioxidant-metabolizing enzymes such as: glutamate cysteine synthetase cysteine/glutamate exchange transporter (Wild et al, 1999), glutathione S-transferase, nicotinamide adenine dinucleotide phosphate quinone oxidoreductase-1 (NQO1), HO-1 (Alam et al, 1999) and thioredoxin (Ishii et al, 1999). Catalase, SOD and GPx are also dependent on Nrf2 (Kawachi et al, 2008). Overexpression of Nrf2 was shown to protect the cells from Fas-induced apoptosis (Kotlo et al, 2003) because it reduce the export of glutathione from apoptotic cells and increase intracellular GSH levels (Morito et al, 2003). In addition, the Nrf2–Keap1 pathway inhibit activation of activator protein 1 (AP-1) and nuclear factor kappa B (NF-kB) pathways, transcription factors involved in the inflammatory processes (Ichihashi, 2003; Li & Nel, 2006). A recent study indicated that p53, which is a key molecule in UV-induced apoptosis, suppressed the Nrf2-dependent transcription of antioxidant response genes (ARE) (Faraonio et al., 2006). Several cytosolic kinases such as protein kinase C (PKC)(Huang et al, 2002), mitogen-activated protein kinase (MAPK), p38 (Alam et al, 2000), and phosphatidylinositol-3-kinase (PI3K) (Kang et al, 2002) have been shown to modify Nrf2 and participate in the mechanism of signal transduction from antioxidants to the ARE. ROS also affect regulation of the gene expression of signaling molecules such as MAPKs and interrelated inflammatory cytokines as NF-κB and AP-1 (Katiyar & Mukhtar, 2001). MAPKs are components of kinase cascades that connect extracellular stimuli to specific transcription factors, thereby converting these signals into cellular responses. In mammalian systems, there are three subgroups of MAPKs: extracellular-signal-regulated kinases (ERKs), Jun N-terminal Kinases (JNKs), and p38 mitogen activated protein kinase (Chang & Karin, 2001). Once activated, these serine/threonine kinases translocate to the nucleus and phosphorylate AP-1 and NF-kB (Bode & Dong, 2003). AP-1 regulates the expression of some cellular cycle regulatory proteins, such as cycline D1, p53, p21, p19 (Aggarwal & Shishodia, 2006). The activation of NF-kB increases the expression of some pro-inflammatory cytokines, cyclooxygenase-2 (COX-2) and inducible nitric oxide synthase (iNOS) (Baldwin, 2001). Several reports published within the last decade showed that activation of NF-kB promoted cell survival and proliferation and down-regulation of NF-kB sensitized the cells to apoptosis induction (Dorai & Aggarwal, 2004). The genes NF-kB up-regulated including antiapoptotic proteins (Bcl-2, Bcl-XL), inhibitor of apoptosis (cIAP), survivin, TNF receptor-associated factors (TRAF1, TRAF2) have been reported to block apoptosis pathway (Garg & Aggarwal, 2002). ROS generated by UV radiation also induce matrix metalloproteinases (MMPs) and inactivate their tissue inhibitors, resulting in increased levels of matrix degrading enzymes, a key feature of photoaged skin. A cellular mechanism for the elimination of UV-damaged skin cells is to initiate apoptosis. Apoptosis is controlled by two signaling pathways, the extrinsic or death receptor-mediated pathway and the intrinsic or mitochondrial-mediated pathway. The death receptor-mediated pathway is initiated by the interaction of the ligand with its receptor, which leads to the activation of caspase 8 and 3. In contrast, the intrinsic pathway of apoptosis relies primarily on the permeabilization of mitochondrial membranes, with associated release of cytochrome c, leading to activation of caspase 9 and cleavage of caspase 3, 6, or 7. These downstream caspases induce in turn the cleavage of protein kinases and cytoskeletal proteins affecting cytoskeletal structure, the cell cycle regulatory effect and the related signaling pathways. DNA fragmentation, chromatin condensation, membrane blebbing cell shrinkage finally occurs. Recent studies indicate a third option to induce apoptosis namely one mediated by the endoplasmic reticulum. Strong stressing agents such as: UV radiation, chemotherapy, and peroxinitrite, determine the overexpression of DNA damage-inducible gene 153 (GADD153) and induce dephosphorylation of the pro-apoptotic protein Bad and down-regulation of Bcl-2 expression, enabling apoptosis (Tagawa et al, 2008). The extrinsic and intrinsic apoptotic pathways are regulated by several proteins such as NF-κB, Bcl-2 family proteins and the inhibitors of apoptosis (IAPs). An important component of IAP is survivin, the overexpressed protein in embryonic tissues and in tumors (Altieri, 2003). Because its level correlates with tumor angiogenesis, chemoresistance, tumor relapse and poor prognosis is considered as a potential molecular target for cancer therapy. The tumor suppressor protein p53 is a transcription factor that plays an essential role in the cellular response to UV. By blocking the cell cycle in cells which have suffered an excessive DNA damage, p53 prevents replication of damaged DNA as long as it has not been repaired. In case of unsuccessful reparation, p53 induces apoptosis via induction of p21waf1/cip1, Bax, apoptotic protease activating factor-1 (Apaf-1) and the caspase cascade (Amin et al, 2009).

In the process of carcinogenesis, the immunosuppressive effect of the UV radiation has to be taken into account. UV-induced inflammation is considered an early event in tumor promotion and/or tumor development (Katiyar, 2008). Similar to many chemical tumor promoters, UV also elicits NF-kB-mediated inflammation and changes in the expression of genes associated with cell proliferation and differentiation, as well as prostaglandin and cytokine production. Pro-inflammatory cytokines such as interleukin IL-1β, IL-6, IL-10 and tumor necrosis factor-α (TNF-α) impair the antigen presenting abilities of Langerhans cells which may result in suppression of the immune response (Susan et al, 2007). The inflammatory cells produce ROS and IL-10 which increase DNA oxidative damage and induce tumor promotion (Mukhtar H & Elmets, 1996). In addition, the UV radiation decreases the number of circulating T lymphocytes and the T helper/T suppressors' ratio and it alters the immune function of tumor cells (Patrick & Noah, 2007). Several studies showed using various experimental models of tumorigenesis that TNF-α and IL are involved in tumor promotion (Surh, et al, 2005). As a response to inflammatory stimuli and under the influence of COX, prostaglandins (PG) are produced in the skin, especially PGE2 and PGF2, molecules that play a role in tumor promotion (Narisawa et la, 1997). Another inflammation mediator is NO. NO released by iNOS is involved in tumor promotion; this fact is supported by the suppressive effect of aminoguanidine, an iNOS inhibitor on tumor promoter 12-O-tetradecanoylphorbol 13-acetate (TPA)-induced mouse skin tumor formation (Chun et al, 2004). It was showed that CPDs induced immunosuppression through cytokines production such as IL-10 or through the inhibition of transcription factors (Amerio et al, 2009). Photoisomerization of urocanic acid, which is found in high concentrations in the stratum corneum, may play a role in skin immunosuppresion. For this reason, the prevention of UV-induced immunosuppresion represents an important strategy in the management of skin cancers. Considering that UV induces oxidative stress-mediated adverse effects in the skin, the regular intake or topical application of antioxidants is suggested to be a useful way to reduce the harmful effects of UV radiation. These agents could prevent the formation of initiated cells or eliminate the initiated cells reducing the risk of cancer development.

2. Chemoprevention in skin cancers

The continue increase in the incidence of skin neoplasia, especially the non-melanoma ones, justifies the permanent preoccupation of the medical world to find an optimal solution for prevention. Chemoprevention, defined as "the use of agents capable of ameliorating the adverse effects of UVB on the skin" by natural compounds, represents a new concept in the attempt to control the carcinogenesis process (Zhao et al, 1999). This concept may be understood as a way to control tumor development by which the tumor evolution is slowed down or stopped; this control is realized by natural products or synthetic chemical compounds. The beginning of chemoprevention date back to 1920 but it was relaunched in 1970 by the research performed by Sporn (Sporn et al, 1976). The fruits, vegetables and plants with different pharmacological properties present rich sources of chemical substances with a chemopreventive role (Zhao et al, 1999). In fact, the role of chemoprevention is to interrupt the cascade of aberrant cellular signals and to stop the carcinogenic process. It seems that more than one dietary product has a chemopreventive role by modulating one or more signaling pathways in the cellular proliferation process. Exploring of the action mechanism of these compounds through *in vivo* studies to identify the target molecules and signaling pathways is critical in order to evaluate their clinical applicability. Taking into account the epidemiological data and the studies on animal models we can state that there are 30 new categories of clinical substances included in clinical trials as photochemopreventive agents. Some of them are antioxidants (vitamin E, ascorbic acid, polyphenols, isoflavonoids), which protect the skin from the oxidative effects; others interfere with the process of DNA repair or modulate the immunosuppresion induced by UV radiation.

2.1 Signaling pathways and target molecules involved in chemoprevention

The cell signaling pathways activated by natural dietary agents are numerous and different for different agents. The inhibitory effects of natural compounds in skin carcinogenesis have been attributed mainly to the biologic activities of the polyphenolic fractions. Polyphenols have antioxidant effects; they reduce the DNA oxidative damage, formation of lipid peroxides and carbonyl proteins and inhibit UVB-induced oxidative stress-mediated phosphorylation of MAPK signaling pathways. Polyphenols are known to inhibit the protein tyrosine kinase activities of epidermal growth factor (EGF), platelet-derived growth factor (PDGF) and fibroblast growth factor (FGF), inhibit UVB-induced phosphatidylinositol-3-kinase (PI3K) activation, blocked cell cycle progression at G1 phase and inhibited the activities of CDK-2 and CDK-4 in a dose-dependent manner. Also, blocked the activation of NF-kB and AP-1 and inhibited expression of COX-2 and iNOS. All these qualities make polyphenols an important option in chemoprevention. In the following sections we will focus on the mechanisms involved in the antiproliferative activity of natural products in skin cancer. The figure 1 presents the molecular targets of natural compounds in chemoprevention.

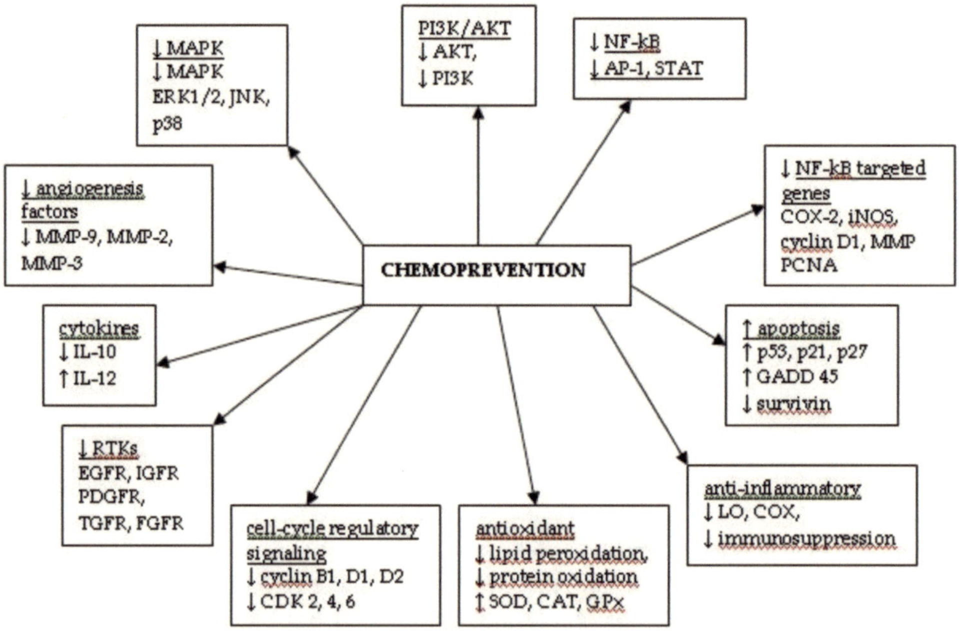

Fig. 1. Molecular targets of natural compounds in chemoprevention. The effects of natural compounds in skin carcinogenesis are variable: reduce inflammation, angiogenesis and oxidative stress, inhibit DNA damage, immunosuppresion and modulate the signaling pathways involved in the development of skin cancers. Abbreviations: MAPK - mitogen activated protein kinase, ERK1/2 - extracellular-signal-regulated kinases, JNK - Jun N-terminal Kinase, p38 - p38 mitogen activated protein kinases, AP-1 – activator protein 1, NF-kB – nuclear factor kappa B, COX-2 – cyclooxigenase 2, AKT - serine/threonine protein kinase, PI3K - phosphatidylinositol-3-kinase, MMP- metalloproteases, IL– interleukin, RTKs – receptor tyrosine kinases, EGFR - epidermal growth factor receptor, PDGFR - platelet-derived growth factor receptor, FGFR - fibroblast growth factor receptor, TGFR - transforming growth factor receptor, IGFR - insulin-like growth factor receptor, SOD – superoxid dismutase, CAT – catalase, GPx – glutathione peroxidase, IKK – IkB kinase, CDK - cyclin-dependent kinases, LO – lipooxigenase, iNOS - inducible nitric oxide synthase, PCNA – proliferating cell nuclear antigen, GADD45 - growth arrest and DNA damage, p53- tumor suppressor protein, p21, p27 - cyclin-dependent kinase inhibitors.

2.1.1 Receptor tyrosine kinases signaling

Receptor tyrosine kinases (RTKs) are important regulators involved in controlling cell proliferation, differentiation, survival, migration and metabolism (Schlessinger & Lemmon, 2006). The RTKs families include EGFR, PDGFR, FGFR, transforming growth factor receptors (TGFR), insulin-like growth factor receptors (IGFR). About 15 years back, curcumin, a natural agent, was reported to inhibit EGFR intrinsic kinase activity in human epidermoid carcinoma A431 cells (Korutla & Kumar, 1994). In *in vitro* assay, EGCG also strongly inhibited the protein tyrosine kinase activities of EGFR, PDGFR and FGFR (Lin, 2002). On another *in vitro* experimental model, EGCG could reduce the autophosphorylation level of EGFR and blocked of EGF binding to its receptor. Nomura et al. demonstrated that EGCG inhibited also the activation of PI3K and AKT phosphorylation UVB-induced in epidermis of mice (Nomura et al, 2001). Based on these findings it could be concluded that modulation of RTKs signaling might be involved in antiproliferative effects of natural compounds.

2.1.2 Signal transducers and activators of transcription pathway

Signal transducers and activators of transcription (STAT) proteins function as downstream effectors of signaling, which control cell proliferation, survival, apoptosis and differentiation (Kundu et al, 2009). STAT-1, STAT-3 and STAT-5 can be considered as molecular markers for early detection of certain types of tumors, as well as prognostic factors and predictors of response to various types of therapy (Buettner et al, 2008). Several dietary agents, such as green tea, resveratrol and curcumin have been shown to suppress STAT activation in tumor cells. So, green tea reduced the binding of STAT-1 to ADN by reducing the phosphorylation of protein I without involving its antioxidant role (Tedeschi et al, 2004). EGCG has also been shown to down-regulate the phosphorylation of STAT-3 (Masuda et al, 2001) while curcumin inhibited IL-6-induced STAT-3 and IFN-α-induced STAT-1 phosphorylation (Schnyder et al, 2002). These data provide further arguments in favor of the therapeutic effect of natural agents which suppress STAT activation.

2.1.3 Cell-cycle regulatory signaling

Several dietary agents including curcumin, resveratrol, genistein, dietary isothiocyanates, apigenin, and silibinin have been shown to interfere with the abnormal progression of cell cycle regulation in cancer cells (Lapenna & Giordano, 2009; Schwartz & Shah, 2005). Curcumin has been shown to inhibit progression of the cell cycle by down-regulating the expression of cyclin D1 at the transcriptional and posttranscriptional level, most probably by suppressing the activity of NF-kB (Aggarwal & Shishodia, 2006). As a consequence, it inhibited cell proliferation and induced apotosis. Resveratrol inhibited UV-mediated increase in proliferating cell nuclear antigen (PCNA), CDK 2, 4 and 6, cyclins (D1 and D2), and the MAPKs in SKH-1 hairless mice. On cell lines of epidermoid carcinoma (A431) Ahmad et al. showed that resveratrol induced the blocking of the cellular cycle in the G1 phase and apoptosis *via* modulations in CDKIs-cyclin-CDK machinery (Ahmad et al, 2001). The authors showed that a retinoblastoma (Rb)-E2F/DP pathway was part of this mechanism. On SK-Mel-28 human melanoma cells, Larrosa et al. showed that resveratrol induced apoptosis, S phase arrest and up-regulation of cyclins A, E, and B1 (Larrosa et al, 2003). Another compound, carnosol, a phenolic diterpenes, present in rosemary, induced G2/M cell cycle arrest through altering the levels of cyclin A and cycle B1 (Pan & Ho, 2008). Honokiol, a biphenolic compound and constituent of the bark and leaves of Magnolia plant species, caused cell cycle arrest in tumor cells by stimulating Kip1/p27 and Cip1/p21 and it reduced the protein levels of CDK 2, CDK 4 and CDK 6, cyclin D1, D2 and E (Vaid et al, 2010). These studies indicate that natural products can exert their antiproliferative effect by modulating CDKIs-cyclin-CDK complex.

2.1.4 Apoptotic regulators

Many natural chemopreventive agents induce cell cycle arrest or apoptosis by activating p53 and its target genes. Ahmad et al. performed the first studies regarding the role of EGCG in the apoptosis of tumor cells in 1997 (Ahmad et al, 1997). They observed that EGCG protected the normal cells by reducing the number of keratinocytes that were sunburned. In precancer lesions (papillomas) and invasive squamous carcinoma EGCG stimulated apoptosis (Chung et al, 2003). Several studies showed that green tea administered orally in hairless SKH-1 mice increased the number of p53 and p21 positive cells in epidermis after irradiation (Khan et al, 2006; Yusuf et al, 2007). Also, it was noticed that polyphenols induced nuclear condensation, the activation of caspase 3 and the cleavage of poly (ADP)-ribose polymerase. They determined the oligomerization of Bax and the depolarization of the mitochondrial membrane, realising the cytochrome c into the cytosol. These findings were supported by the fact that adding catalase to the cellular system prevented the apoptosis generated by EGCG (Khan et al, 2006). Babli et al. have shown that treatment with different concentrations of theaflavins and thearubigins from black tea on A375 cells reduced of Bcl-2 protein expression, and increased the Bax expression (Babli et al, 2008). The increased ratio of Bax/Bcl-2 proteins may be responsible for the induction of apoptosis in these cells.

Huang et al reported that resveratrol induced apoptosis in cells expressing wild-type p53, but not in p53-deficient cells (Huang et al, 1999). Resveratrol also, activated the expression of p21, p27, BAX, PUMA, MDM2, and cyclin G, all important downstream targets (Shankar et al, 2007). She et al. found that, in the JB6 mouse epidermal cell line, resveratrol activated ERK1/2, JNK, and p38 MAPK and induced serine-15 phosphorylation of p53 (She et al, 2001). In addition, resveratrolul modulated the function of survivin, a biomarker of tumor promotion and a negative regulator of apoptosis (Bhardwaj et al, 2007). Several studies have shown that topical treatment with silymarin to SKH-1 hairless mice inhibited solar UV radiation-induced skin tumorigenesis. The compound inhibited the proliferation of epidermis cells by inducing the expression of p53 and p21/cip 1 in cells (Dhanalakshmi et al, 2004). It was shown that curcumin, another natural compound, induced apoptosis in human basal cell carcinoma by increasing the expressions of p53, p21Waf1 and GADD145 proteins. It seems that the most important effect of curcumin is the anticarcinogenic one mainly due to the reduction of cellular proliferation and induction of apoptosis in the tumor cells and less due to its antioxidant and antiinflammatory effect (Pan & Ho, 2008). Naringenin, a flavanone present in orange peel, is believed to contribute to the activation of phase II detoxifying enzymes by protecting against UVB-induced apoptosis in keratinocyte HaKaT cells. In addition, naringenin induces apoptosis in various cancer cells (El-Mahdy et al, 2008).

Most of the natural chemopreventive agents including curcumin, resveratrol, EGCG, lycopene, genistein, and luteolin act as inhibitors of NF-kB pathways (Aggarwal & Shishodia, 2006; Amin et al, 2009; Singh & Aggarwal, 1995). These compounds may block one or more steps in the NF-kB signaling pathway such as: inhibition of the most upstream growth factor receptors that activate the NF-kB signaling cascade, translocation of NF-kB to the nucleus, DNA binding of the dimers, or interactions with the transcription. The most known NF-kB target genes influenced by the natural chemopreventive agents include inhibition of Bcl-2, Bcl-xXL, cyclin D1, MMPs and VEGF (Shishodia et al, 2005). It seems that curcumin and curcuminoids mediate their therapeutic effects by modulating NF-kB target genes. Resveratrol inhibited TPA stimulated activation of AP-1 in mouse skin *in vivo* and, applied topically, attenuated NF-kB activation by blocking IKKβ activity (Cooper & Bowden, 2007). Curcumin also, suppressed the TNF-α dependent activation of IKK and as a result it inhibited the translocation of the p65 subunit. Also, it inhibited the activation of NF-kB mediated by phorbol esters and hydrogen peroxide (Singh & Aggarwal, 1995). The same inhibitory effects were induced by resveratrol on epithelial cells (Masuda et al, 2001) or on models of chemical induced carcinogenesis (Manna et al, 2000). Another compound, the caffeic acid, decreased the binding of the p50-p65 complex to ADN while other antioxidants such as sanguinarine and emodin blocked the degradation of IkBa as a response to TNF-α, phorbol esters and IL-1 (Chaturvedi et al, 1997). Yang sc. showed that green tea polyphenols and EGCG inhibited the activation of NF-kB by inhibiting the activity of IKK, a mechanism that explains their antiproliferative effect (Yang et al, 2002).

Ahmad et al. recently reported that EGCG treatment inhibited cell growth and induced apoptosis in human epidermoid carcinoma (A431) cells but not in normal human epidermal keratinocytes (NHEK) (Ahmad et al, 2000). The effect was due to a stronger inhibition of EGCG on tumor cells of TNF-α-mediated NF-κB activation compared to normal cells.

It was shown that green tea polyphenols, quercetin, resveratrol, curcumin and capsaicin inhibited the activation of AP-1 by inhibiting the binding of AP-1 to DNA and as a consequence the transcriptional activation was inhibited. The effects of natural agents differ on the type of cells used. So, on human transformed bronchia cells EGCG inhibited c-Jun and ERK1/2 phosphorylation (Yang et al, 2000) while on normal keratinocytes EGCG increased the response to AP-1, a MAPKinase mediated effect (Balasubramanian et al, 2002). On HaKaT keratinocytes it was observed that EGCG blocked the activation of c-Fos induced by UVB and inhibited the activation of p38 (Chen et al, 1999). Recently, EGCG has been shown to inhibit 12-O-tetradecanoylphorbol-13-acetate or EGF-induced transformation of mouse epidermal cell line JB6 by the inhibition of AP-1 (Lu et al, 1994). *In vitro* it was shown that resveratrol inhibited the TNF-α dependent activation of AP-1 and as a consequence the activation of JNK and MEK kinases (Manna et al, 2000). Curcumin suppressed the expression of c-Jun and c-Fos in CD-1 mouse skin after treatment with TPA and the expression of COX-2 and PGE2 in the same model (Lu et al, 1994). Quercetin, another potent antioxidant, blocked the transcription of TNF-α induced by LPS in macrophages by inhibiting MAPkinases and the binding of AP-1 to DNA (Wadsworth et al, 2001).

The dietary phytochemicals such as curcumin (Cho et al, 2005), resveratrol (Shih et al, 2002), and green tea polyphenols (Katiyar et al, 2001) have been shown to modulate the MAPkinases. The first observations were made *in vitro* on epidermis microsomes from irradiated mice pre-treated with polyphenols. EGCG strong inhibited the tyrosine kinase and MAPK activities in transformed mouse embryonic fibroblast cells without effect in the normal cells (Wang & Bachrach, 2002). Pretreatment of normal human epidermal keratinocytes with EGCG reduced UVB-induced hydrogen peroxide production and its mediated phosphorylation of MAPK signaling pathways (Katiyar, et al., 2001). Thus, EGCG inhibited oxidative stress-mediated phosphorylation of MAPK signaling pathways. During acute UVB exposure, silibinin inhibited the activation of MAPK and AKT, induced p53 and Cip1/p21 expression and suppressed DNA damage in mouse skin (Gu et al, 2005). Resveratrol also, modulated all three MAPKinases, a variable effect depend on the cell type and the dose of resveratrol used. As a result, in some cells it activated MAPKinase and inhibited it in others. Woo et al. showed that resveratrol inhibited MMP-9 expressions PMA-induced by inhibiting JNK (Woo et al, 2004). It seems, that the ability of curcumin to modulate the MAPK signaling pathway, might contribute to the inhibition of inflammation by curcumin. Ursolic acid also, inhibited the activity of lipooxygenasis, the activation of STAT-3, the activation of c-Src, Janus 1, Janus 2 kinases and of the kinases regulated by extra-cellular signal (ERKs) (Hollosy et al, 2000). Another terpene carnosol, found in rosemary and sage leaves, inhibited LPS-induced activation of p38 and p44/42 MAPK and IKK, and reduced LPS-induced iNOS expression (Lo et al, 2002). Moreover, carnosol reduced invasion in B16/F10 melanoma cells, possibly through inhibition of NF-kB and c-Jun, and by blocking MMP-2 and MMP-9 activity (Huang et al, 2005).

2.1.5 Antioxidative effects

Tea polyphenols are strong scavengers against superoxide, hydrogen peroxide, hydroxyl radicals, nitric oxide and peroxynitrite produced by various chemicals and biological systems.

It has been shown that polyphenols from green tea administered topically or in the drinking water reduced the proliferation of experimental tumors in a dose-dependent manner and induced partial regression of skin papillomas in SKH-1 mice (Katiyar et al, 2001). This effect was due to reduction the DNA damage. Polyphenols decreased the generation of CPDs in the skin and protected against UV-induced depletion of antioxidant-defense enzymes. Green tea polyphenols have been reported to induce transcription of ARE (antioxidant-responsive element) dependent reporter genes and also to strongly activate ERK2 and JNK1 (Bode & Dong, 2003). This activation was shown to be associated with increased mRNA levels of the immediate-early response genes, *c-jun* and *c-fos*. EGCG, the most potent compound of green tea, protected against UV-induced depletion of GSH level and GPx activity in human skin (Katiyar et al, 2001), restored detoxification enzymes SOD and CAT on models of chemical-induced carcinogenesis (Saha & Das, 2002). Further more, EGCG treatment inhibited UVB-induced leukocyte infiltration in mouse and in human skin, and thus decreased oxidative stress (Benelli et al, 2002). Topical treatment of EGCG or GTPs inhibited acute or chronic UVB-induced protein oxidation in mice (Vayalil et al, 2004). The same effect was obtained when administered the green tea extract orally. Further more, the positive effect manifested also on skin MMPs suggesting a protective effect against ageing and carcinogenesis (Benelli et al, 2002). Proantocyanidins from grape seeds were more potent antioxidants and scavengers of free radicals than the ascorbic acid or vitamin E (Katiyar, 2008). Previously, our group has shown that topical application of a grape seed extract (Burgund Mare variety, *BM*) to mouse skin before a single UVB exposure (240 mJ/cm^2) markedly decreased UVB-induced production of lipid peroxides and nitric oxide and reduced caspase-3 activity (Filip et al, 2011). Our preliminary data revealed that *BM* extract reduced the UVB-induced increased cytokines (IL-6, TNF-α) levels and afforded protection against UV-induced alteration of GPx and CAT activities (in press). In addition, 24 hrs following irradiation *BM* extract inhibited one dose UVB-induced sunburn cells and CPDs formation (in press). The data showed also that MnSOD activity decreased after multiple UVB exposures and increased after topical application of *BM* extract, close to control and vehicle groups. The lower MnSOD activity observed after UVB irradiation was most likely due to the damage of mitochondria (Denning et al, 2001). In other studies, UVB irradiation of human keratinocytes induced a significant increase in SOD activity and protein level. This increase in SOD was attributed to CuZnSOD (Sasaki et al, 1997). In fact, the literature concerning this antioxidant enzymes activity following UV irradiation are rather contradictory. Sharma et al. reported a decrease in CAT activity after a single UV exposure which was doubled after multiple irradiations (Sharma et al, 2007). *In vitro* experiments have revealed that the dose-dependent decline in CAT activity after UV exposure is mainly due to the direct photodestruction (Afaq & Mukhtar, 2001). Iizawa et al. noticed that chronic UVB irradiation had no effect on CAT activity in mice (Iizawa, et al, 1994). In vitro, on keratinocytes cell lines, proantocyanidins reduce the ROS mediated phosphorylation of MAPKs and the activation of NF-kB. Similar effects were obtained with other natural compounds. Ginkgo biloba extract inhibited lipoperoxidation by quenching the peroxyl radical and decreasing the formation of UVB-induced sunburn cells in skin (Svobodová, et al, 2003). The flowers of *Prunus persica* inhibited UVB-induced DNA damage and lipid peroxidation in skin fibroblasts and delayed UVB-induced tumorigenesis in SKH-1 hairless mice (Svobodová et al, 2003). Curcumin reduced TPA-induced inflammation, hyperplasia, proliferation, activity and expression of ornithine decarboxylase, generation of ROS, and oxidative DNA damage in mouse skin (Huang et al, 1997). Interestingly, although curcumin is considered as antioxidant there is a growing number of evidence that curcumin can act as pro-oxidant under certain conditions, exerting its anticancer activity by inducing ROS generation. In fact, the effect depends on its concentration. Whereas low concentrations of curcumin (<20 µM) decreased ROS production, higher concentrations favored ROS generation (Chen et al, 2005).

2.1.6 Anti-inflammatory activity

It was affirmed that chronic inflammation though the recruitment of inflammatory cells, the release of cytokines and ROS created a micromedium favorable to cellular proliferation and carcinogenesis. On a model of contact hypersensitivity induced in mice by topical or systemic administration of 2,4-dinitrofluorobenzen it was observed that the proantocyanidins had a protective effect on the UVB-induced immunosuppresion. Proanthocyanidins also inhibited carrageenan-induced paw edema in rats and suppressed LPS-induced inflammation (Ho et al, 2007). Quercetin has anti-inflammatory effect due to the inhibition of lipoxygenase, cyclooxygenase, and PKC, resulting in a reduction of the production of pro-inflammatory mediators (Pan & Ho, 2008). More recently, silibinin has been found to inhibit inflammation and angiogenesis in SKH-1 hairless mice and protect from photocarcinogenesis by modulation of cell cycle regulators, MAPK and AKT signaling pathways (Gu et al, 2005).

2.1.7 COX-2

Several dietary components including galangin, luteolin, apigenin, genistein, green tea catechins, curcumin, and resveratrol have been shown to suppress COX-2. The inhibition took place at a transcriptional level. Curcumin was one of the first chemopreventive phytochemicals shown to possess significant COX-2 inhibiting activity through the suppression of NF-kB (Kundu et al, 2009). A similar effect was observed in delphinidin, an anthocyanidin present in dark fruit (Afaq et al, 2007). It inhibited the COX-2 expression by blocking MAPK signaling and NF-kB, AP-1 and C/EBPd nuclear translocation and conferred protection against UVB-mediated oxidative stress and apoptosis in mouse skin. It was found that the treatment with silymarin and green tea extract inhibited UVB-induced sunburn cell formation, COX and ornithine decarboxylase activities and ornithine decarboxylase mRNA expression (Katiyar et al, 1997). Moreover, pretreatment with green tea extract inhibited COX-2 expression induced by TPA in mouse skin and assured a good protection against erythema, immunosuppression and photoageing of the irradiated skin. Also, EGCG treatment reduced UVB-induced production of PG metabolites, such as PGE2, PGF2a and PGD2, molecules involved in tumor promotion. Topical application of oligonol-G, an innovative formulation composed of catechin-type oligomeric polyphenols, lowered chemically induced tumor promotion, UVB-induced lipid peroxidation, and 12-O- tetradecanoylphorbol-13-acetate (TPA) or UVB-induced COX-2 expression in mouse skin (Kundu et al., 2008). The oral administration of oligonol-L or oligonol-G had the same effect as the topical treatment on COX-2 expression in UVB irradiated hairless mouse skin (Kundu et al, 2009). The effect was mediated by the inhibition of ERK1/2 and p38 MAPkinase activation. Pretreatment with caffeine inhibited phosphorylation of AKT and up-regulation of COX-2, two critical oncogenic pathways in skin tumorigenesis. Also, it increased UVB-induced apoptosis in HaKaT cells, and blocked UVB-induced CDK1 phosphorylation (Han et al, 2011).

2.1.8 MMPs

Recent studies have indicated that the MAPkinase signal transduction pathways play an important role in regulating a variety of cellular functions including MMP expression and cell growth (Cho et al, 2007). It was shown that MMP-9 expression was regulated by JNK- and ERK-dependent signaling pathways; the regulatory effect was inhibited by the administration of de green tea polyphenols and black tea extract (Gum et al, 1997). EGCG has been also, reported to inhibit the MMP-2 and MMP-9 and prevent UVB-induced suppression of the immune system in mice. Administered orally, the green tea extract inhibited UV carcinogenesis, reduced the expression of MMP-2 and MMP-9 in parallel with an increase in the expression of the TIMP-1 inhibitor (Mantena et al, 2005). Moreover, it was observed that its effect was accompanied by a reduction in the expression of vascular endothelial cell antigens, such as CD31 and VEGF, in the UVB-induced tumors. Curcumin was shown to down-regulate the expression of MMP-2 and MMP-9 (Heng, 2010). It was known as MMP-2 and MMP-9 are responsible for digestion of collagen IV in basement membranes and subendothelial collagen V, allowing the tumor cells to invade the dermis, as well as penetrate blood vessels.

3. Botanicals antioxidants used in chemoprevention

Of all the chemopreventive agents polyphenols enjoy the most attention as they are found in a great variety of fruits and plants and have proven their complex effects in both *in vivo* and *in vitro* studies. In the table are presented the main phytochemicals used in chemopreventions of skin cancer, the experimental models studied and the mechanisms involved.

Plant	Active principals	Experimental model	Target/Mechanism of action
Curcuma longa	curcumin	DMBA-TPA-induced papillomas	↓ MAPK, ↓ NF-kB (Chun et al, 2003)
		DMBA-induced papillomas	antioxidant (Soudamini & Kuttan, 1989)
		CD-1 mice/TPA	↓ COX (Ishizaki et al, 1996)
		HEC cell	↓ caspases, ↓ cytochrome c (Chan et al, 2003)
		A 431 , HaKaT cell	↓ COX, AP-1, ↑ caspases, cytochrome c (Cho et al, 2005)
Ocimum sanctum	leaf extract	DMBA-induced skin tumors in mice	antioxidant (Prashar et al, 1994)
Ocimum gratissimum	clocimum oil	DMBA-induced skin papillomas	antioxidant, ↑ -SH, ↑cytochrome b5 (Singh et al, 1999).
Zingibe officinale	gingerol	JB6 cells	↓ AP-1 (Bode et al, 2001)
		HaKaT cell	↓ ROS, ↓ caspases, ↓ COX-2, ↓ NF-kB (Kim et al, 2007)
		SKH-1	↓ COX-2, ↓ NF-KB (Kim et al, 2007)
Silybum marianum	silibinin	SENCAR mouse	↓ LPO, ↓ DNA synthesis (Aggarwal et al, 1994)
		SKH-1	↓ tumors, ↓ iNOS, ↓ COX-2, ↓ NF-kB (Gu et al, 2005); ↓ CPDs, ↓ p53 (Dhanalashmi 2004)
		HaKaT	↓ ROS, ↑ GSH (Svobodova et al, 2007)
		C3H/HeN	↓ IL-10, ↓ IL-12, ↓ ROS, ↓ CD 11b+ (Katiyar et al, 2008)
fruits	apigenin	SKH-1	↓ ODC, p53, cell cycle regulatory proteins (Svobodova et al, 2003)
Rosemarinus officinalis and Salvia officinalis	carnusol, acid ursolic	mouse	↓ DMBA-initiation, TPA-promotion, ↓ mARN MMP-1 (Svobodova et al, 2003)
Ginko biloba	ginko biloba extract	mouse	↑ SOD, ↑ CAT in skin (Svobodova et al, 2003)

Plant	Active principals	Experimental model	Target/Mechanism of action
Sanguinaria canadiensis	sanguinarine	A 431	↑ apoptosis (Ahsan et al, 2007)
		SKH-1	↓ edema, ↓ hyperplasia, ↓ PCNA, ↓ ODC (Ahsan et al, 2007)
Soy isofavones	genistein	hairless mice	↓ expression of protooncogene and skin tumorigenesis (Svobodova et al, 2003)
		SENCAR	↓ c-fos, ↓c-jun (Wang et al, 1998)
		SKH-1	↓ H_2O_2, ↓ LPO, ↓ 8-OHdG (Wei et al, 2002)
Prunus persica	kaempferol	in vitro	↓ cytotoxicity, ↓ DNA damage, ↓ LPO (Svobodova et al, 2003)
		guinea pigs	↓ edema
		SKH-1	↓ tumor development
Punica granatum	delphinidin	HaKaT	↓ LPO, ↓ PCNA, ↓ 8-HOdG (Afaq et al, 2005)
		SKH-1	apoptosis, ↓ CPDs (Afaq et al, 2007)
Vitis vinifera	proanthocyanidins	DMBA-TPA-induced skin tumorigenesis	↓ ODC, ↓ myeloperoxidase, ↓ PKC (Bomser et al, 2000)
	polyphenols	DMBA-TPA-induced skin carcinogenesis	antioxidant (Zhao, et al, 1999)
	resveratrol	SKH-1	↓ survivin,↑ Smac/DIABLO (Aziz, et al, 2005) ↓ edema, ↓ H_2O_2, ↓ infiltration of leucocytes, ↓ COX, ↓ NF-kB (Afaq et al, 2003) ↓ROS, ↓ MAPK, ↓ NF-kB (Katiyar 2008)
		NHEK	↓ NF-kB (Adhami et al, 2003)
		in vitro	antioxidant, antiinflamamtory, antiproliferative (Dong, 2003)
Withania somnifera	root extract	DMBA-induced papillomas in mice	antioxidant (Prakash et al, 2002)
Camellia sinensis	EGCG, polyphenols	SKH-1	antioxidant (Vayalil, et al, 2003), ↑ p53, ↑ NER (Lu et al, 2000)
		Balb/c	↓ incidence, multiplicity and volume of tumors (Katiyar et al, 2001)
		C3H/HeN	↓ LPO, protein oxidation, ↑ GSH, ↓ CD 11b+ cells (Afaq et al. 2005, Matsumura and Anastawamy, 2004)
		C3H/HeN mice	↑ IL-12 and prevent immunosuppression UV-induced (Ahmad et al, 2000)

Abbreviations: ↓down-regulation, ↑up-regulation, NHEK - normal human epidermal keratinocytes, LPO – lipid peroxidation, ODC – ornithine decarboxylase, PCNA- proliferating cell nuclear antigen, MAPkinase- mitogen activated kinase, Smac - second mitochondria-derived activator of caspase, AP-1 – activator protein 1, NF-kB – nuclear factor kappa B, COX-2 – cyclooxigenase 2, SOD – superoxid dismutase, CAT – catalase, iNOS - inducible nitric oxide synthase, p53- tumor suppressor protein, MMP- metalloproteases, IL– interleukin, DIABLO - Direct IAP binding protein of low PI, ROS – reactive oxygen species, NER - nucleotide excision repair, 8-OHdG - 8-hydroxy-20-deoxyguanosine, GSH- glutathione reduced, TPA - 12-O-tetradecanoyl-phorbol-13-acetate , DMBA - 7,12-dimethylbenz-alpha- anthracene, c-fos, c-jun - protein of AP-1

Table 1. Molecular mechanisms involved in chemopreventive activity of natural products.

4. Clinical trials

Due to the growing literature on natural compounds efficacy against a variety of cancers, several human trials using these agents have been conducted in the recent years. Epidemiological studies support a protective role of flavonoids, lycopene, lutein and various nutrient combinations administered orally or topically against DNA-damage. However, the data are not entirely consistent. Linden et al. used topical epigallocatechin gallate in a randomized, double-blind, placebo-controlled phase II clinical trial in the prevention of nonmelanoma skin cancer (Linden et al, 2003). Other dietary compounds, including silibinin, genistein, curcumin and resveratrol, have been recognized as cancer chemopreventive agents but their role in humans is still limited.

5. Conclusions and perspectives

UV irradiation of skin causes a number of cellular and pathological changes, including DNA damage, cell-cycle arrest, formation of sunburn cells (apoptosis), depletion of the antioxidant defense system, release of proinflammatory cytokines and immunosuppressive effects. The combination of these events can lead to cancer development. Epidemiologic and animal studies have identified the associations between certain diets and modulation of cancer risk. Diet/nutrition can exacerbate or interfere with carcinogenesis through genetic and epigenetic modulation, leading to altered cellular phenotypes and differing cancer outcomes. Thus, dietary intervention appears to be a promising strategy to prevent carcinogenesis. Further more, the natural compounds are non toxic agents and their using in therapy may also decrease the systemic toxicity caused by chemotherapy or radiotherapy. Understanding the molecular mechanisms of their action and effects on cellular signaling processes, as well as their structure-activity relationships is necessary for the generation of new, more effective derivatives. Further investigation of optimal doses and mechanism of protection are needed to better target and prevent photodamage with dietary and/or topical treatments.

6. Acknowledgment

This work was supported by the Ministry of Education, Research and Youth by PN II Program (42-104/2008)

7. References

[1] Adhami, V M. Afaq, F. Ahmad, N. (2003). Suppression of ultraviolet B exposure-mediated activation of NF-κB in normal human keratinocytes by resveratrol. *Neoplasia*, 5:74-82

[2] Afag, F. Mukhtar, H. (2001). Effects of solar radiation on cutaneous detoxification pathways. *J. Photochem. Photobiol, B* 63 61–9, ISSN.

[3] Afaq, F. Malik, A. Syed, D. Maes, D. Matsui, M S., Mukhtar, H. (2005). Pomegranate fruit extract modulates UV-B-mediated phosphorylation of mitogen-activated protein kinases and activation of nuclear factor κ B in normal human epidermal keratinocytes. *Photochem and Photobiol*, 81, 38–45.

[4] Afaq, F. Adhami, V M. Ahmad, N. (2003). Prevention of short-term ultraviolet B radiation-mediated damages by resveratrol in SKH-1 hairless mice. *Toxicol and Applied Pharmacol*, 186, 28-37.

[5] Afaq, F. Syed, D N. Malik, A. Hadi, N. Sarfaraz, S. Kweon, M H. Khan N, Zaid, M A. Mukhtar, H. (2007). Delphinidin, an anthocyanidin in pigmented fruits and vegetables, protects human HaCaT keratinocytes and mouse skin against UVB-mediated oxidative stress and apoptosis. *J. of Investig. Dermatol*, 127, 222–232.

[6] Agarwal, R. Katiyar, S K. Lundgren, D W. Mukhtar, H. (1994). Inhibitory effect of silymarin, an anti-hepatotoxic flavonoid, on 12-O-tetradecanoylphorbol-13-acetate-induced epidermal ornithine decarboxylase activity and mRNA in SENCAR mice. *Carcinogenesis*, 15, 1099-1103.

[7] Aggarwal, B B. Shishodia, S. (2006). Molecular targets of dietary agents for prevention and prevention and therapy of cancers. Biochem Pharmacol, 71, 1397- 1421.

[8] Ahmad, N. Gupta, S. Mukhtar, H. (2000). Green tea polyphenol epigallocatechin-3-gallate differentially modulates nuclear factor kappa B in cancer cells versus normal cells. *Arch Biochem Biophys*, 376, 338–46.

[9] Ahmad, N. Adhami, V M. Afaq, F. Feyes, D K. Mukhtar, H. (2001). Resveratrol causes WAF-1/p21-mediated G (1)-phase arrest of cell cycle and induction of apoptosis in human epidermoid carcinoma A431 cells. *Clin Cancer Res*, 7, 1466-1473.

[10] Ahmed, N U. Ueda, M. Nikaido, O. Osawa, T. Ichihashi, M. (1999). High levels of 8-hydroxy-2'-deoxyguanosine appear in normal human epidermis after a single dose of ultraviolet radiation. *Br. J. Dermatol*, 140, 226–231.

[11] Ahsan, H. Reagan-Shaw, S. Eggert, D M. Tan, T C. Afaq, F. Mukhtar, H. Ahmad, N. (2007). Protective effect of sanguinarine on ultraviolet B-mediated damages in SKH-1 hairless mouse skin: implications for prevention of skin cancer. *Photochem and Photobiol*, 83, 986-993.

[12] Alam, J. Stewart, D. Touchard, C. Boinapally, S. Choi, A M. Cook, J L. (1999). Nrf2, a Cap'n'Collar transcription factor, regulates induction of the heme oxygenase-1 gene. *J Biol Chem*, 274, 26071–8.

[13] Alam, J. Wicks, C. Stewart, D. Gong, P. Touchard, C. Otterbein, S. Choi, A M. Burow, M E. Tou (2000). Mechanism of heme oxygenase-1 gene activation by cadmium in MCF-7 mammary epithelial cells. Role of p38 kinase and Nrf2 transcription factor. *J Biol Chem*, 275, 27694-27702.

[14] Altieri, D C. (2003). Validating survivin as a cancer therapeutic target. *Nat Rev Cancer*, 3, 46-54.

[15] Amerio, P. Carbone, A. Auriemma, M. Varrati, S. Tulli, A. (2000). UV Induced Skin Immunosuppression. *Anti-Inflammatory & Anti-Allergy Agents in Medicinal Chemistry*, 8, 3-13.

[16] Amin ARMR, Kucuk O, Khuri FR, Shin DM, (2009) Perspectives for Cancer Prevention With Natural Compounds, *J Clin Oncol*, 27, 2712-2725.

[17] Aziz, M H. Reagan-Shaw, S. Wu, J. Longley, B J. Ahmad, N. (2005). Chemoprevention of skin cancer by grape constituent resveratrol: relevance to human disease? *The FASEB Journal*, 19, 1193-5.

[18] Babli, H. Udayan, B. Sibabrata, M. Ashok, K G. (2008). Molecular mechanism of black tea polyphenols induced apoptosis in human skin cancer cells: involvement of Bax translocation and mitochondria mediated death cascade. *Carcinogenesis*, 29, 129–38.

[19] Balasubramanian, S. Efimova, T. Eckert, R L. (2002). Green tea polyphenol stimulates a Ras, MEKK1, MEK3, and p38 cascade to increase activator protein 1 factor-dependent involucrin gene expression in normal human keratinocytes. *J Biol Chem,* 277(3), 1828–36.

[20] Baldwin, A S. (2001). Control of oncogenesis and cancer therapy resistance by the transcription factor NF-kB. *J Clin. Investig,* 107, 241-246.

[21] Basset-Seguin, N. Moles, J P. Mils, V. Dereue O. & Guillou J J. (1994) P53 tumor suppressor gene and skin carcinogenesis *J. Invest. Dermatol,* 103, 102S–106S.

[22] Bartsch, H. Nair, J. (2004). Oxidative stress and lipid peroxidation-derived DNA lesions in inflammation driven carcinogenesis. *Cancer Detect. Prev,* 28, 385–91.

[23] Benelli, R. Vene, R. Bisacchi, D. Garbisa, S. & Albini, A. (2002). Anti-invasive effects of green tea polyphenol epigallocatechin-3-gallate (EGCG), a natural inhibitor of metallo and serine proteases. *Biol Chem,* 383, 101–105.

[24] Bhardwaj, A. Sethi, G. Vadhan-Raj, S. Bueso-Ramos, C. Takada, Y. Gaur, U. Nair, A S. Shishodia, S. Aggarwal, B B. (2007). Resveratrol inhibits proliferation, induces apoptosis, and overcomes chemoresistance through down-regulation of STAT3 and nuclear factor-kappa B regulated antiapoptotic and cell survival gene products in human multiple myeloma cells. *Blood,* 109, 2293-2302.

[25] Bode, A M. Ma, W Y., Surh, Y J. Dong, Z. (2001). Inhibition of epidermal growth factor-induced cell transformation and activator protein 1 activation by [6]-gingerol. *Cancer Research,* 61, 850-853.

[26] Bode, A. Dong, Z. (2003). Signal Transduction Pathways: Targets for Green and Black Tea Polyphenols, *Journal of Biochemistry and Molecular Biology,* 36, 1, 66-77

[27] Bode, A M. Dong, Z. (2003). Mitogen-activated protein kinase activation in UV-induced signal transduction. *Sci Stke,* 167:1–15.

[28] Bomser, J. Singletary, K. Meline, B. (2000). Inhibition of 12-Otetradecanoyl phorbol-13-acetate (TPA)-induced mouse skin ornithine decarboxylase and protein kinase C by polyphenolics from grapes. *Chem Bull,* 127, 43–59.

[29] Bowden, G T. (2004). Prevention of non-melanoma skin cancer by targeting ultraviolet-B-light signaling. *Nat Rev Cancer,* 4, 23–35.

[30] Brash, D E. Ziegler, A. Jonason, A S. Simon, J A. (1996). Sunlight and sunburn in human skin cancer: p53, apoptosis and tumor promotion. *J Investig Dermatol Symp Proc,* 1, 136–42.

[31] Buettner, R. Mora, L B. Jove, R A. (2002). Activated STAT signaling in human tumors provides novel molecular targets for therapeutic intervention. *Clin Cancer Res,* 8, 945-54

[32] Chang, L, Karin, M. (2001). Mammalian MAP-kinase signaling cascades. *Nature,* 410, 37-40.

[33] Chaturvedi, M M. Kumar, A. Darnay, B G. Chainy, G B. Agarwal, S. Aggarwal, B B. (1997). Sanguinarine (pseudochelerythrine) is a potent inhibitor of NF-kappaB activation, IkappaBalpha phosphorylation, and degradation. *J Biol Chem,* 272(48), 30129–34.

[34] Chen, F. Castranova, V. Shi, X. (2001). New insights into the role of nuclear factor-_B in cell growth regulation. *Am J Pathol,* 159, 387– 397.

[35] Chen, J. Wanming, D. Zhang D, Liu, Q. Kang, J. (2005). Water-soluble antioxidants improve the antioxidant and anticancer activity of low concentrations of curcumin in human leukemia cells. *Pharmazie,* 60, 57-61.

[36] Chen, W. Dong, Z. Valcic, S. Timmermann, B N. Bowden, G T. (1999). Inhibition of ultraviolet B-induced c-fos gene expression and p38 mitogen-activated protein kinase activation by (_)-epigallocatechin gallate in a human keratinocyte cell line. *Mol Carcinogen,* 24(2), 79–84.

[37] Cho, J W. Park, K. Kweon, G R. Jang, B C. Baek, W K. Suh, M H. et al. (2005). Curcumin inhibits the expression of COX-2 in UVB irradiated human keratinocytes (HaCaT) by inhibiting activation of AP-1: p38 MAP kinase and JNK as potential upstream targets. *Exp Mol Med,* 37(3), 186–92.

[38] Chun, K S. Keum, Y. Han, S S. *et al.* (2003). Curcumin inhibits phorbol-ester induced expression of OX-2 in mouse skin through suppression of extracellular signal regulated kinase activity and NF-kappa B activation. *Carcinogenesis,* 24, 1515–24.

[39] Chun, K S. Cha, H H. Shin, J W. Na, H K. Park, K K. Chung, W Y. Surh, Y J. (2004). Nitric oxide induces expression of cyclooxygenase-2 in mouse skin through activation of NF-kB. *Carcinogenesis,* 25, 445–54.

[40] Cooper, S J. Bowden, G T. (2007). Ultraviolet B Regulation of Transcription Factor Families: Roles of Nuclear Factor-kappa B (NF-κB) and Activator Protein-1 (AP-1) in UVB-Induced Skin Carcinogenesis. *Curr Cancer Drug Targets,* 7(4), 325–334.

[41] Denning, M F. Wang, Y. Tibudan, S. Alkan, S. Nickoloff, B J. Qin, J S. (2002). Caspase activation and disruption of mitochondrial membrane potential during UV radiation-induced apoptosis of human keratinocytes requires activation of protein kinase. *C Cell Death Differ,* 9, 40–52.

[42] Dhanalakshmi, S. Mallikarjuna, G U. Singh, R P. Agarwal, R. (2004). Silibinin prevents UV 100 radiation-caused skin damages in SKH-1 hairless mice via decrease in thymine dimmer positive cells and an up-regulation of p53-p21/Cip1 in epidermis. *Carcinogenesis,* 25, 1459-1465.

[43] Dong, Z. (2003). Molecular mechanism of the chemopreventive effect of resveratrol. *Mutation Research,* 523-524, 145-160.

[44] Dorai, T. Aggarwal, B. (2004). Role of chemopreventive agents in cancer therapy *Cancer Lett.* 25, 215(2), 129-40.

[45] Droge, W. (2002). Free radicals in the physiological control of cell function. *Physiol. Rev.* 82, 47–95.

[46] Elmets, C A. Singh, D. Tubesing, K. *et al.* (2001). Cutaneous photoprotection from ultraviolet injury by green tea poliphenols. *J Am Acad Dermatol,* 44, 425–32.

[47] Faraonio, R. Vergara, P. Di Marzo, D. Pierantoni, M G. Napolitano, M. Russo, T et al. (2006) .p53 suppresses the Nrf2-dependent transcription of antioxidant response genes. *J Biol Chem,* 281, 39776–84.

[48] Filip, A. Daicoviciu, D. Clichici, S. Mocan, T. Muresan, A. Postescu, I D. (2011).Photoprotective effects of 2 Natural Products on Ultraviolet B-Induced Oxidative Stress and Apoptosis in SH-1 Mouse Skin. *J Med Food,* 2011, 14(7-8), 761-766.

[49] Fischer, S M. Pavone, A. Mikulec, C. Langenbach, R. Rundhaug, J E. (2007). Cyclooxygenase-2 Expression Is Critical for Chronic UV-Induced Murine Skin Carcinogenesis. *Mol Carcinog,* 46(5), 363-371.

[50] Garg, A. Aggarwal, B B. (2002). Nuclear transcription factor-kB as a target for cancer Drug Development. *Leukemia,* 16, 1053-1068.

[51] Gu, M. Dhanalakshmi, S. Moha,n S. Sing,h R P. Agarwal, R. (2005). Silibinin inhibits ultraviolet B radiation-induced mitogenic and survival signaling, and associated biological responses in SKH-1 mouse skin. *Carcinogenesis,* 26, 1404–13.

[52] Gum, R. Wang, H. Lengyel, E. Juarez, J. Boyd, D. (1997). Regulation of 92 kDa type IV collagenase expression by the jun aminoterminal kinase- and the extracellular signal-regulated kinase-dependent signaling cascades. *Oncogene,* 14, 1481–1493.

[53] Halliday, G M. (2005). Inflammation, gene mutation and photoimmunosuppression in response to UVR-induced oxidative damage contribute to photocarcinogenesis. *Mutat. Res.* 571, 107–120.

[54] Han, W. Ming, M. He, Y Y. (2011). Caffeine promotes UVB-induced apoptosis in human keratinocytes without complete DNA repair. *JBC Papers,* doi/10.1074/jbc.M111.222349

[55] Heng, M. (2010). Curcumin targeted signaling pathways: basis for anti-photoaging and anti-carcinogenic therapy. *Int J of Dermatol* 49, 608–622.

[56] Heck, D E. Vetrano, A M. Mariano, T M. Laskin, J D. (2003). UVB Light Stimulates Production of Reactive Oxygen Species. Unexpected role for catalase. *J. of Biol. Chem.* 278, 25, 22432–22436.

[57] Ho, S C. Hwang, L S. Shen, Y J. Li,n C C. (2007). Suppressive effect of a proanthocyanidin-rich extract from longan (Dimocarpus longan Lour.) flowers on nitric oxide production in LPS-stimulated macrophage cells. *J. Agric. Food Chem.,* 55, 10664-70.

[58] Hollosy, F. Meszaros, G. Bokonyi, G. et al. (2000). Cytostatic, cytotoxic and protein tyrosine kinase inhibitory activity of ursolic acid in A431 human tumor cells. *Anticancer Res,* 20, 4563–70.

[59] Huang, C. Ma, W Y. Goranson, A. et al (1999). Resveratrol suppresses cell transformation and induces apoptosis through a p53-dependent pathway. *Carcinogenesis,* 20, 237-242.

[60] Huang, H C. Nguyen, T. Pickett, C B. (2002). Phosphorylation of Nrf2 at Ser-40 by protein kinase C regulates antioxidant response element-mediated transcription. *J Biol Chem,* 277, 42769-42774.

[61] Huang, S C. Ho, C T. Lin-Shiau, S Y. Lin, J C. (2005). Carnosol inhibits the invasion of B16/F10 mouse melanoma cells by suppressing metalloproteinase-9 through down-regulating nuclear factor-kappa B and c-Jun. *Biochem. Pharmacol,* 69, 221.

[62] Ichihashi, M. Ueda, M. Budiyanto, A. Bito, T. Oka, M. Fukunaga, M. et al. (2003). UV-induced skin damage. *Toxicology,* 189, 21–39.

[63] Iizawa, O. Kato, T. Tagami, H. Akamatsu, H. Niwa, Y. (1994). Long-term follow-up study of changes in lipid peroxide levels and the activity of superoxide dismutase, catalase and glutathione peroxidase in mouse skin after acute and chronic UV irradiation. *Arch.of Dermatol Research,* 286, 47-52.

[64] Ishii, T. Itoh, K. Sato, H. Bannai, S. (1999). Oxidative stress-inducible proteins in macrophages. *Free Radic Res,* 31, 351–5.

[65] Ishizaki, C. Oguro, T. Yoshida, T. Wen, C Q. Suekei, H. Iijima, M. (1996). Enhancing effect of ultraviolet A on ornithine decarboxylase induction and dermatitis evoked

by 12-O-tetra-decanoylphorbol-13-acetate and its inhibition by curcumin in mouse skin. *Dermatology*, 193, 311-317.

[66] Jurkiewicz, B A. Bissett, D L. Buettner, G R. (1995). Effect of topically applied tocopherol on ultraviolet radiation-mediated free radical damage in skin. *J. Invest. Dermatol*, 104, 484-88

[67] Kane, A B. Kumar, V. (1999). Environmental and nutritional pathology. In: Cotran RS, Kumar V, Collins T. (Eds.) Robbins pathologic basis of disease. Philadelphia: WB Saunders Company: 403–58.

[68] Kang, K W. Lee, S J. Park, J W. Kim, S G. (2002). Phosphatidylinositol 3-kinase regulates nuclear translocation of NF-E2-related factor 2 through actin rearrangement in response to oxidative stress. *Mol Pharmacol*, 62, 1001-1010.

[69] Katiyar, S K. Norman, N J. Mukhtar, H. Agarwal, R. (1997). Protective Effects of Silymarin Against Photocarcinogenesis in a Mouse Skin Model, *J Natl Cancer Inst*, 89 (8), 556-565.

[70] Katiyar, S K. Afaq, F. Azizzudin, K. et al. (2001). Inhibition of UVB-induced oxidative stress-mediated phosphorylation of mitogen-activated protein kinase signaling pathways in cultured human epidermal keratinocytes by green tea polyphenol (-)-epigallocatechin-3-galate. *Toxicol Appl Pharmacol*, 2001, 178, 110-7.

[71] Katiyar, S K. Elmets, C A. (2001). Green tea antioxidants and skin photoprotection. *Int J Oncol*, 18, 1307–1.

[72] Katiyar, S K. Mukhtar, H. (2001). Green tea polyphenol (-)-epigallocatechin-3-gallate treatment to mouse skin prevents UVB-induced infiltration of leukocytes, depletion of antigen cells and oxidative stress. *J Leukoc Biol*, 69, 719–26.

[73] Katiyar, S. (2008). Grape seed proanthocyanidines and skin cancer prevention: onhibition of oxidative stress and protection of immune system. *Mol Nutr Food Res*, 52 (Suppl 1), S71–6.

[74] Kawachi, Y. Xu, X. Taguchi, S. Sakurai, H. Nakamura, Y. Ishii, Y. Fujisawa, Y. Furuta, J. Takahashi, T. (2008). Attenuation of UVB-Induced Sunburn Reaction and Oxidative DNA Damage with no Alterations in UVB-Induced Skin Carcinogenesis in Nrf2 Gene-Deficient Mice. *J of Investig Dermatol*, 128, 1773–1779.

[75] Khan, H. Afaq, F. Saleem, M. Ahmad, N. (2006). Targeting multiple signaling pathways by green tea polyphenol (-)-epigallocatechin- 3-gallate. *Cancer Res*, 66, 2500–5.

[76] Kim, J K. Kim, Y. Na, K M., Surh, Y J. Kim, T Y. (2007). Gingerol prevents UVB-induced ROS production and COX-2 expression in vitro and in vivo. *Free Radical Research*, 41, 603-614.

[77] Klatt, P. Lamas, S. (2000). Regulation of protein function by S-glutathiolation in response to oxidative and nitrosative stress. *Eur J Biochem, 267*, 4928-4944.

[78] Klaunig, J.E. Kamendulis, L M. (2004). The role of oxidative stress in carcinogenesis. *Annu Rev Pharmacol. Toxicol, 44*, 239-267.

[79] Korutla, L. Kumar, R. (1994). Inhibitory effect of curcumin on epidermal growth factor receptor kinase activity in A431 cells. *Biochim Biophys Acta*, 1224, 597-600.

[80] Kotlo, K U. Yehiely, F. Efimova, E. Harasty, H. Hesabi, B. Shchors, K. et al. (2003). Nrf2 is an inhibitor of the Fas pathway as identified by Achilles' Heel Method, a new function-based approach to gene identification in human cells. *Oncogene*, 22, 797–806.

[81] Kundu, K J. Choi, K S. Fujii, H. Sun, B. Surh, Y J. (2009). Oligonol, a lychee fruit-derived low molecular weight polyphenol formulation, inhibits UVB-induced cyclooxygenase-2 expression, and induces NAD(P)H:quinine oxidoreductase-1 expression in hairless mouse skin. *J of Functional Food.* 1, 98-108.

[82] Lapenna, S. Giordano, A.(2009). Cell cycle kinases as therapeutic targets for cancer. *Nat Rev Drug Discov*, 8, 547-66

[83] Larrosa, M. Tomas-Barberan, F A. and Espin, J C. (2003). Grape Polyphenol Resveratrol and the Related Molecule 4- Hydroxystilbene Induce Growth Inhibition, Apoptosis, S-Phase Arrest, and Upregulation of Cyclins A, E, and B1 in Human SK-Mel-28 Melanoma Cells. *J Agric Food Chem*, 51, 4576- 4584.

[84] Li, N. Nel, A E. (2006). Role of the Nrf2-mediated signaling pathway as a negative regulator of inflammation: implications for the impact of particulate pollutants on asthma. *Antioxid Redox Signal*, 8, 88–98.

[85] Lin, J K. (2002). Cancer Chemoprevention by Tea Polyphenols Through Modulating Signal Transduction Pathways. *Arch of Pharm Res*, 25, 5 561-571.

[86] Linden, K G. Carpenter, P M, Mc Laren, C E. Barr, R J. Hite, P. Sun, J D. Li, K T. Viner, J L. Meyskens, F L. (2003). Chemoprevention of nonmelanoma skin cancer: experience with a polyphenol from green tea. *Recent Results Cancer Res*, 163, 165-71.

[87] Lo, A H. Liang, Y C. Lin-Shiau, S Y, Ho, C T. Lin, J K. (2002). Carnosol, an antioxidant in rosemary, suppresses inducible nitric oxide synthase through down-regulating nuclear factor-kappaB in mouse macrophages. *Carcinogenesis*, 23, 983.

[88] Lopez-Torres, M. Thielle, J J. Shindo, Y. (1998). Topical application of α-tocopherol modulates the antioxidant network and diminishes ultraviolet-induced pxidative damage in murine skin. *Br J Dermatol*, 138, 207–15.

[89] Lu, Y P. Chang, R L. Lou, Y R. Huang, M T. Newmark, H L. Reuhl, K R. Conney, A H. (1994). Effect of curcumin on 12-O-tetradecanoylphorbol-13-acetate- and ultraviolet B light-induced expression of c-Jun and c-Fos in JB6 cells and in mouse epidermis. *Carcinogenesis*, 15, 2363–70.

[90] Lu, Y P. Lou, Y R. Li, X H., Xie, J G. Brash, D. Huang, M T. Conney, A H. (2000). Stimulatory effect of oral administration of green tea or caffeine on ultraviolet light-induced increases in epidermal wild-type p53, p21(WAF1/CIP1), and apoptotic sunburn cells in SKH-1 mice. *Cancer Res*, 60, 4785-4791.

[91] Luo, J L. Tong, W M. Yoon, J H. *et al.* (2001).UV-induced DNA damage and mutations in Hupki (human p53 knock-in) mice recapitulate p53 hotspot alterations in sun-exposed skin. *Cancer Res*, 61, 8158–62.

[92] El-Mahdy M A. Zhu, Q. Wang, Q E. Wani, G. Patnaik, S. Zhao, Q. Arafa, E S. Barakat, B. Mir, S N. Wani A A. (2008). Naringenin protects HaCaT human keratinocytes against UVB-induced apoptosis and enhances the removal of cyclobutane pyrimidine dimers from the genome. *Photochem. Photobiol*, 84(2), 30716.

[93] Manna, S K. Mukhopadhyay, A. Aggarwal, B B. (2000). Resveratrol suppresses TNF-induced activation of nuclear transcription factors NF-kappa B, activator protein-1, and apoptosis: potential role of reactive oxygen intermediates and lipid peroxidation. *J Immunol* 64(12), 6509–19.

[94] Mantena, S K. Meeran, S M. Elmets, C A. Katiyar, S K. (2005). Orally Administered Green Tea Polyphenols Prevent Ultraviolet Radiation- Induced Skin Cancer in Mice

through Activation of Cytotoxic T Cells and Inhibition of Angiogenesis in Tumors. *J Nutr,* 135, 2871–287.
[95] Masuda, M. Suzui, M. Weinstein, I B. (2001). Effects of epigallocatechin-3-gallate on growth, epidermal growth factor receptor signaling pathways, gene expression, and chemosensitivity in human head and neck squamous cell carcinoma cell lines. *Clin Cancer Res,* 7(12), 4220–9.
[96] Matsumura, Y. Ananthaswamy, H N. (2004). Toxic effects of ultraviolet radiation on the skin. *Toxicol and Applied Parmacol,* 195, 298-308.
[97] Mitchell, D L. Rudiger, G. de Gruijl, F R. Guikers, K L H. Breitbart, E W. Byrom, M. Gallmeier, M M. Lowery, M G. Volkmer, B. (1999). Effects of chronic low-dose ultraviolet B radiation on DNA damage and repair in mouse skin. *Cancer Res,* 59. 2875–2884.
[98] Mlakar, V. Glava, D. (2007). DNA microarrays and their use in dermatology. *Acta Dermatoven APA,* 16, 1, 7-12.
[99] Morito, N. Yoh, K. Itoh, K. Hirayama, A. Koyama, A. Yamamoto, M. et al. (2003). Nrf2 regulates the sensitivity of death receptor signals by affecting intracellular glutathione levels. *Oncogene,* 22, 9275–81.
[100] Mukhtar, H. Elmets, C A. (1996). Photocarcinogenesis mechanisms, models and human health implications. *Photochem Photobiol,* 63, 355-447.
[101] Murakami, T. Fujimoto, M. Ohtsuki, M. et al. (2001). Expression profiling of cancer-related genes in human keratinocytes following non-lethal ultraviolet B irradiation. *J Dermatol Sci* 2, 121–9.
[102] Narisawa, T. Takahashi, M. Niwa, M. Fukaura, Y. Wakizaka, A. (1987). Involvement of prostaglandin E2 in bile acid-caused promotion of colon carcinogenesis and anti-promotion by the cyclooxygenase inhibitor indomethacin. *Jpn J Cancer Res,* 78, 791-798.
[103] Nomura, M. Kaji, A. He, Z. et al. (2001). Inhibitory mechanisms of tea polyphenols on the ultraviolet B-activated phosphadytilinositol-3-kinase-dependent pathway. *J Biol Chem,* 276, 46624–31.
[104] Pan, M H. Ho, C T. (2008). Chemopreventive effects of natural dietary compounds on cancer development. *Chem Soc Rev,* 37, 2558–2574.
[105] Patrick, E. Noah, S. (2007). A review of DNA repair and possible DNA- repair adjuvants and selected natural anti-oxidants. *Dermat Online J,* 13, 10
[106] Prashar, R. Kumar, A. Banerjee, S. *et al.* (1994). Chemopreventive action by an extract from Ocimum Sanctum on mouse skin papillomagenesis and its anhancement of skin glutathione-Stransferase activity and acid soluble sulfhydryl level. *Anticancer Drugs,* 5, 567–72.
[107] Prakash, J. Gupta, S K. Dinda, A K. (2002). Withania Somnifera root extract prevents DMBA-induced squmous cell carcinoma of skin in Swiss albino mice. *Nutr Cancer,* 42: 91–7.
[108] Robinson, J K. (2005). Sun exposure, sun protection, and vitamin D. *JAMA,* 294, 1541-43.
[109] Saha, P. Das, S. (2002). Elimination of Deleterious Effects of Free Radicals in Murine Skin Carcinogenesis by Black Tea Infusion Theaflavins Epigallocatechin Gallate. *Asian Pac J Cancer Prev,* 3:225–30.

[110] Sasaki, H. Akamatsu, H. Horio, T. (1997). Effects of a single exposure to UVB radiation on the activities and protein levels of copper-zinc and manganese superoxide dismutase in cultured human keratinocytes. *Photochem. Photobiol*, 65, 707–13.

[111] Schafer, F Q. Buettner, G R. (2001). Redox environment of the cell as viewed through the redox state of the glutathione disulfide/glutathione couple. *Free Radic Biol Med, 30*, 1191-1212.

[112] Schnyder, B. Schnyder-Candrian, S. Panski, A. Bommel, H. Heim, M. Duschl, A. et al. (2002). Phytochemical inhibition of interleukin-4-activated Stat6 and expression of VCAM-1. *Biochem Biophys Res Commun*, 292(4), 841–7.

[113] Schwartz, G K. Shah, M A. (2005). Targeting the cell cycle: a new approach to cancer therapy. *J Clin Oncol*, 23, 9408-21

[114] Shae, C R. Parrish, J A. (1991). Nonionizing radiation and the skin. In: LA, G., editor. Physiology, biochemistry and molecular biology of the skin. Oxford University Press; New York: 910-927.

[115] Shankar, S. Siddiqui, I. Srivastava, R K. (2007). Molecular mechanisms of resveratrol (3,4,5-trihydroxytrans- stilbene) and its interaction with TNF-related apoptosis inducing ligand (TRAIL) in androgeninsensitive prostate cancer cells. *Mol Cell Biochem*, 304:273-285.

[116] Sharma, R.Yang, Y. Sharma, A. Awasthi, S. Awasthi, Y C. (2004). Antioxidant role of glutathione S-transferases: protection against oxidant toxicity and regulation of stress-mediated apoptosis. *Antioxid. Redox Signal*, 6, 289–300.

[117] Sharma, S D. Meeran, S M. Katiyar, S K. (2007). Dietary grape seed proanthocyanidins inhibit UVB-induced oxidative stress and activation of mitogen-activated protein kinases and nuclear factor-kB signalling in in vivo SKH-1 hairless mice. *Mol Cancer Ther*, 6, 3: 995-1005

[118] She, Q B. Bode, A M. Ma, W Y. Chen, N Y. Dong, Z. (2001). Resveratrolinduced activation of p53 and apoptosis is mediated by extracellular-signal-regulated protein kinases and p38 kinase. *Cancer Res*, 61(4), 1604–10.

[119] Shih, A. Davis, F B. Lin, H Y. Davis, P J. (2002). Resveratrol induces apoptosis in thyroid cancer cell lines via a MAPK- and p53- dependent mechanism. *J Clin Endocrinol Metabol*, 87(3), 1223–32.

[120] Shishodia, S. Sethi, G. Aggarwal, B B. (2005). Curcumin: getting back to the roots. *Ann NY Acad Sci*, 1056, 206–17.

[121] Singh, S. Aggarwal, B B. (1995). Activation of transcription factor NF-kappa B is suppressed by curcumin (diferuloylmethane). *J Biol Chem*, 270, 24995-25000.

[122] Singh, A. Singh, S P. Bamezai, R. (1999). Modulatory potential of Clocimum oil on mouse skin papillomagenesis and the xenobiotic detoxication system. *Food Chem Toxicol*, 37, 663–70.

[123] Soudamini, K K. Kuttan, R. (1989). Inhibition of chemical carcinogenesis by curcumin. *J Ethnopharmacol*, 27, 227–33.

[124] Sporn, M B. Dunlop, N M. Newton, D I. Smith, J M. (1976). Prevention of chemical carcinogenesis by vitamin A and its synthetic analogs (retinoids). *Fed Proc*, 35: 1332-1338

[125] Surh, Y I. Kundu, J K. Na, H K. Lee, J S. (2005). Redox-Sensitive Transcription Factors as Prime Targets for Chemoprevention with Anti-Inflammatory and Antioxidative Phytochemicals, *J Nutr*, 29, 135, 2993S–3001S.

[126] Svobodová, A. Psotová, J. Walterová, D. (2003). Natural phenolics in the prevention of UV-induced skin damage. *A review Biomed. Papers*, 147(2), 137–145.

[127] Svobodová, A. Zdarilová, A. Walterová, D. Vostálová, J. (2007). Flavonolignans from *Silybum marianum* moderate UVA-induced oxidative damage to HaCaT keratinocytes. *J of Dermatol Science*, 48, 213-24.

[128] Taylor, C R. Stern, R S. Leyden, J J. Gilchrest, B A. (1990). Photoaging/photodamage and photoprotection. *J Am Acad Dermatol*, 22: 1–15.

[129] Tedeschi, E. Menegazzi, M. Yao, Y. Suzuki, H. Forstermann, U. Kleinert, H. (2004). Green tea inhibits human inducible nitricoxide synthase expression by down-regulating signal transducer and activator of transcription-1alpha activation. *Mol Pharmacol* 65(1), 111–20.

[130] Unna, P. (1894). Die Histopathologie der Hautkrankheiten. In: Orth J, ed. *Lehrbuch der speziellen pathologischen Anatomie*. 8. Berlin, Germany: A Hirschwald.

[131] Vaid, M. Sharma, S D. Katiyar, S K. (2010). Honokiol, a phytochemical from the Magnolia plant, inhibits photocarcinogenesis by targeting UVB-induced inflammatory mediators and cell cycle regulators: development of topical formulation. *Carcinogenesis*, 31 (11), 2004-2011.

[132] Vayalil, P K. Mittal, A. Katiyar, S K. (2004). Proanthocyanidins from grape seeds inhibit expression of matrix metalloproteinases in human prostate carcinoma cells, which is associated with the inhibition of activation of MAPK and NFkB. *Carcinogenesis*, 25, 6, 987-995.

[133] Wadsworth, T L. McDonald, T L. Koop, D R. (2001). Effects of Ginkgo biloba extract (EGb 761) and quercetin on lipopolysaccharide-induced signaling pathways involved in the release of tumor necrosis factor-alpha. *Biochem Pharmacol*, 62(7), 963–74.

[134] Wang, Y. Zhang, X S. Lebwohl, M. Deleo, V. Wei, H C. (1998). Inhibition of ultraviolet B (UVB)-induced c-Fos and c-Jun expression *in vivo* by a tyrosine kinase inhibitor genistein. *Carcinogenesis*, 19, 649-654.

[135] Wang, Y C. Bachrach, U. (2002). The specific anti-cancer activity of green tea (_)-epigallocatechin-3-gallate (EGCG). *Amino Acids*, 22(2), 131–43.

[136] Wei, H. Zhang, X. Wang, Y. Lebwohl, M. (2002). Inhibition of ultraviolet light induced oxidative events in the skin and internal organs of hairless mice by isoflavone genistein. *Cancer Letters*, 185, 21-29.

[137] Wild, A C. Moinova, H R. Mulcahy, R T. (1999). Regulation of gammaglutamylcysteine synthetase subunit gene expression by the transcription factor Nrf2. *J Biol Chem*, 274, 33627-36.

[138] Woo, J H. Lim, J H. Kim, Y H. Suh, S I. Min, D S. Chang, J S. et al. (2004). Resveratrol inhibits phorbol myristate acetate-induced matrix metalloproteinase-9 expression by inhibiting JNK and PKC delta signal transduction. *Oncogene*, 23(10), 1845–53.

[139] World Health Organization. (2004). *Skin cancer facts and figures*. Retrieved April 3, 2008, from www.who.int/uv/faq/skincancer/en/index1.html

[140] Tagawa, Y. Hiramatsu, N. Kasai, A. Hayakawa, K. Okamura, M. Yao Y. Kitamura, M. (2008). Induction of apoptosis by cigarette smoke via ROS-dependent endoplasmic reticulum stress and CCAAT/enhancer-binding protein-homologous protein (CHOP). *Free Radical Biol Med*, 45, 1, 50–59.

[141] Trouba, K J. Hamadeh, H K. Amin, R P. Germolec, D R. (2002). Oxidative stress and its role in skin disease. *Antioxid Redox Signal*, 4, 665–673.

[142] Yang, G Y. Liao, J. Li, C. Chung, J. Yurkow, EJ. Ho, C T. et al. (2000). Effect of black and green tea polyphenols on c-jun phosphorylation and H(2)O(2) production in transformed and non-transformed human bronchial cell lines: possible mechanisms of cell growth inhibition and apoptosis induction. *Carcinogenesis*, 21(11), :2035–9.

[143] Yang, C S. Maliakal, P. and Meng, X. (2002). Inhibition of carcinogenesis by tea. *Annu Rev Pharmacol Toxicol*, 42, 25-54.

[144] Yusuf, N. Irby, C. Katiyar, K S. et al. (2007). Photoprotective effects of green tea polyphenols. *Photodermatol Photoimmunol Photomed*; 23: 48-56.

[145] Zhao, J. Wang, J. Chen, Y. Agarwal, R. (1999). Anti-tumor-promoting activity of a polyphenolic fraction isolated from grape seeds in the mouse skin two-stage initiation-promotion protocol and identification of procyanidin B5-3/-galalte as the most effective antioxidant constituent. *Carcinogenesis*, 20, 9, 1737-1745.

10

Photodynamic Therapy in Skin Cancer

Simona Clichici and Gabriela Adriana Filip
Department of Physiology, University of Medicine and Pharmacy, Cluj-Napoca
Romania

1. Introduction

In the last decades the improvements in cancer treatments were an important challenge both for physicians and researchers. The major aim was to obtain a targeted therapy that selectively destroys tumor cells, without affecting the normal tissues. For a very long period of time, the classical methods of treatment were surgery, chemotherapy and radiotherapy. Nevertheless, in most cases, the classical therapies are efficient only in the incipient stages and the solid tumors are often resistant to treatment. Two thirds of the patients are discovered in advanced stages of the disease. Even treated, their death occurs because of relapses and metastases. A quarter of the patients with a tumor in an operable stage can not benefit from the treatment because of their age and co-morbidities. They can only receive palliative therapy with a high relapse percentage.

The concept of cellular death determined by the interaction of light with certain drugs was developed a century ago. The first to describe this process was Oscar Raab, in 1900. von Tappeiner and a dermatologist, Jesionek, used a combination between topically applied eosin and white light for the treatment of cutaneous tumors. In fact, Hermann von Tappeiner was the one who introduced the term "Photodynamic Therapy" (PDT) in clinical use, demonstrating the necessary presence of oxygen for the photosensitizing reaction to take place. In 1942, Auler and Banzer injected hematoporphyrin in tumor-bearing animals and observed that, after exposure to a halogen lamp fluorescence, the tumor necrosis appeared. The purification of hematoporphyrin, the use of its derivatives, and especially the introduction of LASER as a light source by Maiman led to improvements in the effects of this therapy.

The modern era of PDT began in 1960 with the studies of Lipson and Schwartz, when they observed the red fluorescence of neoplasic lesions after the injection of hematoporphyrin compounds. Since then, considerable efforts have been made to improve the effects of this therapy. 5-aminolevulinic acid was used in 1990 by Kennedy and represented a major advancement in PDT. The first approved photosensitizer to be used on humans was Photofrin.

Today, PDT is a non-invasive cancer therapy that associates the use of three components: the photosensitizer (PS), the light, and oxygen. PDT consists of the administration of a PS which accumulates in the lesion and the irradiation of the affected area with light in order to activate the drug. Thus, PDT becomes a treatment with double specificity. On one hand, PS accumulates selectively in the tumor, on the other hand the irradiation is targeted at the tumor. Several factors favor the selective accumulation of PS in tumor cells, including their high proliferation rate, the increased number of low density lipoprotein receptors, the increased vascular permeability, and the production of collagen which can bind the PS (Nowis et al, 2005).

2. Photosensitizers

The main classes of photosensitizers are porphyrin derivatives, chlorines, phtalocyanines and porphycenes.
One of the gold standards for the PDT is to find the ideal PS. This should comply with some criteria: to be chemically pure; to have chemical and physical stability; to be activated only in the presence of light , with no dark toxicity; to have the absorption peak at a wavelength >630 nm, where it presents an optimal tissue penetration; to have a high absorption coefficient; to be rapidly and predominantly retained in the tumor tissue; to be rapidly eliminated from the organism, so as to prevent the risk of prolonged systemic photosensitivity; to have a clearance from the tumor tissue slower than that of normal cells; to generate cytotoxic reactive oxygen species (Gomer & Henderson, 1998). To these desiderata some principles that must be followed should be added for the effectiveness of PDT responses and depend on the localization of the PS: the wavelength of the light used for the PDT must correspond to the PS's absorption peaks; adequate time must be considered following PS administration in order to allow the substance to penetrate the targeted cells. Nevertheless, the risk of skin cancer after the UV irradiation should be taken into consideration. To minimize this risk, the wavelength of the light used for the PDT treatment must be longer than those in the UV spectrum.
None of the PS used until now complies with all these criteria and this is the reason why new PS are being studied in the search for one with superior properties.
The most studied PS are porphyrins. These are a group of pigments that have in their structure a tetrapyrrolic macrocycle and a metal ion that mediate the biological reactions of oxidation. There are natural porphyrins synthesized by live matter. One of the best known porphyrin structures is the heme ring, a tetrapyrrolic macrocycle with iron that is produced by the mitochondria with the help of an enzymatic complex formed by 8 enzymes. The synthetic porphyrins are heterocycle macrocycles characterized by the presence of some modified pyrrolic subunits interconnected at the level of carbon atoms by methyl bridges (=CH-) and have the hydrogen atoms substituted in the meso-position. The structure contains 18 electrons that can form bonds with metal ions (Kral et al, 2006). The first synthesized porphyrin by Rothmund in 1936 was tetraphenylporphyrin (TPP). Since then, numerous porphyrins have been synthesized, both symmetric and asymmetric ones. The study of synthetic proteins was started in 1960, and the first isomer was synthesized by Vogel in 1986, porphycene. There were synthesized porphyrins with contracted molecules, (e.g. corrole), but also expanded ones. Texaphyrins have a peak of absorption in infrared, at 730-770 nm, which allows a high penetration in the tissues and might be used in the treatment of thick tumors or of melanomas (Kral et al, 2006).
Under the influence of light, the photosensitizer passes from ground to the excited singlet state. From this phase, the PS may either decay to the ground state, or pass to the triplet excited state. From this last condition, the PS can react with the oxygen molecules in 2 ways: a direct reaction with a substrate, mediated by hydrogen or electron transfer (type I photooxidation), or energy transfer to nearby molecules of oxygen (type II). During the type I reaction free oxygen radicals are formed, while during the type II reaction singlet oxygen is formed. All the generated oxygen species (ROS) can attack the susceptible surrounding substrates. However, singlet oxygen is considered to be the main cytotoxic agent in PDT (Triesscheijn et al, 2006).
There are different criteria in order to classify the PS. According to their water solubility, the photosensitizers (PS) are hydrophobic, hydrophilic and amphophilic. The hydrophobic PS

don't have electric charges in the periphery and are not soluble in water or alcohol. The hydrophilic PS have 3 or more peripheral substitutes that are electrically charged and they dissolve in water at a physiological pH. The amphophilic PS have 2 or less than 2 peripheral substitutes and are soluble in water or alcohol at physiological pH (Boyle & Dolphin, 1996). According to the modality of administration, PS can be administered systematically or topically, as a prophotosensitizer.

The systemic photosensitizers include porfimer, benzoporphyrin derivative monoacid ring A (BPD-MA), metatetrahydroxyphenylchlorin (mTHPC, temoporfin) and tin ethyl etiopurpurin (SnET2). After their administration, a long-lasting photosensitivity can persist, because they are retained in tissue macrophages and tumor cells.

The prophotosensitizers have a low-molecular weight, are hydrophilic and are topically administered on the skin surface. These include 5-delta-aminolevulinic acid (ALA) and methyl-esterified ALA (MAL). In fact, the topical application of ALA became the most common used technique in dermatology (Torpe & Bhardwaj, 2008).

The most extensive way of studying PS is to describe them in the chronological manner in which they entered in use. We can describe PS of first, second, third generation. The first generation of PS includes: hematoporphyrin (HdP), hematoporphyrin derivatives and the commercial purified compound Porfimer sodium or Photofrin. Photofrin is a mixture of hematoporphyrin products with different absorption peaks and it is the active purified fraction of HpD. It was the first PS approved for PDT for recurrent, superficial papillary bladder cancer. HpD is an effective tumor killer in red light PDT. HpD was the first prophyrin used in clinical practice not only on patients with bladder cancer, but also skin cancer. At 630 nm, the wavelength most used in the clinic to activate porfimer sodium, it present a weak absorption (1,170 cm^{-1} mol^{-1} l^{-1}). The skin photosensitivity after PDT with porfimer sodium lasts for 4-12 weeks (Triesscheijn et al, 2006). To obtain similar results with PS of the second generation, the first generation ones must be used in high quantities and with a high fluence rate. This stimulated the research for new PS (Nowis et al, 2005).

From the second generation of PS, ALA is the most used. Applied topically, it increases the concentration of protoporphyrin IX (PpIX) in the tumor cells. Actually, the PS based on ALA are not intrinsic photoactive but they accumulate preferentially in the tumor cells and are metabolized by the pathway of heme biosynthesis becoming a photosensitizing porphyrin. If the cells don't undergo PDT the porphyrines are metabolized to heme, which is photodynamically inactive for 24-48h. Protoporphyrin IX (PpIX) is a porphyrinic compound with photodynamic activity, which can be synthesized by all the nucleated cells. When activated by light, at 630 nm, PpIX emits red fluorescence. ALA is a natural precursor of heme. Two molecules of ALA form porphobilinogen (PBG). Four molecules of PBG form uroporphyrinogen, which is then converted into coproporphyrinogen. Inside the mitochondria, the latest is converted into protoporphyrinogen IX, and under the action of protoporphyrinogene oxidase, this is converted into PpIX. In the end, under the action of ferrochelatase, the Fe^{+2} is incorporated into the tetrapyrrol ring, and the PpIX is converted into heme. The tumor cells have a lower ferrochelatase activity than normal cells (Calzavara Pinton et al, 2007, Kondo et al, 1993). After the administration of ALA, the capacity of ferrochelatase is exceeded, and PpIX accumulates into the tumor. The accumulation of PpIX depends on the activity of ferrochelatase and the Fe^{+2} availability. The Fe^{+2} source is represented by mitochondrial reserve and the simultaneous administration of ALA and iron chelators (EDTA, desferrioxamine) increases the rate of accumulation of porphyrins. If the level of iron decreases, the ferrochelatase may incorporate Zn in the PpIX leading to the formation of fluorescent protoporphyrines with Zn. ALA can be administered systemically (orally, intravenously, inhalatory) or topically. PpIX is detected in the epidermis within 3-8 hours after systemic administration of ALA. In general, PpIX is eliminated from the blood 24-48 hours after the topical or systemic administration of ALA. The peak in the plasma of PpIX is detected 8-12 hours after the oral administration (60 mg/bw), 4,1 hours after inhalatory administration (500 mg) and 2,9 hours after the instillation into the bladder (Rick et al, 1997). For that reason, the risks of prolonged sensitivity are minimal. After the topical application of ALA on the skin neither ALA nor PpIX can be detected in the blood stream. ALA has been approved for PDT treatment since 1999.

The use of ALA has advantages as compared to porfimer sodium. First of all, skin sensitivity lasts only 1-2 days due to the more rapid clearance. On the other hand, it can be applied both topically, for the treatment of skin cancer, but also systematically, for cancer in the oral cavity, or digestive tract, with a good selectivity for the tumor cells.

The major disadvantage of ALA is that it traverses the cellular membrane with difficulty because of its hydrophilic profile and it may accumulate with difficulty in the tumor cells. This process is dependent on energy, pH and temperature and is slow, although in the tumor cells it is more rapid than in healthy ones.

From our studies on Walker tumor in rats (Filip et al, 2008), the concomitant administration of ALA with chitosan increased the level of PpIX in tumor significantly after one hour as compared to the sole administration of ALA. Six hours after administration PpIX disappears from the plasma. The administration of chitosan favors the plasmatic clearance and the concentration in the tumor of the active porphyrin.

On the contrary, the alkyl esters of ALA can penetrate easily into the cells. MAL, the esterified derivative of ALA (methyl ester of ALA), is lipophilic and with an increased selectivity for tumor cells as compared to ALA. The transmembranary transport of MAL is made by mechanisms of facilitated diffusion, being more efficient in tumor cells. Due to their increased permeability, the selectivity of MAL for tumor cells is greater as compared to ALA. After entering the cell MAL is demethylated to ALA and the next steps to PpIX are similar. Prior to MAL topical application, the stratum cornosum of the skin is removed by superficial curettage.

Second generation PS like meso-tetrahydroxyphenylchlorine (MTHPC) or benzoporphyrin derivative monoacid A ring (Verteporfin) have a limited cutaneous photosensibility. They were administered systemically for the treatment of basal cell carcinoma and Bowen's disease. mTHPC (temoporfin, Foscan) has an absorption peak at 652 nm with a better penetration of the light in the tissues as compared to ALA and porfimer sodium. Foscan was approved in 2001 in EU for the palliative treatment of head and neck cancer (Triesscheijn et al, 2006).

In the search for newer PS numerous third generation PS were developed. These are generally activated by higher wavelengths, have an increased tumor specificity and the generalized photosensitivity is shorter. The most studied are tin ethyletiopurpurin (SnET2), mono-L-aspartyl chlorine e6 (Npe6), benzoporphyrin derivative (BPD), lutetium texaphyrin (Lu-Tex).

To improve the effects of PDT, some methods to increase the efficacy of existing PS were researched and new PS were tested. Phthalocyanines are macrocyclic compounds and have a major disadvantage for the clinical application which reduces their efficiency in PDT: they have a strong tendency to form oligomers, especially dimers. Zinc phthalocyanines' incorporation into liposomes decreases their aggregation degree (Garcia et al, 2011). In vitro and in vivo studies have been conducted with new PS. For example, phtalocyanine-polyamine conjugates proved a high phototoxicity against human colon adenocarcinoma HT29 cells and hamster ovary cells. They have high affinity toward the lysosomes, but not the mitochondria, and they inhibit the growth of the tumor without toxicity for the normal cells (Jiang et al, 2010). N-heterocyclic (NHC) - pyridine complexes incorporating a carbene unit as an ancillary ligand were synthesized (Chen et al, 2011), chlorine compounds with conjugated substituents such as vynil groups and carboxylic acids (Eriksson & Eriksson, 2011), cyanine HM 118. Also, chlorine e6 (Ce6) - conjugated glycocol chitosan nanoparticles seem to have potential for PDT (Lee et al, 2011) as well as tumor-targeting albumin nanoparticles containing Ce6 (Jeong et al, 2011). The use of nanomaterials as carriers for the PS tends to improve some of the PDT disadvantages. For example, a folic acid conjugated graphene oxide loaded with Ce6 can accumulate in the tumor cells and shows a great potential for PDT (Huang et al, 2011). Also, glycoconjugated fullerene has a potential use in PDT (Otake et al, 2010).

3. Light sources

An efficient PDT requires not only the appropriate delivery of the light from the source to the target, but also a homogeneous light distribution. The intensity of the irradiation should be verified at the treated point using light detectors. There are four kinds of detectors used in optics: thermopile needed for the measurement of temperature, pyroelectric detector that measures the electric current produced by a crystal when its temperature is modified, photomultiplier tube and the integrative sphere (Sibata et al, 2000). The ideal irradiation during PDT is given by the optimization of the distribution of the light so that is appropriate for its geometric distribution of the PS and matches the optical properties of the targeted tissue so that the effects on the neighboring zones are minimal. A good evaluation of the effect of the PS can be made by dosing the concentration of PS in target tissue. The ideal dosimetry optimizes the distribution of the light dose to the treated volume by selecting the best geometry for irradiation (Jacques, 1998). Techniques of measuring the quantity of PS in vivo non invasively by using elastic scattering were developed (Mourant et al, 1999). The types of interaction of light to the tissue depend on the wavelength and the properties of the irradiated volume. There are five types of interactions: photochemical, thermal, photoablation, plasma induced ablation and photodisruption. For the clinical use of PDT only the photochemical and sometimes thermal interactions are important. It was shown that PDT is synergic to sub-lethal hyperthermia (Chen et al, 1996). In preclinical trials PDT with low power was used to avoid the thermal interactions.

The PDT wavelength ranges between 600 and 1000 nm. Increased wavelength correlates with increased tissue penetration. The minimum threshold was established at 600 nm because hemoglobin absorbs under 600 nm. The penetration depth is given by the thickness of the tissue where the intensity of the incident light decreases by half. It is at about 2-3 mm for 630 nm and increases to 5-6 mm for 700-800 nm. Endogenous chromophores, such as melanin, can interfere with the PS for the absorption of light. This is important in the treatment of patients with a dark phototype or when treating the hyperpigmented lesions of metastatic melanoma.

In PDT red light is generally used (580-700 nm) in a dose of 100-150 J/cm^2, and the intensity of the light dose does not surpass 200 mW/cm^2 to avoid the hyperthermic effects (Clark et al, 2003). For inflammatory skin disorders red light in a dose of 10-40 J/cm^2 and an intensity of 50-70 mW/cm^2 is used in more than one session (Babilas et al, 2006). Porphyrins exhibit typical absorption with the highest peak at 405 nm, called the Soret-band. There are also several Q-bands, the last having the absorption peak at 635 nm, this wavelength is used for irradiation in PDT. It is also possible to use blue light in combination with 5-ALA hydrochloride (Levulan) for the treatment of actinic keratosis.

Visible light from 2 types of light sources is used: noncoherent, conventional or coherent (laser).

The incoherent, broad spectrum light sources are simple, cheap and easy to use both for in vivo and in vitro studies. Such devices are halogen, tungsten, xenon or fluorescent lamps. To select the different wavelengths they are used together with optical filters. Their disadvantages are represented by an important thermal effect, the low light intensity and the difficulty to control the dose of light.

Light emitting diodes (LED) are also incoherent sources available for PDT. LED may generate high energy light with the needed wavelength. LED with a large surface are used for irradiating extended lesions. The usual doses are 37-50 J/cm^2 and the power output is up to 150 mW/cm^2.

LASERS emit a precise wavelength, monochromatic, with high power but are expensive and need high level technical support (Triesscheijin et al, 2006). An important development in PDT is the availability of LASERS with diodes at wavelengths compatible with the most used PS (Wilson, 1998). This system has a low electric power and a cooling system similar to that of a LASER. The advantage of diode LASER is the low cost of acquisition and maintenance, small dimensions and portability (Sibata et al, 2000).

4. Mechanisms involved in PDT effects

The mechanisms involved in PDT's effects are very complex and not entirely understood. The key effect achieved using PDT is the damage of the tumor cells; this can be obtained both directly and indirectly. The direct antitumor effect implies the cellular destruction by apoptosis or necrosis. The indirect effects of PDT consist, on the one hand, in the stimulation of the immune response of the host and, on the other hand, in the damage produced to the vasculature, with consecutive disruption in the tumor micromedium. The contribution of each mechanism in the occurrence of cell death is hard to be established and depends on the type of photosensitizer (hydrophilic or hydrophobic), the light fluence rate, the timing of illumination following photosensitizer administration, the depth of the tumor localization. The type of photosensitizer influences its subcellular localization and the organelles that are primarily damaged. The lipophilic PS enter the cell through receptor mediated endocytosis (Marcus & McIntyre, 2002) and accumulate in the lipophilic compartments of the cell: plasma, mitochondria, endoplasmic reticulum, cellular membrane and lysosomal ones (Schneider et al, 2005). The effects appear a few hours from the treatment and they include: the inactivation of the membrane enzymes, the increase in its permeability, the formation of vesicles, the ceasing of the cellular respiration and the cellular death through apoptosis or necrosis. The hydrophilic PS administered i.v. bind to the plasma proteins and enter the tumor tissue. Due to the fact that they have a reduced capacity to traverse the cellular membrane they will mainly affect the tumor vasculature leading to ischemia and consecutively hypoxia (Canti et al, 2002). Another modality of modulating the effects of PDT is through the light dose and the photosensitizer used. When low doses of PS are used, the cells remain viable, but the intracellular signaling pathways, the cytokine formation and the receptor expression are altered. When using high doses of light and/or PS cellular necrosis is triggered through the lesions in the membrane of the cell and organelles, with the subsequent formation of an inflammatory status. When using intermediate doses apoptosis is favored. The apoptotic process is mainly triggered by PS that accumulate preferentially in the mitochondria such as phtalocyanines, porphycenes, verteporfin, hypericin (Calzavara-Pinton et al, 2007), Photofrin, protoporphyrin IX (Kessel & Luo, 1999).

4.1 The effects of PDT on ROS

As described before, under the influence of light, the PS lead to ROS generation, the main cytotoxic agent being singlet oxygen. It has a short life (30-180 nanoseconds) and it diffuses on short lengths (<50 nm) (Niedre et al, 2002), so that, in the end, the localization of the PS in the cell will dictate the cellular structure that will become a target for the singlet oxygen (Peng et al, 1996). For example the PS which will incorporate into mitochondria will determine Bcl-2 lesions that will induce the apoptosis of the tumor cells. Foscan fixes in the endoplasmic reticulum inactivating cytocromoxidase -NADPH and also in the Golgi apparatus inactivating UDP-galactosyltransferase (Teiten et al, 2003).

It seems that the singlet oxygen can interact with more than one cellular structure. Firstly, singlet oxygen can attack the cellular membrane lipids leading to the formation of lipids hydroxyperoxides, that can initiate the oxidation chain of unsaturated lipids and continue to determine effects on other cellular structures (Gutteridge & Halliwell, 2000). Secondly, the membrane and plasma protein may become the target of the toxicity mediated by singlet oxygen with the modification of the aminoacid chains especially at the level of cysteine, histidine, methionine, tryptophan and tyrosine (Schafer & Buettner, 1999). The modification of tyrosine as result of the interaction with ROS is highly important leading to the formation of the tyrosyl radical which dimerises and forms dityrosine (Pfeiffer et al, 2000). Tyrosine is normally involved in the intracellular signal transduction on the tyrosine phosphorilation pathway. The oxidation of tubulin is also important because it leads to lesions of the microtubules determining their inactivation and this makes the photosensitized cells unable to divide blocking the cell cycle in the G2/M phase (Berg & Moan, 1997).

The photo-oxidation of lipids and proteins in the cellular membrane activates the membrane phospholipase leading to the degradation of the altered phospholipids, the modification of the membrane fluidity and the loss of cellular integrity. The alterations affect the membrane enzymes but also the cellular receptors. The membrane depolarization and the ionic equilibrium are also altered.

The effects of ROS manifest themselves also at the level of the mitochondrial and lysosomal membranes. Apoptosis as a result of PDT is a consequence of the release of cytocrome c, the apoptosis induction factor and activation of caspase (Pogue et al, 2001; Rancan et al, 2005). The attack of singlet oxygen at the level of the lysosomes leads to the release of the lysosomal enzymes which determines extensive cellular damage leading to a late apoptosis and/or relocation of the sensitizer in another area of the cell. On the other hand, the effects upon the DNA are rare and the mutagenicity seems to be reduced (Ben-Hur et al, 1987).

Photodymanic therapy induces oxidative stress but also the release of nitric oxide (NO) in the tumor area (Hirst & Flitney, 1997). It determines vasodilatation and increases the blood flow to the tumor facilitating tumor growth and metastasis (Gomes et al, 2002). The tumors that generate low amounts of NO are susceptible to PDT as compared to those that generate high ones. The production of a high amount of NO stops the inflammatory reaction that arises after PDT and also it blocks the effects seen normally after PDT on the blood flow such as vascular occlusion and ischemia. These phenomena are explained by NO capacity to prevent platelet aggregation and endothelial adhesion, and to stop the neutrophil accumulation. NO also inhibits the expression of adhesion molecules and mast cell degranulation (Korbelik et al, 2000). NO has a double function. During treatment it determines vasodilatation and favors ROS generation and after treatment it favors the formation of ischemia/reperfusion lesions, cell apoptosis and the immune reaction with an antitumoral effect (Dougherty et al, 1998; Korbelik et al, 1998).

NO has a cytoprotector effect through a mechanism dependent of cGMP. The protection of tumor cells is realised by inhibiting caspase activation by S-nitrosylation (Gomes et al, 2002) and the modulation of the gene expression through a cGMP dependent mechanism or S-nitrosylation. NO blocks the lipid peroxidation chain by the neutralization of ROS generated by PDT. NO is a scavenger of the superoxide anion but also of the alcoxyl and peroxyl radicals (Rubbo et al, 1994). Through the reaction of NO with the superoxide anion the peroxynitrite anion is generated ($ONOO^-$), which decomposes to form strong oxidants that can provoke tissular damage. Once more NO has a dual role being at the same time a cytoprotector and an aggressor for the cells. It is possible that NO and iNOs have a role in the induction of apoptosis by disturbing the membrane potential and increasing the permeability of the mitochondrial membrane (Thor et al, 1985).

The photodestruction determined by ROS may by partially prevented by the antioxidant enzymatic system: superoxide dismutase (SOD), catalase (CAT) and glutathione peroxidase (GPx). It seems that the activity of SOD increases during PDT as a result of ROS generation in the cell (Saczko et al, 2007), therefore SOD is considered to be an inductible antioxidant enzyme that regulates the sensitivity of tumor cells to PDT (Huang et al, 2000). Nonetheless it seems that just MnSOD is important for the cell response to PDT and the alteration of the mitochondrial function is a critical factor for phototoxicity so that MnSOD may be a molecular target that could modulate the cell sensisivity to PDT (Haylett et al, 2003). The inhibition of SOD activity in tumor cells potentiates the PDT cytotoxic effect and the transitory transvection of MnSOD gene but not the CuZnSOD gene reduces the efficiency of PDT.

The studies made on an experimental model of Walker carcinosarcoma (Daicoviciu et al, 2008), showed that PDT with 5-ALA determines a decrease in the antioxidant enzymes from erythrocytes especially CAT and GPx and the activity of MnSOD increase in tumor homogenates. The behavior of erythrocyte and tissue SOD is adaptive as a result of post-PDT ROS generation. The reduction of the antioxidant enzymes from the erythrocyte after PDT is explained by the lesions in the erythrocyte's membrane and the alteration of the structural protein under the influence of ROS (El-Missiry & Abou-Seif, 2000).

4.2 The effects of PDT on angiogenesis and extracellular matrix

The lesions to the vascular endothelium are part of the indirect mechanisms by which PDT can determine the destruction of tumor cells. The plasmatic concentration of the PS may be a good indicator of the PDT efficiency (Triesscheijin et al, 2006). The complete obliteration of the vessels that feed the tumor is essential for long term good results. PDT damages the cytoskeleton of the endothelial cells (Chaudhuri et al, 1987; Sporn & Foster, 1992), it increase the adhesion and activation of platelets, the secondary release of eicosanoids, especially tromboxane that mediates vasoconstriction and the formation of thrombus (Fingar, 1996). The damage to the endothelial cells leads to the release of leukotrienes which increase the cellular permeability and the interstitial pressure determining consecutive vasoconstriction. Together, the vasoconstriction, the high interstitial pressure and the thrombus lead to ischemia and tissue necrosis. The phenomena are extremely complex because the tissue hypoxia is a triggering factor for tumor angiogenesis. So PDT may be considered proangiogenic because the oxidative stress and the hypoxia consecutive to PDT may activate angiogenic growth factors and an inflammatory adaptive response which, in turn, will initiate tumor angiogenesis (Dougherty et al, 1998). In the meantime, the extracellular matrix (ECM) serves as structural support and provides informational guidance for developing vasculature.

Matrix metalloproteinases (MMPs) are a heterogeneous group of endopeptidases that are synthesized in a latent state. Their activation through photolytic cleavage of -NH_2 terminal prodomain was correlated with the mechanisms involved in PDT. Cytokines, growth factors, oncogenes and, also, ROS are potent factors involved in the activation of MMPs (Overall &Lopes-Otia, 2002). In return, the activity of MMPs on growth factors, chemokines, growth factor receptors, adhesion molecules and apoptosis mediators is essential for the rapid cellular responses critical for angiogenesis and is also involved in mediating tumor growth and progression (Coussens et al, 2002). A large variety of cells, including endothelial cells, fibroblasts, inflammatory cells, can produce MMPs (Werb, 1997). It appears that MMP-2 and MT-1 MMP are essential for the tumor angiogenesis. MMP-2 together with MMP-9 is part of the initial phases of tumor angiogenesis, for the formation of the microvasculature and in the late stages of the process, for the involution, regression, and re-absorption of the neo-vasculature. The most important functions of MMP-2 and MMP-9 are the proteolysis of EMC, the proteolysis of the cell surface the release of growth factors and the activation of cytokines/chemokines (Davidson et al, 2003). The MMPs activity is modulated by the tissular inhibitors (TIMP), an unbalance between the expression or activity of MMPs and TIMP leading to tumor growth. PDT increase the MMPs expression in tumors and the association with MMPs inhibitors increases the therapeutic effect (Ferraio et al, 2004). There may be a connection between the inflammatory process after PDT, as it will be discussed, and the activation of MMPs, one proof being the increase in expression of MMP-1 an MMP-3 dependent on Il-1α released from the fibroblasts exposed to 5-ALA PDT (Karrer et al, 2004). Il-1α is a good NF-kB inducer and it seems that this transcription factor may modulate the activity of proteases (Matroule et al, 2006).

From our own experience regarding 5-ALA PDT on Walker carcinosarcoma, we observed the increase of MMP-2 activity in the tumor 1 hour after PDT. The association between chitosan and 5-ALA in biocomposite modifies the effect of MMP-2, the chitosan increases the curative effect of the antitumoral treatment probably by improving the host immune response (Filip et al, 2008). On the same experimental model PDT with 5,10,15,20-tetrasulfonato-phenyl-porphyrina (TSPP), showed the increase in MMP-2 activity 3 hours after the treatment. The increased values were also observed 14 days after treatment (Clichici et al, 2010).

At the level of the extracellular matrix , PDT also affects the proteoglycans, which have a role in the integrity of ECM (Lopes et al, 2006). Studies regarding this issue are still relatively few. The decrease of versican, a proteoglycan involved in the cellular proliferation was highlighted after PDT with methylene blue (Wight, 2002). At the same time it seems that PDT has effects on ICAM-1 (the intercellular adhesion molecule 1), VCAM-1 (the adhesion molecule to vascular cells), PECAM-1 (the adhesion molecule of the platelet to the endothelial), these adhesion molecules having as a result the extravasations of circulating

tumor cells and metastasis (Kobayashi et al, 2007). The results are contradictory, some studies showed a decrease in the ICAM-1 and VCAM-1 expression after PDT (Volanti et al, 2004), while other studies showed the increase of ICAM-1 expression on the surface of leucocytes in tumors treated with PDT (Castano et al, 2005).
One of the most important regulators of angiogenesis is the vascular endothelial factor (VEGF). Among the factors which determine the release of VEGF from the hypoxic cells are MMPs (Lee et al, 2005). VEGF promotes the proliferation, migration and survival of endothelial cells through action on the VEGFR-2 receptor, but also the secretion of some specific tissue factors through action on VEGFR-1, among which is the tissue plasminogen activator, urokinase, growth factors, and MMP-9 (Ferrara, 2004). The over-expression of VEGF associates with the progression of the tumor which leads to poor prognosis for the patients (Way et al, 2004). That is why combining anti-angiogenic therapy with special irradiation techniques, for example high-frequency ultrashort pulsed laser, can represent a progress as a vasculature-disrupting therapeutic modality for cancer treatment (Choi et al, 2011)

4.3 PDT and immunity

An important desiderate for an antitumoral therapy is to increase the capacity of the host immune system to recognize and destroy tumor cells, including the residual post-therapy cells, both at the site of the tumor and at distance (Castano et al, 2006). PDT can activate or suppress the immune system depending on the type of PS and the light dose. It seems that PDT activates both the non-specific inflammatory system and the specific one, with the involvement of the antigen presenting cells and lymphocytes (Korbelik, 1996, 2006). The degree of the immune response of the host depends on the chemical nature of the PS, its concentration and subcellular localization, the characteristics of the light source, light fluence and fluence rate, oxygenation level and tumor type (Firczuk et al, 2011).
The tumor treated with PDT becomes massively infiltrated with cells, mostly neutrophils mast cells and macrophages. In the mean time it increases the proinflammatory cytokines IL-1β, TNF-α, Il-6, the macrophages inflammatory proteins (MIP-1, MIP-2) and the cell adhesion molecules E-selectin and ICAM (Dougherty et al, 1998).
The neutrophils accumulated in the vasculature of the tumor, destroy the vascular endothelium, release chemotactic factors for other inflammatory cells and also oxygen metabolites with a role in damaging the tumor tissue. The activated neutrophils play also an important role in the long term suppression of tumor growth. In the initial phases, after PDT, the activation of phagocytosis or the massive destruction of the tumor cells, creates optimal conditions for macrophages, dendritic cells and the antigen presenting cells to process the tumor antigens allowing the specific antitumoral immunity to arise (Krosi et al, 1996). The bigger the amount of cellular detritus the better the processing of the tumor antigens by macrophages (recruited at the tumor site) is facilitated with the recognition of the specific epitopes and the activation of lymphocytes (LT), capable to eliminate the remaining cell after the treatment (Hunt & Chan, 1999).
The macrophages are considered by some authors (Korbelik, 1996) to play a central role in the immunological changes that occur after PDT because they have a tumoricid effect and are also involved in the release of pro- and antiinflammatory cytokines. The association of PDT with granulocyte-macrophage colony-stimulating growth factor enhances the effects of PDT (Krosi et al, 1996).

As we have already discussed, PDT will determine a specific immune reaction with an important role in the long term control of the tumor development, a type of immunity that resembles to that obtained after bacterial vaccines (Korbelik & Dougherty, 1999). The antigen presenting cells will process the tumor antigens and will present them on the surface of the membrane together with the major histocompatibility complex class II. This is followed by the activation of LT helper and consecutively cytoxic LT. CD4 and CD8 clone T cells are formed, they are capable of recognizing the tumor cells, they expand rapidly and get activated and generate a strong immune response (Van Duijnhoven et al, 2003). In addition the LB and NK cells are activated contributing to the immune response after PDT.

PDT can modulate the expression of Il-6 and IL-10 in the normal tissue and the tumor one mediated by the transcription of AP-1 (Dougherty et al, 1998). IL-6 has an important role in PDT because it inhibits the cellular proliferation and by this it potentiates the therapeutic effect of PDT. Blocking the function of this cytokines decreases the effect of PDT (Dougherty et al, 1998). Il-6 also has an inductor effect on the Th-17 subset of lymphocytes that produces Il-17 a cytokine with a role in the amplification of the production of chemokine, proinflammatory cytokines and matrix metalloproteinases capable of mediating the infiltration and destruction of the tissue (Wei et al, 2007). In addition, the hyperproduction of Il-6 accentuates the effect of PDT of inhibiting cell proliferation by perturbing the cell cycle progression at G1/S check point (Ahmad et al, 1999). Nevertheless TNF-α, Il-1β, Il-2, IL-6, Il-8 and Il-10 may represent criteria of evaluation for response to PDT (Yom et al, 2003). PDT amplifies the host immune response; this may explain the regression of untreated tumor metastasis after PDT applied on the primary tumor (Van Duijnhoven et al, 2003). Because lymphocytes act not only on tumor cells from the primary site but also on the metastasis, PDT may be considered a systemic therapy.

The immune response after PDT cannot be discussed without talking about the NF-kB factor. There are two pathways of activating NF-kB namely the classical pathway and the alternative one (Bonizzi& Karin, 2004). The reactive oxygen species generated by PDT lead to the activation of NF-kB, the first observations regarding this phenomenon were made on leukemia cells L1210 treated with Photofrin (Ryter & Gornerr, 1993). In 1995 it was observed that using methylene blue as a PS on monocites and lymphocytes latently infected with HIV-1 it increases the production of singlet oxygen and the activity of NF-kB leading to the activation of the virus (Matroule et al, 2006). It seems that NF-kB has a primordial role in recruiting neutrophils during PDT and it favors the apoptosis in lymphocytes by expressing the Fas ligand (Lin et al, 1999). It also has an antiapoptotic role by promoting the expression of genes that protect against apoptosis (Karin & Lin, 2002). It was observed that NF-kB mediates COX-2 expression; the inhibition of these enzymes improves the response to PDT (Matroule et al, 2006).

In conclusion, the inflammatory reaction is a response that is due to the cytotoxic effects exerted on the tumor cells by PDT, but also due to the vascular changes with the release of vasoactive and proinflammatory mediators and in the meantime the induction of signaling cascades and transcription factors that trigger secretion of cytokines, MMP2 and adhesion molecules (Gollnick et al, 2003; Firczuk et al, 2011).

4.4 PDT effect on COX-2

The cyclooxigenase 2 (COX-2) catalyzes the conversion of the arahidonic acid into prostaglandins and it is an important mediator of angiogenesis due to the production of VEGF and the stimulation of sprouting, migration and formation of vascular tubes (Gately

& Li, 2004). In PDT with photofrin it was shown an increase in the expression of COX-2 (Ferrario et al, 2002). The prolonged administration of COX inhibitors before irradiation increases the response to the antitumoral therapy (Makowski et al, 2003). The COX-2 inhibitor may act as an angiogenic factor which enhances the effects of PDT. The expression of COX-2 increases 30 minutes after PDT and it remains at the same level 12 and even 72 hours. It seems that the oxidative stress generated after PDT activates a cascade of proteinkinases including p38, with a role in increasing the expression of COX-2. The molecular mechanisms that modulate the expression of COX-2 in tumor cells involve the NF-kB dependent transcription of the COX-2 gene, without the involvement of other mechanisms of post-transcriptional regulation (Hendrickx et al, 2003; Volanti et al, 2005).

4.5 The cytotoxic effect of PDT

Apoptosis is a type of cellular death encountered most frequently in PDT because most of the PS accumulate in the mitochondria (Kessel & Luo, 1999). It appears quickly, at about 30 minutes after the photolesion (Oleinick et al, 2002). When the PS is located outside the mitochondria or high doses of PS are given, the type of triggered cellular death is necrosis (Almeida et al, 2004).

Two types of apoptotic process are being described, one is mediated by the mitochondria (the intrinsic pathway) and the other is receptor mediated (the extrinsic pathway) (Almeida et al, 2004). The malignant cells manifest a defective apoptosis; this explains their resistance to chemotherapy (Ahmad et al, 1999). Nonetheless PDT is efficient in the tumors resistant to cytostatics. PDT apoptosis may be influenced by other intracellular signaling pathways, including calcium, ceramides and MAP-kinases.

4.5.1 The mitochondria mediated apoptosis

The first event taking place on the intrinsic pathway of apoptosis is the interruption in the membrane potential and the release of the c cytocrom in the cytosol by opening the high conductance channels from the mitochondrial membrane or the so called mitochondrial permeability transition pore (MPTP). This is a big protein complex formed from at least three transmembranary subunits.

On tumor cell lines of human epidermoid carcinoma A 431 the administration of cyclosporin A and trifluoperazine, potent inhibitors of the MPTP opening, prevents the loss of the mitochondria transmembrane potential and the release of cytocrom c (Lam et al, 2001). The mechanism by which PDT opens the MPTP is not completely understood but it seems that a subunit of MPTP named adenine nucleotide translocator (ANT) is the target of PDT (Belzacq et al, 2001). There are data that support the association between MPTP and other proteins such as Bax, Bcl-2 and enzymes involved in the energetic metabolism such as the mitochondria hexokinase and creatinkinase.

There are also data that support the hypothesis that apoptosis mediated by mitochondria is independent on the opening of the MPTP because in some experimental models using PDT with Hypericin or Hypocrellin, the administration of inhibitors of MPTP did not prevent the changes in the transmembrane mitochondrial potential (Chaloupka et al, 1999). Some authors state that the release of the cytocrom c may be due to the peroxidation of the cardiolipin from the mitochondria (Kriska et al, 2005). The cytocrom c once released into the cytosol is bound by Apaf-1 and procaspase–9 forming a complex called the apoptosome. This self activation leads to the cleavage of caspase 9 that in its turn activates procaspase 3.

The activation of caspases 2, 3, 6, 7, 8 determines the cleavage of cellular proteins, the fragmentation of the DNA and cell death (Almeida et al, 2004).
The family of Bcl-2 proteins regulates the apoptosis induced by stimuli that act especially at the level of the mitochondria. The proteins with an antiapoptotic role from this family include Bcl-2, Bcl-xL, Bcl-w, Mcl-1, Al and Boo and the ones with a proapoptotic role Bax, Bad, Bok, Bcl-xS, Bak, Bid, Bik, Bim, Krk and Mtd (Antonsson & Martinnou, 2000). In the absence of a proapoptotic signal this protein family is sequestered by elements of the cytoskeleton or by other proteins in the cytoplasm. Members of the Bcl-2 proteins are present in the mitochondria membrane, in the nuclear envelop and the endoplasmic reticulum (Gross et al, 1999). The cleavage of Bcl-2 inactivates the protein and promotes apoptosis (Oleinik et al, 2002). Members of the Bcl-2 protein family may initiate apoptosis and favor the release of cytocrom c or inhibit the apoptosis through Bid and Bcl-xL protein that in their turn inhibit the activation of caspase (Gross et al, 1999; Reed, 1998). The rapport between the proapoptotic and antiapoptotic proteins controls the cell death or survival (Adams & Cory, 1998).
Cathepsins are proteases released from the lysosomes that can cleave Bid and initiate apoptosis by releasing proapoptotic proteins from the mitochondria or cleave caspase 3 and by this blocking apotosis. Lesions to the endoplasmic reticulum after PDT determine the release of calcium ions that may initiate apoptosis (Oleinick et al, 2002).
Data regarding the role of the Bcl-2 family in post-PDT apoptosis are controversial. Some authors state that Bcl-2 promotes apoptosis and others that it has no effect on apopstosis (Klein et al, 2001). It seems that the over-expression of Bcl-2 perturbs the mitochondrial transmembrane potential and as a consequence it affects the release of cytocrom c into the cytosol. This phenomena may be explained by the increase in the expression of the proapoptotic protein Bax in the cells that over-express Bcl-2 (Nowis et al, 2005). PDT determines a decrease Bcl-2 without affecting Bax, this rending the cells more sensitive to apoptosis (Kim et al, 1999). It seems that Bcl-2 protein is directly altered by PDT. In the activation of caspase an important role is attributed to singlet oxygen which is produced in high quantities during PDT. The singlet oxygen scavengers such as alpha tocopherol and L-histidine inhibit the lipid oxidation after PDT and also inhibit the activation of caspase. In this respect in the PDT experiments on A 431 cell line pre-incubated with or without alpha tocopherol and L-histidine because the singlet oxygen was scavenged, the caspase-3 was inhibited (Chan et al, 2000). Also, the generation of singlet oxygen is necessary for the activation of JNK in skin fibroblasts (Klotz et al, 1997), proving that singlet oxygen is a common mediator for JNK activation in the cells that undergo oxidative stress due to variations in micromedium. It is not well understood how JNK is activated, but a possible scenario could be: JNK is phosphorylated and activated by SEK 1, that in its turn may be phosphorylated and activated by MEKK 1, the latter being controlled by singlet oxygen. This JNK activation mechanism is not mandatory for cells to enter apoptosis; the apoptotic process may be initiated by an extrinsic mechanism mediated by Fas or dexamethasone (Assefa et al, 1999; Lenczowski et al, 1997).

4.5.2 Receptor mediated apoptosis

The cellular death through apoptotic mechanisms mediated by receptor appears when the PS affects the cellular membrane of the targeted cells and it determines the polymerization of the receptors from the cellular membrane, especially the receptors belonging to the TNF super-family. In fact, there are apoptotic mechanisms initiated by TNF on the one hand, on the other hand by the Fas-Fas ligand, but both of them involve the family of TNF receptors coupled with the signals of the extrinsic pathway. TNF is a cytokine produced especially by macrophages and it represents the major extrinsic pathway of apoptosis. For TNF there are two receptors, R1 and R2, that initiate the activation of caspase using the following membrane proteins: TRADD (tumor necrosis factor receptor type 1-associated Death Domain) and FADD (Fas-Associated protein with Death Domain). The binding of TNF to the receptors leads to the activation of transcription factors with a role in the survival of the cell and its inflammatory response. The Fas receptor also known as Apo-1 or CD 95 is a trans membranary protein that is a part of the TNF family. After its binding to the Fas ligand (FasL), a complex signal inductor of cellular death named DISC that contains FADD, caspase 8 and 10 is formed. In some cellular types (type I) the activation of caspase 8 leads to the activation of a cascade of caspase and the initiation of apoptosis. In other types of cells (type II) the Fas-DISC complex contributes to the release of proapoptotic factors from the mitochondria and finally to the activation of caspase 8 (Chen & Goeddel, 2002).

The caspase 8 might play the role of a trigger for the intrinsic pathway for PS that bind to the membrane. The inhibition of caspase 8 reduces the release of cytocrom c and the activation of caspase 3 in cells photosensitized with Rose Bengal (Zhuang et al, 1999). This effect is probably mediated by the Bid protein that is activated through proteolyses by caspase 8 and promotes the efflux of cytocrom c from the mitochondrial membrane.

5. Clinical results

PDT went beyond the stage of experiments. MAL is approved for use in Europe and United States in combination with red light for treating actinic keratosis (AK), superficial and nodular basal cell carcinoma (BCC) and in-situ squamous cell carcinoma (SCC) or Bowen's disease. A combination of an alcohol-containing ALA solution in a special applicator (Levulan Kerastick) and blue light is also approved in United States for the treatment of AK. The range of possible indications is expanding continuously, including non-malignant conditions and even premature skin aging due to sun exposure. For therapy of multiple lesions or in immunodeficient patients, PDT may be the first choice (Kalka et al, 2000). PDT is also indicated for patients with important comorbidities when surgery and radiotherapy are contraindicated. It may be used for palliative care in combination with chemo or radiotherapy for advanced tumors with skin metastases.

PDT in the dermatological pathology has some clear advantages, as compared to the conventional treatments: radiotherapy, chemotherapy and surgery. Maybe the most valuable advantage of PDT is represented by the limited duration of the treatment. In the majority of cases, one dose of PS followed by one irradiation are needed. In comparison, the radiotherapy must be performed daily for more than one week, the chemotherapy may take months, and surgery, although it consists of one procedure, the hospitalization period is long. To this, the cost-efficiency relation is added, PDT being a low cost therapy but with increased efficiency. The fact that it is a local treatment, at the level of the lesion, without affecting the surrounding healthy tissue is highly important. At the level of the lesion, necrosis may appear, but the tissue regeneration is adequate, because the collagen and elastin fibers are not destroyed. The cosmetic results are excellent. Not to be forgotten the possibility of applying the therapy again on the same region in case of recurrence, which is highly difficult when using the other classical therapies.

The side effects of PDT are relatively scarce. An important side effect is prolonged generalized photosensitivity, which led to the development of local application of PS. As a local side effect we can mention erythema, mild edema and pain. A stinging or burning sensation can occur, and that may influence patient's compliance.After a few days crusts and superficial erosions may appear and very rare, ulcerations. To reduce the pain, general anesthesia may be used, most often when treating children or extensive lesions, or local anesthesia and also premedication with opioids. However, the latter proved inefficient (Itkin &Gilchrest, 2004; Oseroff, 2005).

The results of PDT are estimated by the disappearance of the tumor, this occurs normally after 2-3 days. The result is confirmed by histopathological and cytological examinations. A partial regression is registered when only 50% of the tumor volume is reduced or when the tumor is not clinically visible but the histopathological and cytological examinations are positive. The therapy is considered to have failed when the tumor decreases less than 50% or when the patient does not present any local modification.

5.1 Applications for PDT

A particular application is the use of porphyrins for diagnosis in dermatology. After the systemic or topic administration of PS, the damaged tissue is irradiated with blue light and, due to the fluorescence of the substance, a clear delimitation from the normal tissue is observed. This fluorescent detection allows the guided biopsy of the tumor and also the complete resection of the tumor (Szeimies et al, 2005).

5.1.1 Basal cell carcinoma

Numerous studies have been conducted in order to asses the possible benefits for the use of PDT in BCC from different points of view (Richard et al, 2007). First of all, the efficiency of the therapy was taken into consideration. In a comparative study, MAL-PDT versus placebo, conducted on 66 patients with nodular basal cell carcinoma, a complete remission was observed 6 months after 2 PDT sessions in the treated group, as compared to placebo group (Foley, 2003).Other studies, with a follow-up of the patients ranging from 1 to 36 months, also reported a clearance rate for PDT in superficial BCC up to 100% (Marmur et al, 2004).

When studying the long term effects of PDT with MAL on 350 basal cell carcinoma it was observed that, after a previous curettage of the lesions and incubation with MAL for 3 hours followed by irradiation in a dose of 50-200 J/cm^2, the tumors were completely cured in 79% of the cases (monitored for 2-4 years) with excellent or good cosmetic results in 98% of the cases (Soler et al, 2001). Second, the efficiency of the PDT was compared to that obtained through classic methods. For the superficial BCC, PDT leads to remission rates comparable to cryotherapy, at 48 months follow-up (22% for PDT, 19% for cryotherapy), as well as at 60 months follow-up (75% for PDT, 74% for cryotherapy) (Lehmann, 2007). The results of 2 sessions of PDT with MAL for superficial BCC were compared to surgical excision in 196 patients. Three months after the therapy, the remission rates were 87,4% for the MAL-PDT and 89,4% for surgical excision (Klein et al, 2008). However, when regarding the recurrence rates, PDT seems to be inferior to surgery. An open, multicenter, randomized study which compared the effects of PDT with MAL to surgery on 101 patients with nodular basal cell carcinomas found a similar cure rate at 3 months (91% versus 98%), but the recurrence rate was significantly different (10% at 24 months for PDT and only 2% for surgery) (Soler et al.

2001). A 5-year follow-up study compared the recurrence rate after PDT with MAL and surgical excision in 97 patients. The recurrence rate was 4% for the surgery group and 14 % for MAL-PDT (Rhodes et al, 2007). The cosmetic result is superior for PDT as compared to surgery and the healing period is shorter. Because BCC have a predilection for the head and face, this could be a significant factor in choosing the modality of treatment.
During a Phase III trial, when comparing the effects of PDT with ALA 20% and cryosurgery on 88 unique superficial and nodular BCC, a clinical recurrence of 5% for ALA PDT and 13% for cryosurgery was observed 3 months after the treatment. The histological evaluation showed a 25% recurrence in the group treated with ALA PDT, and 15% for the group treated with cryosurgery (Wang et al. 2001).
This result draws attention to the insufficient penetration of topical ALA in the profound dermis. In one study, although 69% of the topically ALA-treated tumors, including BCC, SCC in situ and invasive SCC were clinically cured, only 46% of the treated tumors were histologically negative, emphasizing the possibility of recurrence (Lui et al, 1995). Improvements regarding this issue can be obtained through the curettage of the tumors right before the application of ALA or through pretreatment with dimethylsulfoxide (DMSO) or by increasing the incubation time of ALA to 48 hours or through intralesional injections with ALA. These protocols have demonstrated improvements in long term curative effects. Also, for the same purpose, the administration of ALA can be combined with ethylenediaminetetraacetic acid (EDTA) or desferrioxamine to increase the formation of PpIX (Torpe & Bhardwaj, 2008).
In nodular BCC, surgical excision remains the treatment of choice. PDT should be reserved for the patients who cannot undergo surgical therapy (Braathen et al, 2007).
For example, in a multicenter, prospectively not controlled study which included patients with recurrent superficial and nodular basal cell lesions, with a risk of complications, with previously poor cosmetic results, it was found that after two PDT sessions carried out in a one week interval the clinical remission at 3 months was 92% for the superficial forms and 87% for the nodular ones. Histological negative margins was obtained in 85% of the superficial basal cell carcinomas and in 75% of the nodular ones (Horn et al, 2003).
ALA-PDT can be used as adjuvant therapy in Mohs microsurgery for the BCC after the excision of the tumor. Applied peripherally, on a distance of 2-5 cm on 4 patients with extensive BCC, it led to a complete remission of the tumor with excellent cosmetic and clinical results during a follow up period of 27 months. If for the patients with localized lesions the use of systemic PS is not justified because of the generalized photosensitizing, general photosensitizers (Porfimer Sodium or mTHPC) are recommended in the treatment of patients with multiple lesions. The results of a study with Porfimer Sodium on 1400 persons with superficial or nodular BCC showed a cure rate of 91%. PDT with mTHPC is efficient in multiple BCC, its advantage being the short duration of the treatment and the reduced radiation dose (Triesscheijn et al, 2006).

5.1.2 Squamous cell carcinoma

Because of the risk of metastatic disease, the use of PDT is restricted to in situ SCC. Bowen's disease is the pathology with the best response to PDT. There are numerous open, randomized trials assessing the effect of ALA-PDT in Bowen's disease. ALA combined with red light has significantly better results than the ones obtained with 5-fluorouracil or cryotherapy at 12 months follow-up with good or excellent cosmetic outcome (Morton et al,

2002). Comparing the effects of 20% ALA-PDT and fluorouracil therapy, a bicentric randomized trial showed a complete response in 88% of the lesions treated with ALA-PDT and only 67% after treatment with fluorouracil (Salim et al, 2003). However, literature data regarding the effect of PDT in Bowen's disease are controversial, some researchers reporting positive results in 90-100%, while others only in 50% of the cases (Fijan et al, 1995).

5.1.3 Other cutaneous cancers

PDT was also studied on the Kaposi sarcoma and the efficiency is similar to that of other treatments (Kalka et al, 2000). Various clinical studies have shown encouraging results for PDT in cutaneous lympho-proliferations. Still, there are no controlled trials on this matter, only isolated cases, treated topically, which can't, unfortunately, prevent the formation of new lesions. PDT is more of an additional therapy in treatment resistant T cell lymphomas (Kalka et al, 2000; Nayak, 2005). Because of the high melanin content of the melanoma, light penetration is greatly reduced. Less pigmented lesions respond better to treatment but still PDT is not a therapeutic option in melanoma. PDT is used with a palliative purpose in cutaneous metastases from breast cancer with the exception of inflammatory carcinoma which responds poorly to treatment and leads to important complications, like pain and cutaneous necrosis (Kalka et al, 2000;Nayak, 2005). PDT with systemically administered PS was used in the extramammary Paget disease resistant to conventional therapy, in severe lip displasia, and in actinic cheilitis.

5.1.4 Premalignant lesions

When treating AK one has many therapeutic options, such as: 5-Fluorouracil, podophyllin, Imiquimod, PDT, cryotherapy, etc. Numerous studies have demonstrated the effectiveness of PDT in trating AK.The response rate found in studies evaluating especially the AK of the face and skull was between 71-100% after one session of PDT. The best results were obtained when using red light (635nm) or blue light (417nm), the green light does not ensure a deep enough penetration in the lesion. An European multicentric, randomized, prospective study which compared MAL-PDT (one session) with cryosurgery in 193 patients having 699 lesions found no difference at 3 months after the treatment between the efficiency of the two methods (PDT 69% versus cryosurgery 75%) and found a small difference regarding the cosmetic results (96% versus 81%) (Szeimies et al, 2002). A study that took place in Australia involving 204 patients with AK compared the effects of 2 sessions of PDT with one session of cryotherapy and to placebo. At 3 months complete remission was reported in 91% of the patients that underwent PDT, 68% with cryotherapy, and 30% of patients who received placebo. The cosmetic results were excellent in 81% of the patients treated with PDT and in only 51% of the cases that received cryotherapy (Freeman et al, 2003). In the US, a randomized, double-blind, placebo controlled, multicentric study on 80 patients with AK treated with MAL-PDT in two sessions with red light (75 J/cm^2) found a complete remission in 89% of the cases compared to placebo (38%), with excellent cosmetic results in 90% of the cases. Also a randomized, placebo controlled, double-blind study on 17 patients with 129 lesions of AK treated with MAL-PDT showed after 16 weeks a complete response in 13 patients of the total of 17 that entered the study. This method is considered safe and efficient in patients who received a transplant and have a high risk for the transformation of AK into SCC (Dragieva et al, 2004). The incubation period of ALA does not influence the therapeutic effect. A proof in this respect are the results of a study on 18 patients, each with at least 4

lesions of AK, that were followed for 4 months and who had a reduction of 90% of the lesions without significant differences regarding the incubation period of ALA. Often, hyperkeratosis can be a reason for therapeutic insuccess. In this case removing hyperkeratosis through gentle abrasion or non-bleeding curettage is necessary before the topical application of PS (Yang et al, 2003).
To obtain an optimal result the incubation period must be about 14-18 hours. Usually ALA products are applied topically on the lesion using protection for the neighboring tissue, 4 to 6 hours before irradiation. When using MAL unguent a 3 hour incubation period is sufficient because this PS has a high selectivity and is preferentially retained by the tumor (Foley, 2003). A burning sensation or pain may appear , especially during the irradiation or a few hours after (Morton et al, 2002). There are studies that show that PDT with MAL is less painful than PDT with ALA (Wiegell et al, 2003). If the treatment is applied on large surfaces, analgesic treatment may be used or the area can be ventilated using cold air (Szeimies et al, 2005). The use of topical unguents with lidocaine and prilocaine is not recommended because they can interact with ALA and inactivate ALA/MAL due to the local increase of the pH. A small discomfort may appear in the treated area because of erythema, edema or even due to dry necrosis, these symptoms disappear after 10-21 days when a complete re-epithelization is seen (Morton & Burden, 2001; Morton et al, 2002).

5.1.5 Conclusions

PDT is one of the most important advances in skin cancer therapy. This technique is valuable especially when size, site or number of lesions limit the efficacy of conventional therapies. The mechanisms involved in obtaining the effects of PDT are complex and intricate, and the results of the therapy depend on a series of parameters that can be appropriately modulated. Further studies must be carried out in order to improve the efficiency of this modality of treatment.

6. References

Adams, JM & Cory, S. (1998). The Bcl-2 protein family: arbiters of cell survival. Science. 281, pp. 1322–1326

Ahmad, N, Gupta, S & Mukhtar H. (1999). Involvement of retinoblastoma (Rb) and E2F transcription factors during photodynamic therapy of human epidermoid carcinoma cells A431. Oncogene. 18, pp. 1891–1896

Almeida, RD, Manadas, BJ & Carvalho, AP. (2004). Intracelular signaling mechanisms in photodynamic therapy. *Biochim Biophys Acta.* 1704, pp. 59-86

Antonsson, B & Martinou, JC. (2000). The Bcl-2 protein family. *Exp. Cell Res.* 256, 50–57

Assefa, Z, Vantieghem, A, Declercq, W, Vandenabeele, P, Vandenheede, J R, Merlevede, W, de Witte, P & Agostinis P. (1999). The activation of the c-Jun N- terminal kinase and p38 mitogen-activated protein kinase signaling pathways protects HeLa cells from apoptosis following photodynamic therapy with hypericin. *J. Biol.Chem.* Vol. 274, pp. 8788-8796

Babilas, P, Landthaler, M & Szeimies, RM.(2006). Photodynamic therapy in dermatology. *Eur J Dermatol.* Vol.16, No.4, pp. 340-348

Belzacq, AS, Jacotot, E, Vieira, HL, Mistro, D, Granville, DJ, Xie, Z, Reed, JC, Kroemer, G, &Brenner, C. (2001). Apoptosis induction by the photosensitizer verteporfin:

identification of mitochondrial adenine nucleotide translocator as a critical target. *Cancer Res.* No. 61, pp. 1260–1264.

Ben-Hur, E, Fujihara T, Suzuki, F& Elkind, M M. (1987). Genetic toxicology of the photosensitization of Chinese hamster cells by phthalocyanines. *Photochem Photobiol.* Vol. 45, No.2, pp. 227-230

Berg, K & Moan, J. (1997). Lysosomes and microtubules as targets for photochemotherapy of cancer. Photochem. Photobiol. No.65, pp. 403–409

Bonizzi, G & Karin, M. (2004). The two NF-kappa B activation pathway and their role in innate and adaptive immunity, *Trends Immunol,* No. 25, pp. 2195-2224

Boyle, RW & Dolphin, D.1996. Structure and biodistribution relationships of photodynamic sensitizers. Photochem. Photobiol. 64, pp. 469-485

Braathen, LR, Szeimies, RM, Basset-Seguin, N, Bissonnette, R, Foley, P,Pariser, D, Roelandts, R, Wennberg, AM & Morton, CA. (2007). Guidelines on the use of nonmelanoma skin cancer: an international. International Society for Photodynamic Therapy in dermatology. *J Am Acad Dermatol,* 56, pp.125-143

Calzavara-Pinton, PG, Venturini, M & Sala R. (2007) Photodynamic therapy: update 2006, part 1. Photochemistry and photobiology. *JEADV,* no.21, pp. 293-302

Canti, G, De Simone, A & Korbelik, M. (2002). Photodynamic therapy and the immune system in experimental oncology. *Photochem. Photobiol. Sci,* no. 1, pp. 79–80

Castano, A P, Demidova, TN & Hamblin, MR.(2005). Mechanisms in photodynamic therapy: part two-cellular signaling, cell metabolism and modes of cell death. *Photodiagn. Photodyn. Ther.* 2, pp. 1-23

Castano, AP, Mroz, P & Hamblin, MR.(2006). Photodynamic therapy and antitumor immunity. *Nat Rev Cance.* No. 6, pp. 535-545

Chaloupka, R, Obsil, T, Plasek, J & Sureau, F. (1999). The effect of hypericin and hypocrellin-A on lipid membranes and membrane potential of 3T3 fibroblasts. Biochim Biophys Acta. Vol. 1418, pp. 39–47

Chan, WH, Yu, JS & Yang, SD.(2000). Apoptotic signaling cascade in photosensitized human epidermal carcinoma A431 cells: involvement of singlet oxygen, c-Jun N-terminal kinase, caspase-3 and p21-activated kinase 2. *Biochem. J.* Vol. 351, pp. 221-232

Chaudhuri, K, Keck, RW & Selman, S. (1987). Morphological changes of tumour microvasculature following hematoporphyrin derivative sensitised photodynamic therapy. *Photochemistry and Photobiology.* Vol. 46, pp. 823–827

Chen, G & Goeddel, DV. (2002). TNF-R1 signaling: a beautiful pathway. *Science.* Vol. 296, No.5573, pp. 1634-5

Chen, HS, Chang, WC, Su, C, Li, TY, Hsu, NM, Tingare, YS, Li, CY, Shie, JH & Li, WR. (2011). Carbene-based ruthenium photosensitizers. *Dalton Trans,* Epub ahead of print

Chen, Q, Chen, H & Hetyel, EW. (1996). Tumor oxygenation changes post-photodynamic therapy. *Photochemistry and photobiology,* 65, pp. 422-426

Choi, H, Choi, M, Choi, K &Choi, C. (2011). Blockade of vascular endothelial growth factor sensitizes tumor-associated vasculatures to angiolytic therapy with ahigh-frequency ultrashort pulsed laser, *Microvasc Res,* epub ahead of print

Clark, C, Bryden, A & Dawe, R. (2003). Topical 5-aminolevulinic acid photodynamic therapy for cutaneous lesions: outcome and comparison of light sources. *Photodermatol. Photoimmunol. Photomed.* 19, pp. 134-41

Clichici, S, Filip, A, Daicoviciu, D, Ion, RM, Mocan, T, Tatomir, C, Rogojan, L, Olteanu, D& Muresan, A. (2010).The dynamics of reactive oxygen species in photodynamic therapy with tetra sulfophenyl-porphyrin. *Acta Physiologica Hungarica*, Vol.97, No.1, pp.41-51

Coussens, lM, Fingleton, B & Matrisian, LM. (2002). Matrix metalloproteinase inhibitors and cancer: trials and tribulations. *Science*; Vol. 295, pp. 2387-2392

Daicoviciu, D, Filip, A, Clichici, S, Suciu, S, Muresan, A, Decea, N & Dreve, S.(2008). Oxidative effects after photodynamic therapy in rats. *Buletin USAMV-CN*, 2008, Vol. 65, No.1-2, pp.1454-1464

Davidson, B, Goldberg, I, Berner, A, Kristensen, GB & Reich, R. (2003). EMMPRIN (extracellular matrix metalloproteinase inducer) is a novel marker of poor outcome in serous ovarian carcinoma. *Clin. Exp. Metastasis.* 20, pp.161-169

Dougherty, TJ, Gomer, CJ, Henderson, BW, Jori, G, Kessel, D, Korbelik, M, Moan, J & Peng Q. (1998). Photodynamic therapy. *J Natl Cancer Inst* Vol.90,No. 12, pp. 889-905

Dragieva, G, Hafner, J, Dummer R. (2004). Topical photodynamic therapy in the tretament of actinic keratoses and Bowen's disease in transplant reciepients. *Transplantation.* Vol.77, pp. 115-21

El-Missiry, MA& Abou-Seif, M. (2000). Photosensitization induced reactive oxygen species and oxidative damage in human erythrocytes. *Cancer Lett*, 158, pp. 155-163

Eriksson, ES & Eriksson, LA. (2011). Computational design of chlorin based photosensitizers with enhanced absorption properties. *Phys Chem Chem Phys,* Epub ahead of print

Ferrara, N. (2004). Vascular Endothelial Growth Factor: Basic Science and Clinical Progress. *Endocrine Reviews.* Vol. 25, Vo.4, pp. 581–611

Ferrario, A, Chantrain, CF, Von Tiehl, K, Buckley, S, Rucker, N & Shalinsky, DR. (2004).The matrix metalloproteinase inhibitor prinomastat enhances photodynamic therapy responsiveness in a mouse tumor model. *Cancer Res.* 64, pp. 2328-2332

Ferrario, A, von Tiehl, KF, Wong, S, Luna, M & Gomer, CJ.(2002). Cyclooxigenase-2 inhibitor treatment enhances photodynamic therapy-mediated tumor response. *Cancer Res.* 62, pp. 3956-61

Fijan, S, Honigsman, H & Ortel, B. (1995). Photodynamic therapy of epithelial skin tumours using delta-aminolaevulinic acid and desferrioxamine. *Br. J. Dermatol*, Vol. 133, No.2, pp.: 282-8

Filip, A, Clichici, S, Muresan, A, Daicoviciu, D, Tatomir, C, Login, C, Dreve, S & Gherman, C. (2008). Effects of PDT with 5-aminolevulinic acid and chitosan on Walker carcinosarcoma *Exp. Oncol.* Vol. 30, No.3, pp. 212–219

Fingar, VH. (1996). Vascular effects of photodynamic therapy. *J. Clin. Laser Med. Surg.* 14, pp. 323–328

Firczuk, M, Nowis, D & Golab, J. (2011). PDT-induced inflammatory and host responses, Photochem photobiol Sci.Vol. 10, No. 5, pp. 653-63

Foley, P. (2003). Clinical efficacy of methyl aminolevulinate (Metvix) photodynamic therapy. *J. Dermatolog Treat.* 2003; Vol. 14 (Suppl. 3), pp. 15-22

Freeman, M, Vinciullo, C, Francis D. (2003). A comparison of photodynamic therapy using topical methyl aminolevulinate (Metvix) with single cycle cryotherapy in patients with catinic keratosis: a prospective, randomized study. *J. Dermatol. Treta*, 14, pp. 99-106

Garcia, AM, Alacorn, E, Munoz, M, Scaiano, JC,Edxards, AM & Lissi, E. (2011). Photophysical behaviour and photodynamic activity of zinc phthalocyanines associated liposomes. *Photochem Photobiol Sci,*Vol.10, No.4, pp.507-514

Gately, S & Li, WW. (2004). Multiple roles of COX-2 in tumor angiogenesis: a target for antiangiogenic therapy. *Semin. Oncol.* No. 31, pp. 2-11

Gollnick, SO, Evans, SS, Baumann, H, Owczarczak, B, Maier, P & Vaughan, L. (2003). Role of cytokines in photodynamic therapy-induced local and systemic inflammation. *Br J Cancer.* No. 88, pp. 1772-1779

Gomer, C & Henderson, B. (1998). Photodynamic therapy. *J. Natl. Cancer Inst.* Vol. 90, pp. 889-905

Gomes, ER, Almeida, R, Carvalho, AP & Duarte, C B. (2002). Nitric oxide modulates tumor cell death induced by photodynamic therapy through a cGMP-dependent mechanism. Photochemistry and Photobiology, Vol. 76, No. 4, pp. 423-430

Gomes, ER, Almeida, R, Carvalho, AP& Duarte, CB.(2002). Nitric oxide modulates tumor cell death induced by phtodynamic therapy through a cGMP-dependent mechanism. *Photochemistry and Photobiology,* Vol.76, No.4, pp. 423-430

Gross, A, McDonnell, JM & Korsmeyer, SJ. (1999). BCL-2 family members and the mitochondria in apoptosis. Genes Dev. 13, pp. 1899–1911

Gutteridge, JMC & Halliwell, B. (2000) Free radicals and antioxidants in the year 2000. A historical look to the future. *Ann. N.Y. Acad. Sci.* No. 899, pp. 136 - 147

Haylett, AK, Ward, TH & Moore, JV. (2003). DNA damage and repair in Gorlin syndrome and normal fibroblasts after aminolevulinic acid photodynamic therapy: a comet assay study. *Photochem. Photobiol.* 78, pp. 337-341

Hendrickx N, Volanti, C, Moens, U, Seternes, OM, De Witte, P & Vandenheede, JR. (2003). Up-regulation of cyclooxygenase-2 and apoptosis resistance by p38 MAPK in hypericin-mediated photodynamic therapy of human cancer cells. *J Biol Chem,* No. 278, pp. 52231-52239

Hirst, DG & Flitney, FW. (1997). The physiological importance and therapeutic potential of nitric oxide in tumour-associated vasculature. In *Tumour Angiogenesis,* Bicknell R, Lewis CE, Ferrara N, 153–167, Oxford University Press: Oxford.

Horn, M, Wolf, P, Wulf, HC. (2003). Topical methyl aminolevulinate photodynamic therapy in patients with basal cell carcinoma prone to complications and poor cosmetic outcome with conventional treatment. *Br. J. Dermatol.* Vol. 149, pp.1242-9

Huang, P, Feng, L, Oldham, EA, Keating, MJ& Plunkett, W. (2000). Superoxide dismutase as a target for the selective killing of cancer cells. *Nature.* 407, pp. 390-395

Huang, P, Xu, C, Lin, J, Wang, C, Wang, X, Zhang, C, Zhou, X, Guo, S & Cui, D. (2011). Folic acid-conjugated graphene oxide loaded with photosensitizers for targeting photodynamic therapy. *Theranostics,* vol.1, pp. 240-50.

Hunt, D W& Chan, AH. (1999). Photodynamic therapy and immunity. Idrugs. Vol.2, No.3, pp. 231-236.

Itkin, AM & Gilchrest, BA. (2004). σ - aminolevulinic acid and blue light photodynamic therapy for treatment of multiple basal cell carcinomas in two pacients with nevoid basal cell carcinoma syndrome. *Dermatologic Surgery,* vol 30, no 7, pp. 1054-1061

Jacques, SL.(1998). Light distributions from point line and plane sources for photochemical reactions and fluorescence in turbid biological tissues. *Photochemistry and photobiology.* Vol.8, No. 67, pp. 23-32

Jeong, H, Huh, M, Less, SJ, Koo, H, Kwon IC, Jeong, SY, Kim, K. (2011). Photosensitizer-conjugated human serum albumin nanoparticles for effective photodynamic therapy. *Theranostics,* 1, pp. 230-9

Kalka, Merk,H,& Mkhtar H. (2000). Photodynamic therapy in dermatology. *J Am Acad Dermatol.* 42, pp.389-416

Karin, M & Lin, A. (2002). NF-kappa B at the crossroads of life and death. Nat. Immnun. No. 3, pp. 221-227

Karrer, S, Bosserhoff, AK, Weiderer, P & Landthaler, M. (2004). Keratinocyte-derived cytokines after photodynamic therapy and their paracrine induction of matrix metalloproteinases in fibroblasts. *Br. J. Dermatol.* 151, pp. 776-783

Kessel, D &Luo, Y. (1999). Photodynamic therapy: a mitochondrial inducer of apoptosis. Cell Death Differ. Vol. 6, No.1, pp. 28-35

Kessel, D& Luo, Y. (1999). Photodynamic therapy: a mitochondrial inducer of apoptosis. *Cell Death Differ*, vol. 6, no.1, pp. 28-35

Kim, HR, Luo, Y, Li, G & Kessel D. (1999). Enhanced apoptotic response to photodynamic therapy a_er bcl-2 transfection. *Cancer Res. 59*, pp. 3429–3432

Klein, A, Babilas, P, Karrer, S, Landthaler, M & Szeimies, RM. (2008). Photodynamic therapy in dermatology - an update 2008. *J Dtsch Dermatol Ges.* Vol. 6, No. 10, pp. 839-846

Klein, SD, Walt, H, Rocha, S, Ghafourifar, P, Pruschy, M, Winterhalter, KH & Richter, C.(2001). Overexpression of Bcl-2 enhances sensitivity of L929 cells to a lipophilic cationic photosensitiser. *Cell Death Differ.* 8, pp. 204–206

Klotz, LO, Briviba, K & Sies, H. (1997). Singlet oxygen mediates the activation of JNK by UVA radiation in human skin fibroblasts. *FEBS Lett.* Vol. 408, pp. 289-291

Kobayashi, H, Boelte, KC & Lin PC. (2007). Endothelial cell adhesion molecules and cancer progression. *Curr Med Chem,* Vol. 14, No. 4, pp. 377-386

Kondo, M, Hirota, N, Takaoka, T & Kajiwara, M. (1993). Heme-biosynthetic enzyme activities and porphyrin accumulation in normal liver and hepatoma cell lines of rat, *Cell Biol. Toxicol.* 9, 95-105

Korbelik ,M. (2006). PDT-associated host response and its role in the therapy outcome. *Lasers Surg Med,* Vol. 38, No.5, pp. 500-508

Korbelik, M & Dougherty, GJ. (1999). Photodynamic therapy-mediated immune response against subcutaneous mouse tumors. *Cancer Res.* 59, pp. 1941–1946

Korbelik, M, Parkins, CS, Shibuya, H, Cecic, I & Stratford, MR. (2000). Nitric oxide production by tumor tissue: impact on the response to photodynamic therapy. *Br. J. Cancer,* 82, pp.1835-1843

Korbelik, M, Shibuya, H & Cecic, I. (1998). Relevance of nitric oxide to the response of tumors to photodynamic therapy. *Proceedings of SPIE – The International Society for Optical Engineering.* Vol. 3247, pp. 98–105

Korbelik, M. (1996). Induction of tumor immunity by photodynamic therapy. *J. Clin. Laser Med. Surg.* 14, pp. 329–334

Kral, V, Kralova, J, Kaplanek, R, Briza, T& Martasek, P. (2006). Quo vadis porphyrin chemistry? *Physiol. Res.* Vol. 55 (Suppl. 2): S3-S26.

Kriska, T, Korytowski, W& Girotti, AW. (2005). Role of mitochondrial cardiolipin peroxidation in apoptotic photokilling of 5-aminolevulinate-treated tumor cells. *Arch Biochem Biophys*, Vol. 433, pp. 435–446

Krosi, G, Korbelik, M, Krosi, J & Dougherty, TJ. (1996). Potentiation of photodynamic therapy elicited antitumor response by localized treatment with granulocyte-macrophage colony stimulating factor. Cancer Res. 56, pp. 3281-3286

Lam, M, Oleinick, NL & Nieminen, AL. (2001). Photodynamic therapy-induced apoptosis in epidermoid carcinoma cells. Reactive oxygen species and mitochondrial inner membrane permeabilization. *J Biol Chem.* No. 276, pp. 47379–47386

Lee, S, Jilani, SM, Nikolova, GV, Carpizo, D & Iruela-Arispe, ML.(2005). Processing of VEGF-A by matrix metalloproteinases regulates bioavalability and vascular patterning in tumor. *J Cell Biol.* Vol. 169, No.4, pp. 681-91

Lee, SJ, Koo, H, Jeong, H, Huh, MS, Choi, Y, Jeong, SY, Byun, Y, Choi, K, Kim, K, Kwon, IC. (2011). Comparative study of photosensitizer loaded and conjugated glycol chitisan nanoparticles for cancer therapy, *J Control Release,* Epub ahead of print

Lehmann, P. (2007). Methyl aminolaevulinate-photodynamic therapy: review of clinical trials in the treatment of actinic keratosis and nonmelanoma skin cancer. *Br J Dermatol.*156, pp:793-801

Lenczowski, JM, Dominguez, L, Eder, AM, King, LB, Zacharchuk, CM & Ashwell, JD.(1997). Lack of a role for Jun kinase and AP-1 in Fas-induced apoptosis. Mol. Cell. Biol. Vol. 17, pp. 170-181

Lin,BC, Skipp,W, Tao,Y, Schleicher, S, Cano,L L, Duke,R C&cheinman RI. (1999). NF-kappa B functions as both a proapoptotic and antiapoptotic regulatory factor within a single cell type. *Cell. Death. Differ.* No. 6, pp. 570-582

Lopes, CC, Dietrich, CP & Nader, HB. (2006). Specific structural features of syndecans and heparan sulfate chains are needed for cell signaling. *Braz J Med Biol Res,* 39, pp. 157-167

Lui, H, Salasche M & Kollias, N . (1995). Photodynamic therapy of nonmelanoma skin cancer with topical aminolevulinic acid: a clinical and histological study. *Archives of dermatology,* vol.131, no.6, pp.737-738

Makowski, M, Grzela, T, Niderla, J, Lazarczyk, M, Mroz, P & Kopee, M. (2003). Inhibition of cyclooxygenase-2 indirectly potentiates antitumor effects of photodynamic therapy in mice. Clin Cancer Res. No. 9, pp. 5417-5422

Marcus, S L & McIntyre, W R. (2002). Photodynamic therapy systems and applications. *Expert. Opin. Emerg. Drugs,* Vol. 7, no. 2, pp. 321-334

Marmur,E S, Schmults,CDE & Goldberg,DJ. (2004). A review of laser and photodynamic therapy for the treatment of nonmelanoma skin cancer. *Dermatol. Surg.* 30, pp. 264-71

Matroule, JY, Voalnti, C & Plette, J. (2006). NF-kB in photodynamic therapy: Discrepancies of a master regulator. *Photochemistry and Photobiology.* 82, pp. 1241-1246

Morton, CA & Burden, AD. (2001). Treatment of multiple scalp basal cell carcinomas by photodynamic therapy. *Clin Exp Dermatol.* Vol. 26, pp. 33–36

Morton, CA, Brown, SB & Collins, S. (2002). Guidelines for topical photodynamic therapy. Report of a workshop of the British Photodermatology Group. *Br J Dermatol,* Vol. 146, pp. 552–567

Mourant, JR, Johnson, TM, Los, G & Bigio, IJ. (1999). Non-invasive measurement of chemotherapy drug concentrations in tissue: preliminary demonstrations of in vivo measurements. *Physics in Medicine and Biology.* 44, pp. 1397-1417

Nayak, CS. (2005). Photodynamic therapy in dermatology Indian J. Dermatol. Venereol. Leprol. No. 71, pp. 155-60

Niedre, M, Patterson, MS& Wilson, BC. (2002). Direct near-infrared luminescence detection of singlet oxygen generated by photodynamic therapy in cells in vitro and tissues in vivo. *Photochem Photobiol,* vol. 75, no. 4, pp. 382-391

Nowis, D, Makowski, M & Stoklosa, T. (2005). Direct tumor damage mechanisms of photodynamic therapy. *Acta Biochimica Polonica.* Vol. 52, No.2, pp. 339-352

Oleinick, NL, Morris, RL & Belichenko, I. (2002). The role of apoptosis in response to photodynamic therapy: what, where, why, and how. *Photochem Photobiol Sci.* No. 1,pp. 1–21

Oseroff, AR, Shieh, S & Frawley, NP. (2005). Treatment of diffuse basal cell carcinomas and basaloid follicular hamartomas in nevoid basal cell carcinoma syndrome by wide-area 5- aminolevulinic acid photodynamic therapy. *Achives of Dermatology,* vol. 141, no 1, pp 60-75

Otake, E, Sakuma, S, Torii, K, Maeda, A, Ohi, H, Yano, S & Morita, A. (2010). Effect and mechanism of a new Photodynamic therapy with glycoconjugated fullerene. *Photochem. Photobiol.* Vol. 86, No. 6, pp.1356-63.

Overall, CM &Lopez-Otia, C. (2002). Strategies for MMP inhibition in cancer: Innovations for the post-trial era. *Nat. Rev. Cancer.* Vol.2, pp. 657-672

Peng, Q, Moan, J & Nesland, JM. (1996). Correlation of subcellular and intratumoral photosensitizer localization with ultrastructural features after photodynamic therapy. *Ultrastructural Pathology,* no.20, pp. 109-129

Pfeiffer, S, Schmidt, K & Mayer, B. (2000). Dityrosine formation out competes tyrosine nitration at low steady-state concentrations of peroxynitrite. Implications for tyrosine modification by nitric oxide/superoxide in vivo. *J. Biol. Chem.* No.275, pp. 6346–6352

Pogue, BW, Ortel, B, Chen, N, Redmond, RW & Hasan, T.(2001). A photobiological and photophysical-based study ofphototoxicity of two chlorines. *Cancer Res.* No. 61,pp. 717-724

Rancan, F, Wiehe, A, Nöbel, M, Senge, MO, Omari, SA, Böhm, F, John, M& Röder, B.(2005). Influence of substitutions on asymmetric dihydroxychlorins with regard to intracellular uptake, subcellular localization and photosensitization of Jurkat cells. *Photochem. Photobiol.* No.78, pp. 17-28

Reed, JC. (1998). Bcl-2 family proteins. *Oncogene.* 17, pp. 3225–3236

Rhodes, LE, de Rie, MA, Leifsdottir, R, Yu, RC, Bachmann, I, Goulden, V, Wong, GAE, Richard,MA, Anstey, A & Wolf, P. (2007). Five-year follow-up of a randomized, prospective trial of topical methyl aminolevulinate photodynamic therapy vs surgery for nodular baal cell carcinoma. *Arch Dermatol,* 143, pp.1131-1136

Rick, K, Sroka, R, Stepp, H, Kriegmair, M, Huber, RM, Jacob, K & Baumgartner, R. (1997). Pharmacokinetics of 5-aminolevulinic acid-induced protoporphyrin IX in skin and blood, *J.Photochem. Photobiol. B,* 40, pp. 313-319

Rubbo, HR, Radi, R, Trujillo, M, Tellieri, R, Kalyanaraman, B, Barnes, S, Kirk, M &Freeman BA. (1994). Nitric oxide regulation of superoxide and peroxynitrite-dependent lipid peroxidation. Formation of noved nitrogen-containing oxidized lipid derivatives. *J. Biol. Chem.* Vol 269, pp. 26066-26075

Ryter, S &Gornerr,CJ. (1993). Nuclear factor kappa mouse L1210 cells following Photofrin II-mediated photosensitiyation.*Photochem. Photobiol.* 58, pp. 753-756

Saczko, J, Kulbacka, J, Chwilkowska, A, Pola, A, Lugowski, M, Marcinkowska, A, Malarska, A & Banas T. (2007). Cytosolic superoxide dismutase activity after photodynamic therapy, intracellular distribution of Photofrin II and hypericin, and P-glycoprotein localization in human colon adenocarcinoma. *Folia Histochemica et cytobiologica* Vol. 45, No. 2, pp. 93-97

Salim, A , Leman, N J & McColl JH. (2003). Randomized comparison pf photodynamic therapy with topical 5-fluouracil in Bowen's disease. *Br. J. Dermatol.* 148, pp. 539-43

Schafer, FQ & Buettner, GR. (1999). Singlet oxygen toxicity is cell line-dependent: a study of lipid peroxidation in nine leukemia cell lines. *Photochem Photobiol*, no.70, pp. 858-867

Schneider, R, Schmitt, F, Frochot, C, Fort, Y, Lourette, N, Guillemin, F, Muller, JF &Barberi-Heyob, M. (2005). Design synthesis and biological evaluation of folic acid terageted tetraphenylporphyrin as novel photosenstitizers for selective photodynamic therapy. *Bioorg. Med. Chem.* Vol. 13. No. 8, pp. 2799-808

Sibata, CH, Colussi, VC, Oleinick, NL & Kinsella, TJ. (2000). Photodynamic therapy: a new concept in medical treatment. *Braz J Med Biol Res.* Vol. 33, No.8, pp. 869-880

Soler, AM, Warloe,T & Berner, A. (2001). A follow-up study of recurrence and cosmesis in completely responding superficial and nodular basal cell carcinomas treated with methyl 5-aminolaevulinate-based photodynamic therapy alone and with prior curettage.*Br. J. Dermatol.* 145, pp. 467-71

Sporn, LA & Foster, TH. (1992). Photofrin and light induces microtubule depolymerization in cultured human endothelial cells. *Cancer Res.* Vol. 52, pp. 3443-3448

Szeimies,R M, Morton,C A, Sidoroff,A, Braathen,L R. (2005). Photodynamic therapy for melanoma skin cancer. *Acta Derm Venerol;* 85, pp.483–490

Szeimies,RM, Karrer,S &Fijan,SR. (2002).Photodynamic therapy using topical methyl 5-aminolevulinate compared with cryotherapy for actinic keratosis. A prospective, randomized study, *J. Am Acad. Dermatol.* 47, pp. 258-62

Teiten, MH, Bezdetnaya, L & Morliere, P. (2003). Endoplasmic reticulum and Golgi apparatus are the preferential sites of Foscan localizations in cultured tumor cells. *Br. J. Cancer.* no.88, pp. 146 - 152

Thor, H, Hartell, P, Svensson, SA, Orrenius, S, Mirahelli, F, Mnarinoni, V & Bellomo. G. (1985). On the role of thiol groups in the inhibition of liver microsomal Ca^{2+} sequestration by toxic agents. *Biochem. Pharmacol.* Vol.34, pp. 3717-3723

Torpe, WD & Bhardwaj SS, (2008). Photodynamic therapy, in dermatology, JL Bologna, JL Lorizzo, and RP Rapini, Eds, pp 2071-2080, Mosby-Elsevier, Spain, 2nd edition

Triesscheijn, M, Baas, P & Schellens, JHM. (2006). Photodynamic therapy in oncology. *The Oncologist.* Vol. 11, No. 9, pp. 1034-1044

Van Duijnhoven, FH, Aalbers, RI, Rovers, JP, Terpstra, OT & Kuppen, PJ. (2003). The immunological consequences of photodynamic treatment of cancer, a literature review: Immunobiology. Vol. 27, No. 2, pp.105-113

Volanti, C, Gloire, G, Vanderplasschen, A, Jacobs, N, Habraken, Y & Piette, J.(2004). Downregulation of ICAM-1 and VCAM-1 expression in endothelial cells treated by photodynamic therapy. *Oncogene.* 23, pp. 8649-8658

Volanti, C, Hendrickx, N, Van Lint, J, Matroule, JY , Agostinis, P & Piette, J. (2005). Distinct transduction mechanisms of cyclooxygenase 2 gene activation in tumor cells after photodynamic therapy. *Oncogene.* No. 24, pp. 2981-2991

Wang, I, Bendsoe, N & Klinteberg C. A. (2001). Photodynamic therapy vs cryosurgery of basal cell carcinomas: results of a phase III clinical trial. *Br. J. Dermatol.* 144, pp.832-40

Way, JS, Stoeltzing, O & Ellis, LM. (2004). Vascular endothelial growth factor receptors: expression and function in solid tumors. *Clin. Adv. Hematol. Oncol.* No. 2, pp. 37-45

Wei, LH, Baumann, H, Tracy, E, Wang, E, Hutson, A, Rose-John, S & Henderson, BW.(2007). Interleukin-6 trans signalling enhances photodynamic therapy by modulating cell cycling. British Journal of Cancer. 97, pp. 1513–1522

Wiegell, SR, Stender, I M, Na, R & Wulf, H C. (2003). Pain associated with photodynamic therapy using 5-aminolevulinic acid or 5-aminolevulinic acid methylester on tape-stripped normal skin. *Arch Dermatol* , 139, pp.1173–1177

Wight, TN. (2002). Versican: a versatile extracellular matrix proteoglycan in cell biology. *Curr Opin Cell Biol* 14, pp. 617-623

Wilson, BC. (1998). Light sources for photodynamic therapy of photosensitization. *Photodynamic Therapy News.* 1, pp. 6-8

Yang, CH, Lee, JC & Chen,CH. (2003). Photodynamic therapy for bowenoid papulosis using a novel incoherent light-emitting diode device. *Br. J. Dermatol.* 149, pp.1297-9.

Yom, SS, Busch, TM, Friedberg, JS, Wileyto, EP, Smith, D & Glatstein E. (2003). Elevated serum cytokine levels in mesothelioma patients who have undergone pleurectomy or extrapleural pneumonectomy and adjuvant intraoperative photodynamic therapy. *Photochem Photobiol.* No. 78, pp. 75-81

Zhuang, S, Lynch, MC & Kochevar, IE. (1999). Caspase-8 mediates caspase-3 activation and cytochrome *c* release during singlet oxygen-induced apoptosis of HL-60 cells. *Exp Cell Res,* 250, pp. 203–212

11

Topical Administration of Anticancer Drugs for Skin Cancer Treatment

Stephânia Fleury Taveira and Renata Fonseca Vianna Lopez
School of Pharmaceutical Sciences of Ribeirão Preto – University of São Paulo, Brazil

1. Introduction

Skin cancer is the most common type of cancer affecting Caucasian populations. It has a very high rate of incidence, exceeding the sum of all other cancers combined (Simonette et al., 2009). There are three forms of skin tumors that stand out: cutaneous malignant melanoma, basal cell carcinoma (BCC) and squamous cell carcinoma (SCC).

BCC and SCC are classified as nonmelanoma skin cancers, with BCC being the most common and constituting 75% of cases (Anthony, 2000). The incidence of nonmelanoma skin cancers has steadily increased, making them a major challenge in terms of management of public health. Moreover, these cancers can have a huge impact on health care costs. In the United States, it is estimated that there are approximately 3 to 4 million cases annually of BCC and approximately 100,000 cases of SCC. Nonmelanoma skin cancers are not fatal but can destroy facial sensory organs such as the nose, ear and lips (Alam et al., 2011). Therefore, these lesions should preferably be treated using noninvasive techniques.

In contrast, melanoma skin cancers are an aggressive type that can metastasize and cause death. These cancers originate from melanocytes, which are pigment-producing cells, and are associated with chronic exposure to sunlight (Einspahr et al., 2002). Because melanoma has a much higher mortality rate than nonmelanoma skin cancers, different treatments, including invasive interventions, are required (Martinez & Otley, 2001).

There are some well-established treatments for nonmelanoma skin cancer, such as curettage, surgery, cryotherapy and chemotherapy. However, these conventional treatments lead to severe inflammation, pain and unappealing scars (Lopez et al., 2004). Treatments for melanoma, in turn, are primarily surgical because these tumors can be resistant to traditional chemo- and radiotherapies (Davids & Kleeman, 2010). Nonsurgical treatments for melanomas are limited to adjuvant therapies, such as immunotherapy, biochemotherapy, gene therapy and photodynamic therapy (Martinez & Otley, 2001; Davids & Kleeman, 2010).

To increase patient compliance and to reduce surgical costs and undesirable scars, particularly in cases where the cancer has spread over large areas of the body, the topical administration of anticancer drugs has been investigated. The topical administration of anticancer drugs is an interesting alternative for reducing side effects and for increasing drug targeting and therapeutic benefits. The major challenge of this kind of treatment is to increase penetration of the antineoplastic tumor drug in sufficient levels to kill tumor cells.

Several techniques and formulations have therefore been developed to successfully overcome skin barriers and to reach skin malignancies by favoring drug penetration into the deep layers of the epidermis. The use of chemical penetration enhancers is the simplest strategy, causing temporary and reversible disruption of the stratum corneum bilayers and leading to increased anticancer drug penetration into the tumor. Moreover, great interest has been shown in nanoparticle delivery systems that can protect anticancer drugs against degradation and, combined with physical methods, significantly increase the tumor penetration of the drug.

This chapter will briefly discuss skin anatomy, the primary barriers to topical anticancer drugs' skin penetration, and the most studied penetration enhancer methods for topical skin cancer treatment. The aim of this chapter is to provide a basic understanding and description of the strategies that can be used to overcome the skin barrier, such as liposomes, polymeric and lipid nanoparticles, iontophoresis and electroporation. Each of these modalities will be discussed in the context of their application for promoting and targeting the delivery of skin tumor drugs following topical, noninvasive, administration.

2. The skin as a barrier against anticancer drug penetration

The skin is the largest organ of the body and is composed of three primary layers: the epidermis, dermis and hypodermis. The epidermis plays an important role in the penetration of substances into the skin. It is the outer avascular layer of the skin, primarily composed of keratinocytes. Because of cellular differentiation, the epidermis is divided into different layers, which are formed by the division of basal cells from the inner part of the body toward the surface (Figure 1). Hence, basal cells undergo progressive maturation, giving rise to the spinous layer or squamous cells. These cells also differentiate, forming the granular layer and finally the stratum corneum, which is the outermost layer of the skin.

The stratum corneum is the major barrier for the penetration of substances into the skin because of its heterogeneous composition and packed organization of corneocytes and the intracellular lipid matrix. The corneocytes are flat anucleated squamous cells packed primarily with keratin filaments and surrounded by a lipid matrix composed primarily of ceramides, cholesterol, and free fatty acids (Bouwstra et al., 2003).

Two other cell types that are important in the context of skin tumor composition, melanocytes and Langerhans, are embedded between the basal keratinocytes. Melanocytes are dendritic cells capable of melanin production, and Langerhans cells are antigen-presenting cells that are responsible for the immune response in the skin (McGrath & Uitto, 2010) (Figure 1).

Because the skin is a heterogeneous organ, this wide variety of cell types can generate several types of benign and malignant tumors. For instance, SCC and BCC originate from keratinocytes. The development of these tumors is associated with many factors, but most of these cancers are related to excess ultraviolet radiation (UV) exposure. Following sun exposure-induced damage, the stratum corneum of tumor lesions usually presents with hyperkeratinization (Neel & Sober et al., 2006), a factor known to hamper drug penetration. Topical anticancer administration therefore requires a well-designed formulation to increase drug penetration into the thicker stratum corneum and to favor drug penetration into the deep skin layers, where tumors are usually located.

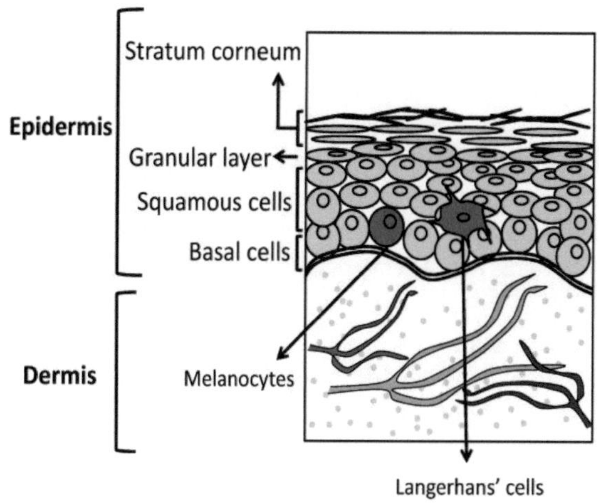

Fig. 1. Schematic representation of the epidermis/dermis and epidermis layers consisting of basal cells, squamous cells, the granular layer and the stratum corneum.

For example, the most superficial malignancy that develops in the epidermis is actinic keratosis, so-named because of the exaggerated production of keratin in the stratum corneum, which causes it to become thicker (Figure 2A and 2B). These lesions can develop into tumors, usually SCCs, which may be nodular (invasive) and hyperkeratotic (Figure 2C). For topical treatment of both actinic keratosis and SCC, anticancer drugs should penetrate the stratum corneum to reach the tumor cells.

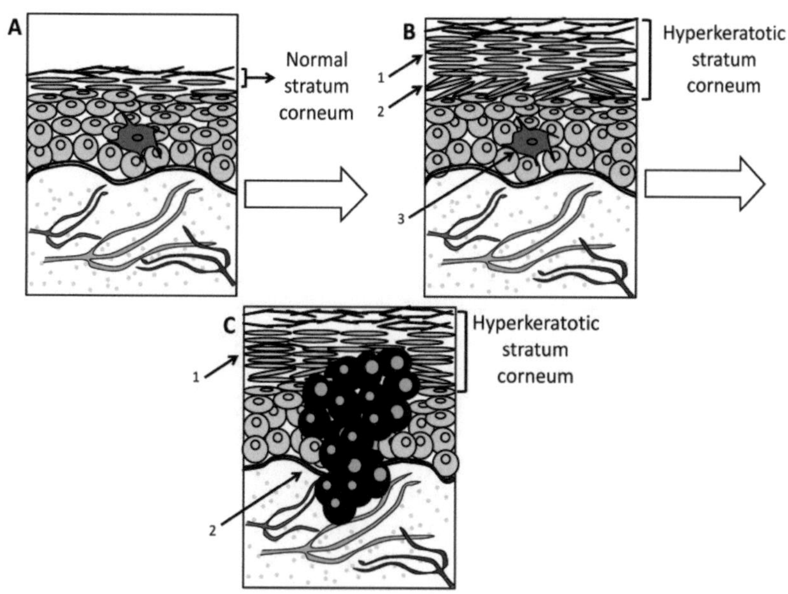

Fig. 2. Schematic representation of the skin layers, especially the stratum corneum, of (A) Normal skin, (B) Actinic Keratosis: (1) hyperkeratosis, (2) atypia of cells, (3) Langerhans cells; (C) Invasive SCC: (1) hyperkeratosis and (2) squamous cells with atypical nuclei (enlarged and hyperchromatic).

Another example for the necessity of drug penetration through the stratum corneum is the use of immunoregulator drugs for the topical treatment of actinic keratosis. To be effective, these drugs need to act in the Langerhans cells to induce the release of proinflammatory cytokines, which stimulate an immune response. To reach Langerhans cells, anticancer drugs must cross the hyperkeratotic stratum corneum (Figure 2B).

Within this context, it is important to understand the mechanisms of drug penetration through the stratum corneum to determine methods or strategies that can increase drug penetration such that the drug reaches sufficient concentrations to kill tumor cells.

2.1 Drug penetration in the skin

Over the past two decades, significant attention has been paid to understanding the mechanisms by which drugs penetrate the skin. It is well known that substances usually penetrate the skin by three different routes: through the stratum corneum between the corneocytes (intercellular route); through these cells and the intervening lipids (intracellular route); or through the skin appendages, such as hair follicles and sweat glands (Moser et al., 2001). Molecules with adequate solubility in water and oil, with a log of oil/water partition coefficients between 1 and 3 (Hadgraft & Lane, 2005) and a molecular weight lower than 0.6 kDa (Schäfer-Korting et al., 2007; Barry, 2001), may penetrate the skin. Therefore, topical administration is limited to hydrophobic and low-molecular weight drugs. Because most anticancer drugs are hydrophilic, have low oil/water partition coefficients, high molecular weights and ionic characters (Souza et al., 2011), they do not easily penetrate the stratum corneum.

Drug permeation through the stratum corneum can be described with Ficks's second law (Williams & Barry, 2004) (Equation 1).

$$J = \frac{\mathrm{Dm}\ \mathrm{Cv}\ P}{\mathrm{L}}, \tag{1}$$

where J is the flux, Dm is the diffusion coefficient of the drug in the membrane, Cv is the drug concentration in the vehicle, P is the drug partition coefficient and L is the stratum corneum thickness.

It can be seen in Equation I that the flux of a drug through the skin is governed by the diffusion coefficient of the drug in the stratum corneum, the concentration of the drug in the vehicle, the partition coefficient between the formulation and the stratum corneum and the membrane thickness. Using this equation, it is a simple matter to determine which parameters can be manipulated to increase drug flux through the stratum corneum. Formulations containing chemical penetration enhancers or the use of physical penetration methods, such as iontophoresis and electroporation, may alter one or more of these parameters to increase drug penetration in the skin. For instance, chemical enhancers can disrupt the stratum corneum barrier and increase the diffusion coefficient of the drug through the altered membranes. Alternatively, enhancers can alter the solvent nature of the skin and improve partitioning between the formulation and the stratum corneum. Nanocarriers can increase drug concentration in the vehicle and so increase drug flux. Physical penetration methods can modify drug penetration routes through the stratum corneum, making it less tortuous, facilitating drug penetration (Williams & Barry, 2004).

In this context, several manuscripts have reported the use of anticancer drugs in combination with penetration-enhancing methods or nanocarriers aimed at obtaining high penetration of the drug through the skin for tumor elimination.

3. Current topical therapies for skin cancer treatment

Current topical treatments for skin cancer include semi-solid formulations of 5-fluorouracil, diclofenac and imiquimod. Another topical treatment also used and approved by the US Food and Drug Administration (FDA) is photodynamic therapy (PDT). These therapies are used to treat nonmelanoma skin cancers and its precursor lesions, such as actinic keratosis. Several studies have discussed the preferred schedules for topical treatment to avoid tumor recurrence. Advantages and disadvantages of each topical treatment will be discussed to give a better understanding of treatment limitations and to propose different approaches that may improve topical skin cancer treatment.

5-fluorouracil has been considered the topical treatment of choice for actinic keratosis since its approval in 1970 by the US FDA (Barrera & Herrera, 2007). It is a structural analogue of thyamine and inhibits the enzyme thymidylate synthetase, blocking DNA synthesis and preventing cell proliferation (Galiczynski & Vidimos, 2011). There are many 5-fluorouracil preparations, and it is available through a variety of trademarks both as creams (5%, 1% and 0.5%) and in solution (5%, 2% or 1%) (Barrera & Herrera, 2007). This medication has some side effects, such as an intense local inflammatory reaction, that result in a lack of patient compliance. Other disadvantages are the relative long treatment period and partial inefficacy of the treatment in the deep layers of skin, such as in cases of hyperkeratotic actinic keratosis (Barrera & Herrera, 2007). These drawbacks emphasize the need for alternative methods or techniques to improve the skin penetration of antineoplastic drugs.

Imiquimod is an immune response modifier that directly and indirectly interacts with the immune system (Perrotta et al., 2011). It was initially approved by the FDA in 1997 for genital and perianal wart treatment but has been used off-label for neoplastic skin treatments (Burns & Brown, 2005). In 2004, the FDA approved the use of imiquimod 5% cream for the treatment of actinic keratosis and superficial BCC in patients for whom surgery is not an option (Perrota et al., 2011). Still, without FDA approval, it has been commonly used for many other cutaneous disorders, such as cutaneous melanoma metastases, BCC, Bowen's disease, SCC and lentigo maligna. Studies have revealed that almost all patients treated with imiquimod exhibit some degree of local inflammation at the application site. In FDA studies, patients presented some degree of erythema, edema, ulceration or erosion (Burns & Brown, 2005).

The formulation of 3% diclofenac gel has been used for the topical treatment of actinic keratosis. At present, it is approved by the FDA and is used only in the US (Berrera & Herrera, 2007). Diclofenac is a nonsteroidal anti-inflammatory drug and has been show to have an antitumor effect by inhibiting arachidonic acid metabolism (Galiczynski & Vidimos, 2011). The examined treatment schedules have been two applications daily for 60 or 90 days, with patients showing complete resolution of actinic keratosis lesions in 47% of cases (Berrera & Herreara, 2007).

PDT is also approved by the FDA for the treatment of nonhypertrophic actinic keratosis of the head and scalp (Galiczynski & Vidimos, 2011). Nevertheless, it has been used off-label to treat various dermatoses, such as superficial and nodular BCC, SCC *in situ* and others (Galiczynski & Vidimos, 2011). PDT involves the administration of a photosensitizing drug or a pro-drug that is converted in a photosensitizer intracellularly (usually 5-aminolevulinic acid, 5-ALA). Subsequent activation by light of a specific wavelength leads to the formation of highly reactive singlet oxygen ($^1O_2$), destroying the cells via chemical, biological and physiological reactions (Araújo et al., 2010). To specifically kill tumor cells, it is therefore important that the photosensitizing drug target the tumor cells at a high concentration. Great efforts have been made to design topical nanocarriers and techniques that can increase the penetration of photosensitizers into the deep skin layers (Souza et al., 2011; Araújo et al, 2010; Gelfuso et al., 2008; Gelfuso et al., 2011) to make topical PDT more effective.

Other clinical trials are underway. The retinoids, or vitamin A analogs, which are commonly used in cosmetic products, have been considered to have certain chemopreventive effects (Berrera & Herrera, 2007). Resiquimod, which is structurally similar to imiquimod but 10–100 times more potent, is another new drug that modulates the immune system (Perrotta et al., 2011) when topically applied. Adequate formulations for both of these drugs still need to be designed for successful skin penetration.

It is interesting to note that the current topical medications approved by the FDA for skin cancer treatment are used primarily to treat superficial skin cancers. This is due to the fact that some skin cancers, such as SCC, can metastasize, and topical therapy is only used for invasive tumors if the patient cannot receive surgical treatments. Moreover, response rates differ for superficial and invasive cancers. For example, Burns (2005) reported that imiquimod was more effective in treating superficial BCC than for nodular BCC. This is likely because nodular BCC occurs deep in the dermis and the drug may not reach the full depth of the tumor invasion.

Again, these limitations highlight the importance of developing new formulations or methods that improve drug penetration of the skin for the treatment of different skin cancers. Several chemical/physical methods and nanocarriers have been studied with the aim of overcoming the above limitations of current treatments and are discussed further.

4. Methods to improve drug skin penetration

Different approaches have been developed to increase skin permeability, such as the use of chemical enhancers, the application of an electric field (e.g., iontophoresis and electroporation) and the use of nanocarriers, such as liposomes and polymeric and solid lipid nanoparticles (Figure 3). These methods have the common goal of overcoming the stratum corneum and targeting tumor cells.

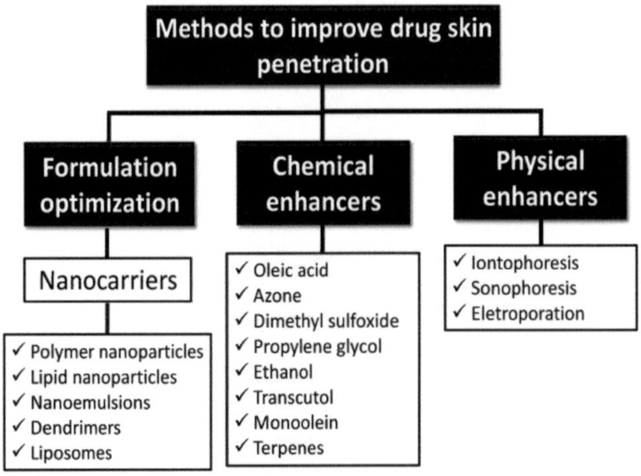

Fig. 3. Methods to improve drug penetration through the skin and examples of each method.

Figure 4 lists the percentage of articles published between 1990 and 2011 that used the most commonly studied nanocarriers and physical/chemical methods to increase the penetration of drugs into the skin. Liposomes are the most frequently studied drug delivery system for topical delivery. Physical penetration methods were used in 22% of the publications, contributing to nearly one quarter of all publications for topical drug delivery (Figure 4). In total, chemical and physical penetration enhancers were employed in nearly half of studies. The other half examined nanocarriers, specifically liposomes and nanoparticles. Other nanocarriers or techniques that have been used to improve topical treatments, such as dendrimers, microemulsions, sonophoresis, etc., were not represented in Figure 4 because they represent a small percentage of studies (less than 10%) when compared to the other systems.

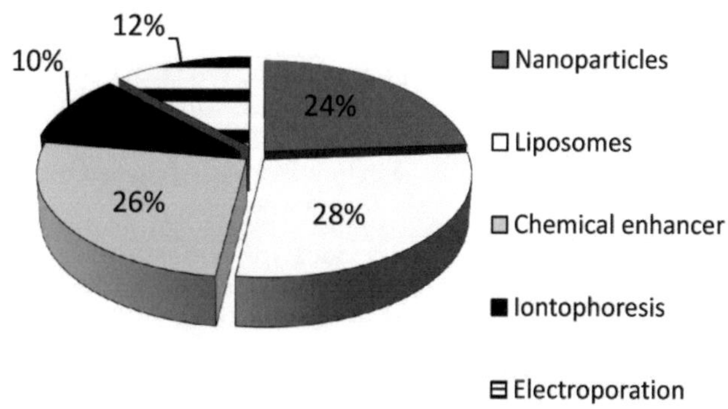

Fig. 4. Percentage of articles published between 1990 and 2011 related to skin-applied liposomes, nanoparticles, chemical enhancers, iontophoresis or electroporation to increase drug penetration ("Science direct®" database, June/2011).

Studies have examined a variety of nanoparticles in the context of improving drug delivery through the skin, including solid lipids, polymeric, gold and silver. Among studies addressing only polymeric or solid lipid nanoparticles, there has been more focus on the former than the latter. This is likely because the studies related to polymeric nanoparticles began around the 1970s, whereas studies related to solid lipid nanoparticles began around the 1990s (Guimarães & Ré, 2011). However, in the last 5 years, articles related to lipid nanoparticles for topical applications have nearly doubled, from 145 to 279 (data available in the "Science Direct" database June 2011).

It is interesting that when considering only publications related to skin cancers that use the strategies outlined in Figure 4, the same distribution of techniques is observed. Specifically, a large number of articles examine the use of liposomes for skin cancer treatment or prevention (33%). Nanoparticles are the second most studied system (20%), followed by chemical enhancers (28%), electroporation (13.5%) and iontophoresis (4.5%). These strategies were therefore chosen for further discussion in this chapter.

4.1 Chemical penetration enhancers

Penetration enhancers have been extensively used in topical formulations. These are chemicals that, when added to the topical formulation, generally promote drug diffusion by 1) reversibly disturbing the structure of the stratum corneum, 2) increasing drug diffusivity and 3) increasing the solubility in the skin (Shah et al., 2000). There are many well known substances

that may act as penetration enhancers. Fatty acids, oleic acid, azone, dimethyl sulfoxide (DMSO) and terpenes all increase the drug diffusion coefficient by disordering the stratum corneum lipid matrix (Moser et al., 2001). Propylene glycol, ethanol, transcutol and N-methyl pyrrolidone act by increasing a drug's solubility in the skin. Monoolein, a frequently studied substance used to enhance the skin penetration of anticancer drugs, causes a temporary and reversible disruption of the stratum corneum, increasing drug penetration.
Table 1 lists studies that employed chemical penetration enhancers for topical anticancer delivery.

Anticancer Drug	Chemical Enhancer	Results	References
5-fluorouracil	Azone, lauryl alcohol and isopropyl myristate	Azone increased drug flux through the skin more than the other penetration enhancers.	Singh et al., 2005.
Doxorubicin	Monoolein and propylene glycol	Increased drug retention in the skin avoiding transdermal delivery.	Herai et al., 2007.
Cisplatin	Monoolein and propylene glycol	Increased drug concentration in the skin by a factor of two when compared to the control.	Simonetti et al., 2009.
Tretinoin	Liposomes combined with decylpolyglucosid , caprylocaproyl macrogol 8-glyceride, ethoxydiglycol and propylene glycol.	Association of the nanocarrier with the penetration enhancers improved drug retention, avoiding transdermal drug delivery.	Manconi et al., 2011.
5-Aminolevulinic acid (5-ALA) and ALA derivatives.	DMSO and DMSO with EDTA	DMSO at 10 and 20% increased the penetration of 5-ALA, a protoporphyrin IX (PpIX) precursor, in hairless mouse skin. These formulations also increased the production and accumulation of PpIX derived from 5-ALA in healthy skin and tumor skin.	De Rosa et al., 2000, Malik et al., 1995.
	Monoolein and propylene glycol	Significantly increased drug penetration and retention in the skin. Results *in vivo* demonstrated that the increase of PpIX was monoolein concentration-dependent.	Steluti et al., 2005.
	DMSO, Caprylic/capric triglycerides PEG-4 esters, triisostearin PEG-6 esters, caprylocaproyl macrogol 8-glyceride, ethoxydiglycol, 1-[2-(decylthio) ethyl]azacyclopentan-2-one (HPE-10)	Penetration enhancers increased the formation of porphyrins in the skin. Caprylic/capric triglycerides PEG-4 esters was less irritating than HPE-10.	Bugaj et al., 2006a. Bugaj et al., 2006b.
	Oleic acid	*In vitro* and *in vivo* studies demonstrated that oleic acid was a potential penetration enhancer of ALA in the skin.	Pierre et al., 2006.

Table 1. Chemical penetration enhancers associated with anticancer drugs for skin cancer treatments.

It can be seen in Table 1 that penetration enhancers generally increase drug penetration and retention into the skin. The most common and extensively studied chemical enhancers for topical chemotherapy are DMSO and monoolein. The lack of toxicity of monoolein compared to DMSO increases the potential use of this penetration enhancer in clinical trials. In addition, monoolein is biodegradable, safe and has been used in different formulations in the pharmaceutical field.

The use of a chemical enhancer to increase the penetration of 5-ALA for topical PDT is another frequently studied strategy. 5-ALA is a prodrug, converted *in situ* by the heme biosynthetic pathway into a highly fluorescent substance, protoporphyrin IX (PpIX), an effective photosensitizer. Thus, for successful PDT therapy, it is important that high concentrations of 5-ALA penetrate the skin for its conversion to PpIX and to facilitate the death of tumor cells when light is applied. Although the FDA has already approved a topical application of ALA for actinic keratosis, extensive efforts have been made to increase 5-ALA penetration into the skin in an appropriate semi-solid formulation. Thus, chemical enhancers appear to be promising for PDT treatment in combination with ALA topical delivery.

4.2 Physical penetration methods

Iontophoresis and electroporation are the most frequently studied physical methods used to improve antineoplastic topical delivery. Both techniques employ an electrical current to overcome the stratum corneum and to increase drug penetration into the skin. In the next sections, the basic principles of iontophoresis and electroporation will be described, and some of the studies that have employed these modalities in the context of skin cancer treatment will be discussed.

4.2.1 Iontophoresis

Iontophoresis is a non-invasive technique that consists of the application of a weak electrical current to increase drug penetration into biologic membranes. It has been extensively studied to increase drug transdermal delivery, i.e., drug penetration across the skin and towards the blood stream. In early 2000, however, iontophoresis began to be used to increase the skin penetration of topical ALA (Gerscher et al., 2000).

To iontophoretically deliver drugs, a constant direct electrical current (usually less than 0.5 mA/cm^2) is applied over the skin using an electrolytic solution containing the drug. A battery or a power supply and two oppositely polarized, insulated electrodes are used to apply this current. The positive electrode is the anode, and the negative electrode is the cathode. When the current is applied, cations from the electrolytic solution in the anode compartment move toward the cathode, whereas anions in the cathode compartment move toward the anode (Figure 5) (Gratieri et al., 2008).

All cations and anions, including ionized molecules (which can be an anticancer drug), are dispersed in the electrolytic solution and transport a fraction of the electrical current, referred to as the transport number (Sieg et al., 2004). The maximum transport number of a specific ion is 1, which is the case when this ion alone carries 100% of the current through the skin. Therefore, several factors related to the electrical properties of the system need to be considered when attempting to increase drug transport by iontophoresis, including the current density and type of electrode. Moreover, the solution/formulation characteristics, such as ionic strength and pH, need to be optimized to increase the fraction of the current (i.e., the transport number) of the drug of interest (Gratieri et al., 2008).

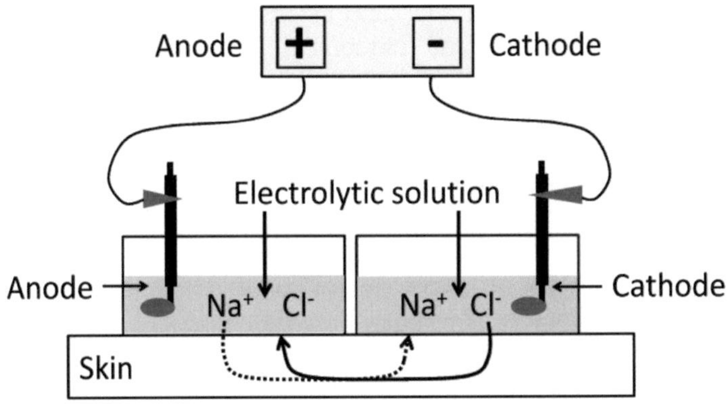

Fig. 5. Schematic representation of an iontophoretic device: cations and anions migrate through the skin during the application of a low-strength electrical current.

The electrode choice has an important influence on the stability of the driving electric current, which is necessary to control drug delivery. Electrodes must guarantee the electroneutrality of the system without changing the pH of the electrolytic solution or altering the drug's properties (Cullander et al., 1993). The most commonly used electrodes are the reversible Ag/AgCl electrodes. This choice is primarily because their electrochemical reactions are rapid and occur at a voltage lower than that required for the water to undergo electrolysis, thereby avoiding variations in the pH of the formulation (Kalia et al., 2004). During the application of the electrical current, Cl^- ions in the electrolyte solution react with the silver electrode, i.e., the anode, donating one electron to the electric circuit ($Ag^o + Cl^- \rightarrow AgCl + e^-$). This electron arrives at the cathode, reducing the AgCl electrode ($AgCl + e^- \rightarrow Ag^o + Cl^-$). To ensure the system's electroneutrality, a cation in the anode moves to the skin or an anion moves from the skin toward the anode. In the cathode, the opposite occurs, i.e., an anion moves to the skin or a cation moves from the skin toward the cathode (Kalia et al., 2004; Chang et al., 2000). Therefore, the electric circuit is completed by the inorganic ions of the skin, primarily Na^+ and Cl^-.

Antineoplastic drugs can be delivered to the skin by iontophoresis through two mechanisms: electromigration and electroosmosis. These mechanisms can act in combination to increase drug skin penetration.

Electromigration refers to the orderly movement of ions in the presence of an electric current. For instance, positively charged antineoplastic drugs, when placed in the positive electrode compartment (anode), migrate away from the electrode with the same polarity into the skin (Tesselaar & Sjöberg, 2011). The same occurs when a negative drug is placed in contact with the cathode compartment. The electromigration contribution to a drug's skin penetration depends on the concentration and the electrical mobility of the drug (ion) (Gratieri et al., 2008). High-molecular weight drugs, which include most antineoplastic drugs, generally have a low electric mobility, decreasing the electromigration contribution for their permeating.

Electroosmosis refers to the solvent flow when an electric potential is applied to the skin. Under physiologic conditions, this flow occurs from the anode toward the cathode due to the skin's cation permselectivity (Figure 6). Specifically, the skin is twice more permeable to cations than to anions (Burnette & Ongpipattanakul, 1987). This is because the skin is negatively charged when in contact with a solution at physiological pH (Merino et al., 1999). As a result, solvent flow occurs in the direction of cation flux, enhancing the transport of cations and slowing the transport of anions (Singh & Mabach, 1996). Electroosmotic flux is the dominant mechanism for macromolecule's skin permeation. This is because the solvent flux pushes the macromolecule and takes advantage of the low-resistance of the skin when iontophoresis is applied (Abla et al., 2005; Pikal, 2001). Hence, neutral and high molecular weight antineoplastic drugs can take advantage of solvent flow and penetrate the skin by iontophoresis. Furthermore, positively charged drugs can penetrate the skin by both electromigration and electroosmotic contributions.

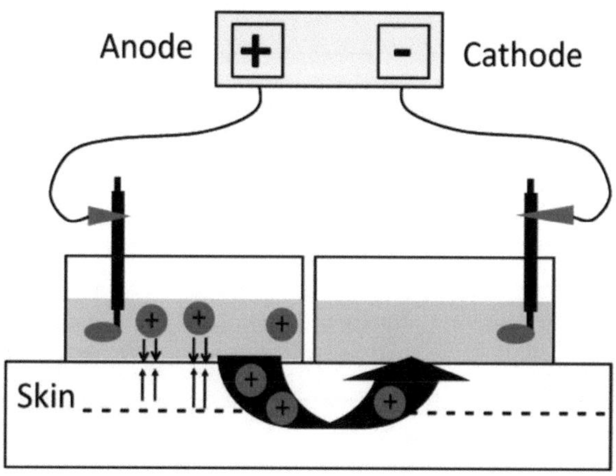

Fig. 6. Schematic representation of the electroosmotic flow that accompanies the electromigration of cations, which is due to the negative charge of the skin at pH 7.

The use of iontophoresis in the topical administration of antineoplastic drugs offers important advantages for tumor drug delivery. Most of these advantages are related to the precise control of drug delivery by electrical current adjustments and formulation characteristics. The applied current density and the short duration of this application, combined with the components and formulation characteristics, may rapidly target the drug to the tumor in high concentrations, avoiding the blood stream (Kalia et al., 2004). As an example of the application of targeted drug delivery using iontophoresis and simple modifications in drug formulation, Taveira et al. (2009) demonstrated that iontophoresis significantly increased skin permeability to doxorubicin. However, because this drug is positively charged at a physiological pH, it interacted with the negatively charged stratum corneum, decreasing its permeation to the deep skin layers. Interestingly however, the authors demonstrated that the incorporation of a cationic polymer (chitosan) in the drug formulation decreased the skin's negatives charge when iontophoresis was applied, releasing doxorubicin from ionic interactions with the skin and improving its diffusion into the deep skin layers.

Despite the obvious benefits that iontophoresis may offer for topical skin tumor treatment, there have been limited studies using this technique to this purpose. Most studies have applied iontophoresis to increase the penetration of ALA and porphyrins for topical PDT (Table 2)

Drug	Skin model	Electrode polarity[a]	Current density (mA/cm²)	Formulation[b]	References
ALA and ester	*In vivo*: human	Anode	0.25	Aqueous solution	Gerscher et al., 2000.
ALA and Ester	*In vivo*: human	Anode	0.25	Aqueous solution	Gerscher et al., 2001.
ALA	*In vitro*: human SC	Anode	0.15 - 0.78	isotonic phosphate buffer (pH 2.1)	Bodde et al., 2002.
ALA	*In vivo*: human	Anode	0.2	Aqueous solution and cream	Choudry et al., 2003.
ALA	*In vivo*: rabbits – oral mucosa	Anode	0.5	Ointment	Tanaka et al., 2003.
ALA	*In vitro*: pig ear	Anode and cathode	0.5	Physiological buffer	Lopez et al., 2003.
ALA and esters	*In vitro:* pig ear	Anode	0.5	Distilled water	Lopez et al., 2003.
ALA and m-ALA	*In vitro*: pig ear	Anode	0.5	Lipid sponge phase and buffer with propylene glycol	Merclin et al., 2004.
ALA and m-ALA	*In vitro*: pig ear	Anode	0.5	Anionic Gel	Merclin et al., 2004.
Meso-tetra-[4-sulfonatophenyl]-porphyrin	*In vitro*: pig ear	Cathode	0.5	Electrolytic aqueous solution	Gelfuso et al., 2008.
ALA	*In vivo*: human	Anode	0.25 - 0.5	Distilled water	Mizutani et al., 2009.
Doxorubicin	*In vitro:* pig ear	cathode	0.5	Non-ionic and cationic gel	Taveira et al., 2009.
zinc phthalocyanine tetrasulfonic acid	*In vitro*: pig ear	Anode and cathode	0.5	Non-ionic gel	Souza et al., 2011.
Meso-tetra-(N-methylpiridinium-4-yl)-porphyrin and meso-tetra-(4-sulfonatophenyl)-porphyrin	*In vitro*: pig ear	Anode and cathode	0.5	Non-ionic Gel	Gelfuso et al., 2011.

[a] Polarity of the electrode in contact with the formulation containing the drug.
[B] Composition of the principal components/ions of the formulation/electrolytic solution that contains the drug.

Table 2. Drugs that have been delivered into the skin using iontophoresis as a skin cancer treatment.

The experiments shown in Table 2 demonstrate that iontophoresis significantly increases drug penetration into and through the skin much more rapidly than passive (no current)

administration. For examples, a 50-fold higher flux over passive transport was observed with iontophoretic delivery of methyl-ALA after 2 h (Lopez et al, 2003). Furthermore, the same amount of ALA delivered passively into the stratum corneum in several hours was delivered in only 10 minutes of iontophoresis application (Bodde et al., 2002). *In vivo* experiments performed with ALA and its esters generally show an increase in the depth and intensity of PpIX fluorescence following administration of the prodrug ALA. However, adjustments of electrical and formulation parameters are still required to improve the performance of iontophoretic delivery *in vivo*. *In vitro*, modifications in the pH and ionic strength of drug formulation have shown extensive improvements in drug delivery. For example, the simple elimination of Na^+ from a gel formulation containing the porphyrin meso-tetra-(N-methylpyridinium-4-yl)-porphyrin at pH 5.5 increased anodal drug iontophoretic transport by approximately 30% (Gelfuso et al., 2011).
In summary, iontophoresis has a huge potential for drug delivery in topical skin cancer therapy. Clearly, more studies should be performed *in vivo* with other antineoplastic drugs and with optimized iontophoretic parameters. Moreover, risks and toxicity for other organs should be evaluated to ensure that antineoplastic drugs accumulate in the tumor without entering the systemic circulation in significant quantities.

4.2.2 Electroporation

Electroporation is the application of high-voltage pulses (100 to 1,500 V) in cells or membranes to increase drug penetration (Prausnitz et al., 1996). When applied in cell culture, the pulses create openings in the cell membrane similar to pores, and non-permeant drugs can access the cytosol (Gothelf et al., 2003). The following sequence of events is believed to take place during electroporation: (1) within nanoseconds to microseconds, new aqueous pathways ('pores') are created in the cell membrane, (2) molecules move through these pathways primarily by electrophoresis and/or electroosmosis due to the local electric field, and (3) following the pulse, the pores remain open for milliseconds to hours (Prausnitz et al., 1996) (Figure 7).

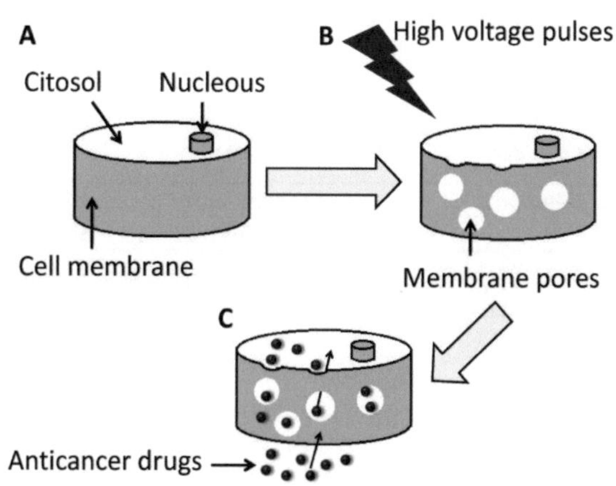

Fig. 7. Schematic illustration of the formation of pathways ('pores') in cell membranes created by electroporation. (A) Schematic representation of a cell, (B) Pathways created in the cell membranes following electroporation, (C) Membrane permeabilization and drug flux into the cells.

When applied to the skin, these high-energy pulses generate transient aqueous pores in the stratum corneum. These pores are responsible for the increase of skin permeability, thereby increasing the penetration of the drugs, especially macromolecules and hydrophilic drugs (Charoo et al., 2010). The electrical pulses are primarily applied using plate electrodes placed on the skin's surface. However, other types of electrodes can be used for different tumors, such as needle electrodes (Gothelf et al., 2003). These may be inserted into the tumor to favor membrane electroporation of the tumor cells. Electroporation has been shown to increase the transdermal delivery of many drugs, such as metoprolol, heparin, fentanyl (Denet et al., 2004), insulin (Murthy et al., 2006), piroxican (Murthy et al., 2004; Guoqiang et al., 2007).

The administration of anticancer drugs followed by electroporation is referred to as electrochemotherapy. The first studies of electrochemotherapy treated subcutaneous tumors by injecting the anticancer drug into the tumor and locally applying high voltage pulses to permeabilize the cells. In clinical trials, bleomycin has been administered by intravenous, intratumoral or intraarterial injection. Different schedules of current application, varying from 8 to 28 minutes, were then performed to define a time window for the administration of electrical pulses and to ensure that the drug reached the tumor (Gothelf et al., 2003).

Most of the electrochemotherapeutic protocols involve the invasive application of the anticancer drug, primarily by intravenous route, followed by the application of the high-voltage pulse over the tumor site. Few studies have examined non-invasive, topical anticancer drug administration. Because the aim of this chapter is the topical administration of anticancer drugs, Table 3 summarizes a subset of the studies that examined topically applied antineoplastic drugs using electroporation.

Drug	*In vitro/ In vivo* model	Pulse Voltage	Time of application	Electrode Type	References
Photosensitizer Methylene blue	*In vitro*: pig ear	0 - 240 V	One pulse per 1 msec for 10-30 min	Ag/AgCl	Johnson et al., 1998.
5-ALA	*In vitro*: pig ear *In vivo*: mice	0 - 240 V	One pulse per 1 msec for 15 min	Ag/AgCl	Johnson et al., 2002.
5-ALA	*In vitro*: pig ear	300 V	one pulse per 30 s, applied for 10 min	Platinum	Fang et al., 2004.
Photosensitizer chlorin and phthalocyanine	*In vitro:* fibroblast cell line	1200V	one pulse per 0.1 ms for 20 min	Ag/AgCl	Labanauskiene et al., 2007.
Ruthenium complex	*In vitro:* melanoma cell line	80 – 240 V	One pulse per 100 μs for 8 s	stainless steel plate	Bicek et al., 2007.

Table 3. Drugs that have been delivered by electroporation into the skin following topical administration.

Table 3 shows that, as with other physical/chemical penetration methods, a great number of studies that use electrochemotherapy are related to PDT and the increase of photosensitizer's permeation through the skin. In each of these studies, electroporation increases drug skin penetration and even drug cytotoxicity (Labanauskiene et al., 2007; Bicek et al., 2007). Combinations of electroporation with other physical methods, such as iontophoresis, often lead to synergistic effects in increasing drug penetration (Johson et al., 2002; Fang et al., 2004). When applied alone, electroporation increases the penetration of the drugs more than iontophoresis. This is because the former creates new pathways through the skin, whereas the later mostly takes advantage of the decreased electrical resistance in existing routes into the skin. In this context, electrochemotherapy is a potential strategy for topical anticancer drug administration. Nevertheless, more studies are required to investigate the side effects and to minimize patient discomfort during the application of the electroporation protocol.

4.3 Nanocarrier systems for topical anticancer drug delivery

Semi-solid conventional formulations, such as creams, ointments and gels, have been used for topical administration of drugs for many years. Simple application of the formulation on the skin's surface, however, is not sufficient to allow the drug to reach the site of action. This means that it is important for the formulation to aid in drug penetration through the different skin layers to reach the tumor site (Schmid & Korting, 1996). Nanocarriers could improve skin targeting, improving the drug's ability to reach and penetrate into tumor cells. Moreover, nanocarriers can improve drug stability and reduce skin irritation by avoiding direct contact of the drug with the skin's surface (Schimid & Korting, 1996).
Different nanocarriers have been used for topical application. This section will discuss the most frequently studied, topically applied carriers for the treatment of skin tumors.

4.3.1 Liposomes

Liposomes are one of the most studied nanocarriers for the treatment of cancer. They are colloidal particles and are biocompatible and biodegradable, consisting primarily of phospholipid vesicles. These vesicles are in turn composed of one or several lipid bilayers (Gratieri et al., 2010). Phospholipids are able to self-assemble into vesicular structures when dispersed in an aqueous medium because of their amphiphilic characteristic. The non-polar tails orient toward non-polar tails of other phospholipid molecules present in the medium in an attempt to avoid the water. This process forms lipid bilayers that are separated by the polar heads of the phospholipids (Figure 8). Because of this special arrangement, liposomes are able to entrap both hydrophilic and hydrophobic compounds in the aqueous compartments or within the lipid bilayer, respectively. Moreover, lipid bilayers are biocompatible with the stratum corneum, increasing the liposome's affinity for the skin and making them able to release drugs directly to this membrane.

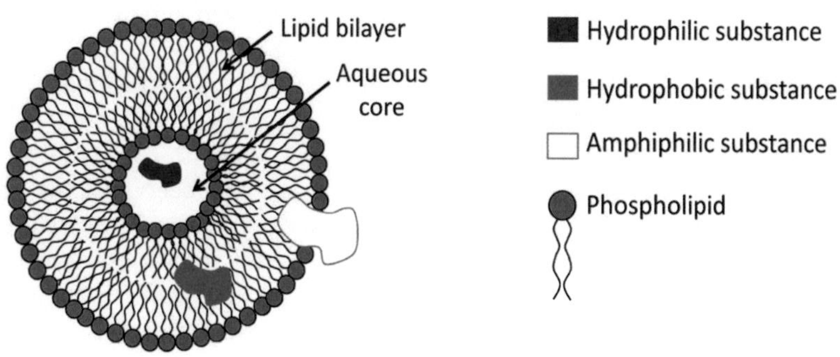

Fig. 8. Schematic representation of liposomes, which are vesicles formed primarily from phospholipids that can self-organize into vesicles in aqueous media. Liposomes have regions capable of encapsulating drugs with different physicochemical characteristics.

Traditional liposomes are composed primarily of phospholipids. Liposomes formed with different components have been developed in an attempt to increase the stability of the vesicles and their ability to penetrate through different membranes, especially the stratum corneum. In this way, elastic liposomes, also called ultradeformable or ultraflexible liposomes, are the new generation of liposomes. These contain surfactants, other amphiphiles or ethanol in their composition, which improve the flexibility of the lipid bilayer. Transfersomes®, niosomes and ethosomes® were the names given to the first, second and third flexible liposome generations, respectively (Santana & Zancheta, 2011). Transfersomes® were introduced by Cevc and Blume (1992) and are composed of phosphatidylcholine and sodium cholate. Ethosomes® consist of a mixture of phosphatidilcoline and ethanol, and niosomes are non-ionic surfactant vesicles (Manconi et al., 2002). The ability of these vesicles to deform gives them the ability to pass through narrow pores, such as the pores present on the skin surface, possibly improving the penetration of drugs carried by these vesicles into the deep skin layers (Manconi et al., 2002, Santana & Zancheta, 2011). These new generations of liposomes have been well studied in the context of topical administration and have also been introduced into the field of topical skin cancer treatments.

Most of the studies involving liposomes in the treatment of cancer have been performed using invasive administration, such as intravenous injections. Liposomes containing doxorubicin (Hosoda et al., 1995; Barenholz et al., 2001), cisplatin (Lasic et al., 1999; Krieger et al., 2010), oxaliplatin (Lila et al., 2010), camptothecin (Watanabe et al., 2008) and others have been shown to increase these drugs cytotoxicity and to reduce side effects because of direct targeting. Some of these liposomes, such as DOXIL®, are already commercially available. This liposomal formulation contains doxorubicin and was approved in the US in 1995 (Barenholz, 2001).

The topical application of anticancer drugs is, once again, primarily related to the administration of the pro-drug ALA for topical PDT. Fang et al. (2008) performed an *in vivo* study of the influence of liposomes and ethosomes in ALA skin penetration. This study showed that the flexible liposomes (ethosomes) increased 5-ALA penetration to a greater degree than did the traditional liposomes, although both formulations increased ALA penetration when compared to the control treatment. Cationic ultradeformable liposomes have also been shown to increase ALA skin permeability *in vitro*. *In vivo*, these liposomes result in persistent ALA retention in the skin and induce the production of high levels of PpIX (Oh et al., 2011). ALA skin retention was also improved when a traditional ALA-containing liposome was examined *in vitro* (Pierre et al., 2001).

In addition to these ALA studies, 5-fluorouracil-loaded niosomes showed an 8-fold improvement of this drug's cytotoxicity and penetration when compared to the aqueous solution (Paolino et al., 2008). It is worth noting that liposomes in combination with other drugs not traditionally used in skin cancer treatments have also been studied. For instance, tretinoin and diclophenac-loaded liposomes (Kitagawa et al., 2006; Zaafarany et al., 2010) showed improvement in these drugs' skin penetration over non-liposomal formulations. These studies, however, were aimed at treating acne, psoriasis and other inflammatory conditions but not skin tumors. These formulations, however, are currently proposed to treat skin cancer malignances.

In summary, liposomes have been shown to increase drugs' penetration into the skin, and it appears that ultradeformable liposomes may have an even stronger effect. However, some reports describe liposome instability and drug leakage during the storage period (Glavas-

Dodov et al., 2005). Therefore, more studies should be performed to develop more stable liposomes. *In vivo* experiments with humans should be performed to demonstrate the potential of flexible liposomes loaded with different anticancer drugs for topical skin cancer treatment.

4.3.2 Polymeric and lipid nanoparticles

Nanoparticle drug carrier systems are potential formulations to improve the therapeutic effectiveness and safety profile of conventional cancer chemotherapies (Wong et al., 2007). Different types of nanoparticles have been investigated for topical delivery. The most commonly studied nanoparticles are solid lipid nanoparticles and polymeric nanoparticles, such as those made from poly(dl-lactic acid) (PLA), poly(lactic-co-glycolic acid) (PLGA) and poly-ε-caprolactone (PCL) (Rancan et al., 2009).

Polymeric nanoparticles can be classified as nanocapsules and nanospheres. Nanospheres have a solid matrix while nanocapsules have a shell that surrounds a core usually oily (Figure 9). Anticancer drugs can be encapsulated inside or be associated with the nanoparticle surface.

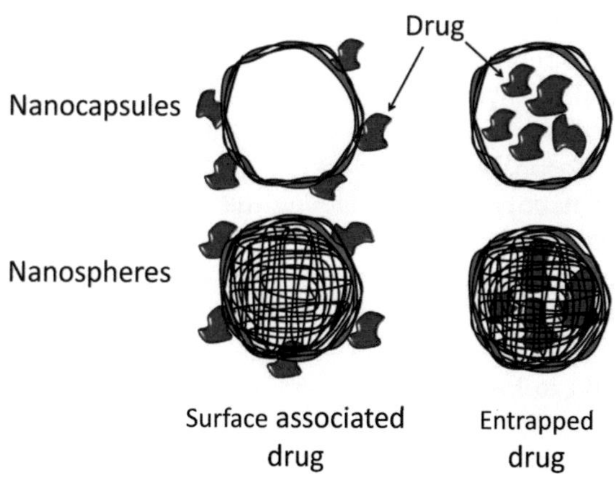

Fig. 9. Schematic representation of polymeric nanoparticles. Nanocapsules have a polymeric shell with an interior phase that is often oily. Also shown are the solid-matrix nanospheres.

Solid lipid nanoparticles (SLNs) have been studied since the 1990s and are considered new relative to liposomes and polymeric nanoparticles. SLNs are primarily composed of lipids, which are solid at room temperature, dispersed in water. They are similar to nanoemulsions, but the inner liquid lipid is replaced with a solid lipid (Gratieri et al., 2010). This structure can improve sustained drug release because drug mobility is lower in SLNs. When compared to liposomes, SLNs exhibit greater stability, prolonged drug release and greater ease in sterilization and in scaling the manufacturing process to an industrial level. The absence of organic solvents in the preparation of SLNs is a huge advantage compared to polymeric nanoparticles. However, low drug loading and drug expulsion during storage can be a limiting factor for some therapeutic treatments.

Both SLNs and polymeric nanoparticles have been shown to promote sustained drug release and protection against drug degradation when topically applied (Teixeira et al., 2010; Marquele-Oliveira et al., 2010). In addition, they allow for modifications to matrix softness and superficial charges, adjustments that may improve skin targeting. The exact mechanism by which these particles increase drug penetration through the skin is not completely understood, but efforts to understand this property have been made by developing and characterizing different nanoparticles (Lopez et al., 2011). It appears that nanoparticles can closely contact the superficial junctions of corneocyte clusters and furrows, possibly favoring drug accumulation for several hours. This would allow for the sustained release of anticancer drugs. However, there are controversies regarding the ideal mean diameter, flexibility and superficial charge of nanoparticles to contribute to skin penetration.

Studies of nanoparticles have not been limited to the examination of cytotoxic cancer drugs; numerous studies have also been performed that use these systems to deliver anti-proliferative drugs. Of studies of the topical administration of anticancer drugs, nanoparticles containing the 5-ALA, 5-fluorouracil and tretinoin are the most common (Prow et al., 2011). Some examples of recent results obtained with these and other drugs encapsulated in nanoparticles are described below. SLNs have been shown to increase tretinoin stability and to decrease drug irritation (Kumar et al., 2007, Mandawgade et al., 2008). Microparticles containing ALA were shown *in vitro* to be capable of temperature-triggered ALA release, enhanced drug stability and improved penetration through keratinized skin (Kassas et al., 2009). *In vivo*, high levels of PpIX were observed in mouse skin treated with ALA-loaded microparticles. This study also demonstrated a reduction in skin tumor growth rate (Donelly et al., 2009). Polymeric micro- and nanocapsules increased porphyrin-induced phototoxicity by a factor of 4 in cultured HeLa cells when compared to a liposomal emulsion of phosphatidylcholine loaded with an equivalent amount of porphyrin (Deda et al., 2009). PLA nanoparticles containing the prodrug 5-fluorouracil demonstrated linear release of this drug for 6 h with no evidence of a burst effect (McCarron et al., 2008). Promising results were found for resveratrol encapsulated in SLNs, a formulation that showed increased cellular uptake (Teskac et al., 2010). Nitrosyl ruthenium complex-loaded SLNs performed well at releasing and protecting the complex against degradation *in vitro*, showing this formulation to be a promising carrier for the topical delivery of nitric oxide (Marquele-Oliveira et al., 2010). Podophyllotoxin-SLNs were demonstrated *in vitro* to increase drug retention on the skin's surface, avoiding transdermal penetration (Prow et al., 2011).

In summary, most studies have described the advantages of drug encapsulation in nanoparticles by demonstrating increased drug stability, sustained release and improved skin penetration and cytotoxicity. Despite such promising results, more studies should be performed to elucidate the mechanisms by which nanoparticles increase the ability of anticancer drugs to penetrate the skin.

5. Conclusion

The penetration of drugs into the skin through the keratinized stratum corneum is a major obstacle to the delivery of high concentrations of anticancer drugs into tumor cells. The use of chemical and physical methods and the development of nanoparticle-based drug delivery systems are very important strategies to improve the ability of drugs to penetrate the skin. Nanocarriers appear to be promising systems because they offer several advantages, such as low skin irritation and increased protection of encapsulated drug. An especially important advantage of these formulations is that they often increase anticancer drug penetration through the skin. Iontophoresis also appears to be a promising technique for improving drug delivery through the skin, especially for PDT, for which high concentrations of the photosensitizer are required for effective treatment. The use of physical methods to improve the penetration of nanocarriers should be considered to increase the anticancer drug's penetration into the skin and to provide for targeted drug release inside tumor cells.

6. Acknowledgements

The authors thank the financial support of FAPESP, CAPES and CNPq.

7. References

Abla, N., Naik, A., Guy, R. H., Kalia, Y. N. (2005). Contributions of electromigration and electroosmosis to peptide iontophoresis across intact and impaired skin. *Journal of Controlled Release*, Vol.108, No.2-3, (November 2005), pp. 319-330, ISSN 0168-3659.

Alam, M., Goldber, L. H., Silapunt, S., Gardner, E. S., Strom, S. S., Rademaker, A. W., Margolis, D. J. (2011). Delayed treatment and continued growth of nonmelanoma skin cancer. *Journal of American Academy Dermatolology*, Vol.64, No.5, (May 2011), pp. 839-848, ISSN 0190-9622.

Anthony, M. L. (2000). Surgical treatment of nonmelanoma skin cancer. *AORN*, Vol.71, No.3, (March 2000), pp. 550-564, ISSN 0001-2092.

Araújo, L. M. P. C., Thomazine, J. A., Lopez, R. F. V. (2010). Development of microemulsions to topically deliver 5-aminolevulinic acid in photodynamic therapy. *European Journal of Pharmaceutics and Biopharmaceutics*, Vol.75, No.1, (May 2010), pp. 48-55, ISSN 0939-6411.

Barenholz, Y. (2001). Liposome application: problems and prospects. *Current Opinion in Colloid & Interface Science*, Vol.6, No.1, (February 2001), pp. 66-77, ISSN 1359-0294.

Barrera, M. V., Herrera, E. (2007). Topical chemotherapy of actinic keratosis and nonmelanoma skin cancer: current options and future perspectives. *Actas Dermo-Sifiliográficas*, Vol.98, No.8, (October 2007), pp. 556-562, ISSN 0001-7310.

Barry, B. W. (2001). Novel mechanisms and devices to enable successful transdermal drug delivery. *European Journal of Pharmaceutical Science*. Vol.14, No.2, (September 2001), pp. 101-114, ISSN 0928-0987.

Bicek, A., Turel, I., Kanduser, M., Miklavcic, D. (2007). Combined therapy of the antimetastatic compound NAMI-A and electroporation on B16F1 tumor cells in vitro. *Bioelectrochemistry*, Vol.71, No.2, (November 2007), pp. 113-117, ISSN 1567-5394.

Boddé, H. E., Roemelé, P. E., Star, W. M. (2002). Quantification of topically deliverd 5-aminolevulinic acid by iontophoresis across ex vivo human stratum corneum. *Photochemistry Photobiology*, Vol.75, No.4, (April 2002), pp. 418-423, ISSN 0031-8655.

Bouwstra, J. A., Ponec, M. (2006). The skin barrier in healthy and diseased state. *Biochimica et Biophysica Acta (BBA) – Biomembranes*, Vol.1758, No.12, (December 2006), pp. 2080-2095, ISSN 0005-2736.

Bugaj, A., Juzeniene, A., Juzenas, P., Iani, V., Ma, L. W., Moan, J. (2006a). The effect of skin permeation enhancers on the formation of porphyrins in mouse skin during topical application of the methyl ester of 5-aminolevulinic acid. *Journal of Photochemistry and Photobiology B: Biology*, Vol.83, No.2, (May 2006), pp. 94-97, ISSN 1011-1344.

Bugaj, A., Juzeniene, A., Juzenas, P., Iani, V., Ma, L. W., Moan, J. (2006b). The effect of dimethylsulfoxide, 1-[2-(decylthio)ethyl]azacyclopentan-2-one and Labrafac(R)CC on porphyrin formation in normal mouse skin during topical application of methyl 5-aminolevulinate: A fluorescence and extraction study. *Photodiagnosis and Photodynamic Therapy*, Vol.3, No.1, (March 2006), pp. 27-33, ISSN 1572-1000.

Burnette, R. R., Ongpipattanakul, B. (1987). Characterization of the permselective properties of excised human skin during iontophoresis. *Journal of Pharmaceutical Science*, Vol.76, No.10, (October 1987), pp. 765-773, ISSN 0022-3549.

Burns, C. A., Brown, M. D. (2005). Imiquimod for the treatment of skin cancer. *Dermatologic Clinics*, Vol.23, (January 2005), pp. 151-164, ISSN 0733-8635.

Chang, S.-L., Hofmann,G. A., Zhang, L., Deftos, L. J., Banga, A. K. (2000). The effect of electroporation on iontophoretic transdermal delivery of calcium regulating hormones. *Journal of Controlled Release*, Vol.66, No.2-3, (May 2000), pp. 127-133, ISSN 0168-3659.

Charoo, N. A., Rahman, Z., Repka, M. A., Murthy, S. N. (2010). Electroporation: An avenue for transdermal drug delivery. *Current Drug Delivery*, Vol.7, No.2, (April 2010), pp. 125-136, ISSN 1567-2018.

Choudry, K., Brooke, R. C. C., Farrar, W., Rhodes, L. E. (2003). The effect of an iron chelating agent on protoporphyrin IX levels and phototoxicity in topical 5-aminolaevulinic acid photodynamic therapy. *British Journal of Dermatology*, Vol.149, (July 2004), pp. 124-130, ISSN 0007-0963.

Cullander, C., Guy, R. H. Routes of delivery: Case studies: (6) Transdermal delivery of peptides and proteins. *Advanced Drug Delivery Reviews*, Vol.8, No.2-3, (March 1992), pp. 291-329, ISSN 0169-409X.

Davids, L. M., Kleemann, B. (2010). Combating melanoma: the use of photodynamic therapy as a novel, adjuvant therapeutic tool . *Cancer Treatment Reviews*, (December 2010), ISSN 0305-7372, doi 10.1016/j.ctrv.2010.11.007.

De Rosa, F. S., Marchetti, J. M., Thomazini, J. A., Tedesco, A. C., Bentley, M. V. L. B. (2000). A vehicle for photodynamic therapy of skin cancer: influence of dimethylsulphoxide on 5-aminolevulinic acid in vitro cutaneous permeation and in vivo protoporphyrin IX accumulation determined by confocal microscopy. *Journal of Controlled Release*, Vol.65, No.3, (April 2000), pp. 359-366, ISSN 0168-3659.

Deda, D. K., Uchoa, A. F., Carita, E., Baptista, M. S., Toma, H. E., Araki, K. (2009). A new micro/nanoencapsulated porphyrin formulation for PDT treatment. *International Journal of Pharmaceutics*, Vol.376, No.1-2, (July 2009), pp. 76-83, ISSN 0378-5173.

Denet, A. –R., Vanbever, R., Preat, V. (2003). Skin electroporation for transdermal and topical delivery. *Advanced Drug Delivery Reviews*, Vol.56, No.5, (March 2004), pp. 659-674, ISSN 0169-409X.

Donnelly, R. F., McCarron, P. a., Al-Kassas, R., Juzeniene, A., Juzenas, P., Iani, V., Woolfson, A. D., Moan, J. (2009). Influence of formulation factors on PpIX production and photodynamic action af novel ALA-loaded microparticles. *Biopharm Drug Dispos*, Vol.30, No.2, (March 2009), pp. 55-70, ISSN 0142-2782.

Einspahr, J. G., Stratton, S. P., Bowden, G. T., Alberts, D. S. (2002). Chemoprevention of human skin cancer. *Critial Reviews in Oncolocy/Hematology*, Vol.41, No.3, (March 2002), pp. 269-285, ISSN 1040-8428.

Fang, J. -Y, Lee, Y. -R., Shen, S-C., Fang, Y. -P., Hu, C, -H. (2004). Enhancement of topical 5-aminolaevulinic acid delivery by erbium: YAG laser and microdermobrasion: a comparison with iontophoresis and electroporation. *British Journal of Dermatology*, Vol.151, (July 2004), pp. 132-140, ISSN 0007-0963.

Fang, Y. -P., Tsai, Y. -H., Wu, P. -C., Huang, Y. -B. (2008). Comparison of 5-aminolevulinic acid-encapsulated liposome versus ethosome for skin delivery for photodynamic therapy. *International Journal of Pharmaceutics*, Vol.356, No.1-2, (May 2008), pp. 144-152, ISSN 0378-5173.

Galiczynski, E. M., Vidimos, A. T. (2011). Nonsurgical treatment of nonmelanoma skin cancer. *Dermatologic Clinics*, Vol.29, (April 2011), pp. 297-309, ISSN 0733-8635.

Gelfuso, G. M., Figueiredo, F. V., Gratieri, T., Lopez, R. F. V. (2008). The effect of pH and ionic strenght on topical delivery of a negatively charged porphyrin (TPPS4). *Journal of Pharmaceutical Science*, Vol.97, (October 2008), pp. 4249-4257, ISSN 0022-3549.

Gelfuso, G. M., Gratieri, T., Souza, J. G., Thomazine, J. A., Lopez, R. F. V. (2011). The influence of positive or negative charges in the passive and iontophoretic skin penetration of porphyrins used in photodynamic therapy. *European Journal of Pharmaceutics and Biopharmaceutics*. Vol. 77, No.2, (February 2011), pp. 249-256, ISSN 0939-6411.

Gerscher, S. Connelly, J. P., Griffiths, J., Brown, S. B., MacRobert, A. J., Wong, G., Rhodes, L. E. (2000). Comparison of the pharmacokinetics and phototoxicity of protoporphyrin IX metabolized from 5-amonolevulinic acid and two derivatives in human skin in vivo. *Photochemistry and Photobiology*, Vol.72, No.4, (October 2000), pp. 569-574, ISSN 0031-8655.

Gerscher, S., Connelly, J. P. (2001). A quantitative assessment of protoporphyrin IX metabolism and phototoxicity in human skin following dose-controlled delivery of the prodrugs 5-amonolaevulinic acid and 5-aminolaevulinic acid-n-pentylester. British Journal of Dermatology, Vol.144, No.5, (May 2001), pp. 983-990, ISSN 0007-0963.

Glavas-Dodov, M., Fredo-kumbaradzi, E., Goracinova, K., Simonoska, M., Calis, S., Trajkovic-Jolevska, S., Hincal, A. A. (2005). The effects of lyophilization on the stability of liposomes containing 5-FU. *International Journal of Pharmaceutics*, Vol. 291No. 1-2, (March 2005), pp. 79-86, ISSN 0378-5173.

Gothelf, A., Mir, L. M., Gehl, J. (2000) Electrochemotherapy: results of cancer treatment using enhanced delivery of bleomycin by electroporation. *Cancer Treatment Reviews*, Vol.29, No.5, (October 2003), pp. 371-387, ISSN 0305-7372.

Gratieri, T., Gelfuso, G. M., Lopez, R. F. V. (2008). Basic principles and applications of iontophoresis for cutaneous penetration of drugs. *Quimica Nova*, Vol.31, No.6, (July 2008), pp. 1490-1498, ISSN 1678-7064.

Gratieri, T., Gelfuso, G. M., Lopez, R. F. V., Souto, E. B. (2010). Current efforts and the potential of nanomedicine in treating fungal keratitis. *Expert Review of Ophthalmology*, Vol.5, No.3 (June 2010), pp. 365-384, ISSN 1746-9899.

Guimarães, K. L., Ré, M. I. (2011). Lipid nanoparticles as carriers for cosmetic ingredients: The first (SLN) and the Second Generation (NLC). In: *Nanocosmetics and Nanomedicines: New approaches for skin care*. Ruy Beck, Silvia Guterres and Adriana Pohlmann, 101-122, Springer, ISBN 978-3-642-19791-8, Retrieved from http://www.springerlink.com/openurl.asp?genre=book&isbn=978-3-642-19791-8.

Guoqiang, J., Dequan, Z., Jia, Z., Fuxin, D. (2007). Transdermal drug delivery of electroporation: the effects of surfactants on pathway lifetime and drug transport. *Chinese Journal of Chemical Engineering*, Vol.15, No.3, (June 2007), pp. 397-402, ISSN 1004-9541.

Hadgraft, J., Lane, M. E. (2005). Skin permeation: The years of enlightenment. *International Journal of Pharmaceutics*, Vol.305, No.1-2, (November 2005), pp. ISSN 0378-5173.

Herai, H., Gratieri, T., Thomazine, J. A., Bentley, M. V. L. B., Lopez, R. F. V. (2007). Doxorubicin skin penetration from monoolein-containing propylene glycol formulations. *International Journal of Pharmaceutics*, Vol.329, No.1-2, (February 2007), pp. 88-93, ISSN 0378-5173.

Hosoda, J., Unezaki, S., Maruyama, K., Tasuchiya, S., Iwatsuru, M. (1995). Antitumor activity of doxorubicin encapsulated in poly(ethylene glycol)-coated liposomes. *Biological & Pharmaceutical Bulletin*, Vol.18, No.9, (September 1995), pp. 1234-1237, ISSN 0918-6158.

Johnson, P. G., Gallo, S. A., Hui, S. W., Oseroff, A. R. (1998). A pulsed electric field enhances cutaneous delivery of methylene blue in excised full-thickness porcine skin. *Journal of Investigative Dermatology*, Vol.111, No.3, (September 1998), pp. 457-463, ISSN 0022-202X.

Johnson, P. G., Hui, S. W., Oseroff, A. R. (2002). Electrically enhanced percutaneous delivery of d-aminolevulinic acid using electric pulses and a DC potential. *Photochemistry and Photobiology*, Vol.75, No.5, (May 2002), pp. 534-540, ISSN 0031-8655.

Kalia, Y.N., Naik, A., Garrison, J., Guy, R. H. (2003). Iontophoretic drug delivery, *Advanced Drug Delivery Reviews*, Vol.56, No.5, (March 2004), pp. 619-658, ISSN 0169-409X.

Kitagawa, S., Kasamaki, M. (2006). Enhanced delivery of retinoic acid to skin by cationic liposomes. *Chemical & Pharmaceutical Bulletin*, Vol. 54, No.2, (February 2006), pp. 242-244, ISSN 0009-2363.

Krieger, M. L., Eckstein, N., Schneider, V., Koch, M., Royer, H. –D., Jaehde, U., Bendas, G. (2009). Overcoming cisplatin resistance of ovarian cancer cells by targeted liposomes in vitro. *International Journal of Pharmaceutics*, Vol.389, No.1-2, (April 2010), pp. 10-17, ISSN 0378-5173.

Labanauskiene, J., Gehl, J., Didziapetriene, J. (2007). Evaluation of cytotoxic effect of photodynamic therapy in combination with electroporation in vitro. *Bioelectrochemistry*, Vol.70, (January 2007), pp. 78-82, ISSN 1567-5394.

Lasic, D. D. (1999). Structure and Structure-Activity Relationships of Lipid-Based Gene Delivery Systems. In: Leaf Huang, Mien-Chie Hung and Ernst Wagner, Editor(s), Nonviral Vectors for Gene Therapy, Academic Press, San Diego, 1999, pp. 69-89, ISBN 978-0-12-358465-6.

Lila, A. S. A., Doi, Y., Nakamura, K., Ishida, T., Kiwada, H. (2010). Sequential administration with oxaliplatin-containing PEG-coated cationic liposomes promotes a significant delivery of subsequent dose into murine solid tumor. *Journal of Controlled Release*, Vol.142, No.2, (March 2010), pp. 167-173, ISSN 0168-3659.

Lopez, R ., Bentley, M. V. B., Delgado-Charro, M. B., Guy, R. H. (2003). Optimization of aminolevulinic acid delivery by iontophoresis. *Journal of Controlled Release*, Vol.88, (February 2003), p. 65-70, ISSN 0168-3659.

Lopez, R. F. V., Bentley, M. V. L. B., Delgado-Charro, M. B., Salomon, D., Bergh, H. D., Lange, N., Guy, R. H. (2003). Enhanced delivery of 5-Aminolevulinic Acid Esters by iontophoresis in vitro. *Photochemistry and Photobiology*, Vol. 77, No. 3, (March 2003), pp. 304-308, ISSN 0031-8655.

Lopez, R. F. V., Lange, N., Guy, R., Bentley, M. V. L. B. (2004). Photodynamic therapy of skin cancer: controlled drug delivery of 5-ALA and its esters. *Advanced Drug Delivery Reviews*, Vol.56, No. 1, (January 2004), pp. 77-94, ISSN 0169-409X. .

Lopez, R. F. V., Seto, J. E., Blankschtein, D., Langer, R. (2011). Enhancing the transdermal delivery of rigid nanoparticles using the simultaneous application of ultrasound and sodium lauryl sulfate. *Biomaterials*, Vol.32, No.3, (January 2011), pp. 933-941, ISSN 0142-9612.

Malik, Z., Kostenich, G., Roitman, L., Ehrenberg, B., Orenstein, A. (1995). Topical application of 5-aminolevulinic acid, DMSO and EDTA: protoporphyrin IX accumulation in skin and tumours of mice. Journal *of Photochemistry and Photobiology B: Biology*, Vol.28, No.3, (June 1995), pp. 213-218, ISSN 1011-1344.

Manconi, M., Sinico, C., Caddeo, C., Vila, A. O., Valenti, D., Fadda, A. M. (2011). Penetration enhancer containing vesicles as carriers for dermal delivery of tretinoin. *International Journal of Pharmaceutics*, Vol.412, No.1-2, (June 2011), pp. 37-46, ISSN 0378-5173.

Manconi, M., Sinico, C., Valenti, D., Loy, G., Fadda, A. M. (2002). Niosomes as carriers for tretinoin. I. Preparation and properties. *International Journal of Pharmaceutics*, Vol.234, No.1-2, (March 2002), pp. 237-248, ISSN 0378-5173.

Mandawgade, S. D., Patravale, V. B. (2008). Development of SLNs from natural lipids: Application to topical delivery of tretinoin. *International Journal of Pharmaceutics*, Vol.363, No.1-2, (November 2008), pp. 132-138, ISSN 0378-5173.

Marquele-Oliveira, F., Santana, D. C. A., Taveira, S. F., Vermeulen, D. M., Oliveria, A. R. M., Silva, R. S., Lopez, R. F. V. (2010). Development of nitrosyl ruthenium complex-loaded lipid carriers for topical administration: improvement in skin stability and in nitric oxide release by visible light irradiation. *Journal of Pharmaceutical and Biomedical Analysis*, Vol.53, No.4, (December 2010), pp. 843-851, ISSN 0731-7085.

Martinez, J-C., Otley, C. C. (2001). The management of melanoma and nonmelanoma skin cancer: a review for the primary care physician. *Mayo Clinic Proceedings*, Vol.76, (December 2001), pp. 1253-1265, ISSN 0025-6196.

McCarron, P.A. , Hall, M. (2007). Incorporation of novel 1-alkylcarbonyloxymethyl prodrugs of 5-fluorouracil into poly(lactide-co-glycolide) nanoparticles. *International Journal of Pharmaceutics*, Vol.348, No.1-2, (February 2008), pp. 115-124, ISSN 0378-5173.

McGrath, J. A., Uitto, J. Anatomy and Organization of Human Skin. In: Rook's *Textbook of Dematology Volume 1*. Tony Burns, Stephen Breathnach, Neil Cox and Christopher Griffiths, pp. 3.1-3.53, Wiley-Blackwell, ISBN 978-1-4051-6169-5, Singapore.

Merclin, N., Bender, J., Sparr, E., Guy, R. H., Ehrsson, H., Egstrom, S. (2004). Transdermal delivery from a lipid sponge phase—iontophoretic and passive transport in vitro of 5-aminolevulinic acid and its methyl ester. *Journal of Controlled Release*, Vol. 100, (November 2004), pp. 191-198, ISSN 0168-3659.

Merclin, N., Bramer, T., Edsman, K. (2004). Iontophoretic delivery of 5-aminolevulinic acid and its methyl ester using a carbopol gel as vehicle. *Journal of Controlled Release*, Vol.98, (July 2004), pp. 57-65, ISSN 0168-3659.

Merino, V., Lopez, A., Kalia, Y. N., Guy, R. H. (1999). Electrorepulsion versus electroosmosis: effect of pH on the iontophoretic flux of 5-fluorouracil. Pharmaceutical Research, Vol.16, No.5, (May 1999), pp. 758-761, ISSN 0724-8741.

Mizutani, K., Watanabe, D., Akita, Y., Akimoto, M., Tamada, Y., Matsumoto, Y. (2009). Photodynamic therapy using direct-current pulsed iontophoresis for 5-aminolevulinic acid application. *Photodermatology, Photoimmunology & Potomedicine*, Vol.25, (October 2009), pp. 280-282, ISSN 0905-4383.

Moser, K., Kriwet, K., Naik, A., Kalia, Y. N., Guy, R. H. (2001). Passive skin penetration enhancement and its qualification in vitro. *European Journal of Pharmaceutics and Biopharmaceutics*, Vol.52, No. 2, (September 2001), pp. 103-112, ISSN 0939-6411.

Murthy, S. N., Zhao, Y. -L., Hui, S. W., Sen, A. (2006). Synergistic effect of anionic lipid enhancer and electroosmosis for transcutaneous delivery of insulin. *International Journal of Pharmaceutics*, Vol.326, No.1-2, (December 2006), pp. 1-6, ISSN 0378-5173.

Murthy, S. N., Zhao, Y. -L., Sen, A., Hui, S. W. (2004). Cyclodextrin enhanced transdermal delivery of piroxicam and carboxyfluorescein by electroporation. *Journal of Controlled Release*, Vol.99, No.3, (October 2004), pp. 393-402, ISSN 0168-3659.

Neel, V. A., Sober, A. J. Other Skin Cancers. In: *Cancer Medicine Volume 7.* Donald W. Kufe, Raphael E. Pollock, Ralph R. Weichselbaum, Robert C. Bast, Ted S. Gansler, James F. Holland and Emil Frei, 1663-1674, DC Decker, ISBN 1-55009-307-X, Colombia.

Oh, E.k., Jin, S-E., Kim, J-K., Park, J-S., Park, Y., Kim, C-K. (2011). Retained topical delivery of 5-aminolevulinic acid using cationic ultradeformable liposomes for photodynamic therapy. European Journal of Pharmaceutical Sciences, (July 2011), ISSN 0928-0987, doi: 10.1016/j.ejps.2011.07.003

Paolino, D., Cosco, D., Muzzalupo, R., Trapasso, E., Picci, N., Freata, M. (2008). Innovative bola-surfactant niosomes as topical delivery systems of 5-fluorouracil for the treatment of skin cancer. *International Journal of Pharmaceutics*, Vol.353, No.1-2, (April 2008), pp. 233-242, ISSN 0378-5173.

Perrotta, E. R., Giordano, M., Malaguarnera, M. (2011). Non-melanoma skin cancers in elderly patients. *Critical Reviews in Oncology/Hematology*, (May 2011), ISSN 1040-8428,doi: 10.1016/j.critrevonc.2011.04.011.

Pierre, M. B., Ticci, E. Jr., Tedesco, A. C., Bentley, M. V. (2006). Oleic acid as optimizer of the skin delivery of 5-aminolevulinic acid in photodynamic therapy. Pharmaceutical Research, Vol.23, No.2, (February 2006), pp. 360-366, ISSN 0724-8741.

Pikal, M. J. (2001). The role of electroosmotic flow in transdermal iontophoresis. *Advanced Drug Delivery Reviews*, Vol. 46, No.1-3, (March 2001), pp. 281-305, ISSN 0169-409X.

Prausnitz, M. R., Lee, C. S., Liu, C. H., Pang, J. C., Singh, T., Langer, R., Weaver, J. C. (1996). Transdermal transport efficiency during skin electroporation and iontophoresis. *Journal of Controlled Release*, Vol.38, No.2-3, (February 1996), pp. 205-217, ISSN 0168-3659.

Prow, T. W., Grice, J. E., Lin, L. L., Faye, R., Butler, M., Becher, W., Wurm, E. M. T., Yoong, C., Robertson, T. A., Soher, H. P., Roberts, M. S. (2011). Nanoparticles and microparticles for skin drug delivery. *Advanced Drug Delivery Reviews*, Vol.63, No. 6, (May 2011), pp. 470-491, ISSN 0169-409X.

Rancan F, Papakostas D, Hadam S, Hackbarth S, Delair T, Primard C, Verrier B, Sterry W, Blume-Peytavi U, Vogt A (2009). Investigation of polylactic acid (PLA) nanoparticles as drug delivery systems for local dermatotherapy. *Pharmaceutical Research*, Vol.26, No.8, pp. 2027-2036, ISSN 0724-8741.

Schäfer-Korting, M.A., Wolfgang, M.B., Korting, H. (2007). Lipid nanoparticles for improved topical application of drug for skin diseases. *Advanced Drug Delivery Reviews*, Vol.59, No. 6, (July 2007), pp. 427-443, ISSN 0169-409X.

Schmid, M. -H., Korting, H. C. (1996). Therapeutic progress with topical liposome drugs for skin disease. *Advanced Drug Delivery Reviews*, Vol.18, No.3, (February 1996), pp. 335-342, ISSN 0169-409X.

Shah, K. A., Date, A. A., Joshi, M. D., Patravale, V. B. (2007). Solid lipid nanoparticles (SLN) of tretinoin: potential in topical delivery. *International Journal of Pharmaceutics*, Vol.345, (December 2007) pp. 163-171, ISSN 0378-5173.

Shah, K. A., Date, A. A., Joshi, M. D., Patravale, V. B. (2007). Solid lipid nanoparticles (SLN) of tretinoin: Potential in topical delivery. *International Journal of Pharmaceutics*, Vol.345, No.1-2, (December 2007), pp. 163-171, ISSN 0378-5173.

Sieg, A., Guy, R. H., Delgado-Charro, M. B. (2004). Electroosmosis in Transdermal Iontophoresis: Implications for Noninvasive and Calibration-Free Glucose Monitoring. *Biophysical Journal*, Vol.87, No.5, (November 2004), pp. 3344-3350, ISSN 0006-3495.

Simonetti, L. D. D., Gelfuso, G. M., Barbosa, J. C. R., Lopez, R. F. V. (2009). Assessment of the percutaneous penetration of cisplatin: the effect of monoolein and the drug skin penetration pathway. *European Journal of Pharmaceutics and Biopharmaceutics*, Vol. 73,No. 1, (September 2009), pp. 90-94, ISSN 0939-6411.

Singh, B. N., Singh, R. B., Singh, J. (2005). Effects of ionization and penetration enhancers on the transdermal delivery of 5-fluorouracil through excised human stratum corneum. *International Journal of Pharmaceutics*, Vol.298, No.1, (July 2005), pp. 98-107, ISSN 0378-5173.

Singh, P., Maibach, H. I. (1996). Iontophoresis: an alternative to the use of carriers in cutaneous drug delivery. *Advanced Drug Delivery Reviews*, Vol.18, No.3, (February 1996), pp. 379-394, ISSN 0169-409X.

Souza, J. G., Gelfuso, G. M., Simão, P. S., Borges, A. C., Lopez, R. F. (2011). Iontophoretic transport of zinc phthalocyanine tetrasulfonic acid as a tool to improve drug topical delivery. *Anticancer Drugs*, Vol. 22, No. 8, (September 2011), pp. 783-93, ISSN 0959-4973.

Steluti, R., De Rosa, F. S., Collett, J., Tedesco, A. C., Bentley, M. V. L. B. (2005). Topical glycerol monooleate/propylene glycol formulations enhance 5-aminolevulinic acid in vitro skin delivery and in vivo protophorphyrin IX accumulation in hairless mouse skin. *European Journal of Pharmaceutics and Biopharmaceutics*, Vol.60, No.3, (August 2005), pp. 439-444, ISSN 0939-6411.

Tanaka, H., Fukuda, H., Kohno, E., Hashimoto, K. (2003). Experimental study on iontophoresis for topical application of 5-aminolevulinic acid to the oral mucosa. *International Congress Series*, Vol.1248, (May 2003), pp. 425-429, ISSN 0531-5131.

Taveira, S. F., Nomizo, A., Lopez, R. F. V. (2009). Effect of the iontophoresis of a chitosan gel on doxorubicin skin penetration and cytotoxicity. *Journal of Controlled Release*, Vol.134, No.1, (February 2009), pp. 35-40, ISSN 0168-3659.

Teixeira, Z., Zanchetta, B., Melo, B. A., Oliveria, L. L., Santana, M. H., Paredes-Gamero, E. J., Justo, G. Z., Nader, H. B., Guterres, S. S., Duran, N. (2010). Retinyl palmitate flexible polymeric nanocapsules: characterization and permeation studies. Colloids and Surfaces B: Biointerfaces, Vol.81, No.1, (November 2010), pp. 374-380, ISSN 0927-7765.

Tesselaar, E., Sjoberg, F. (2011). Transdermal iontophoresis as an in-vivo technique for studying microvascular physiology. *Microvascular Research,* Vol.81, No.1, (January 2011), pp. 88-96, ISSN 0026-2862.

Venosa, G. D., Hermida, L., Fukuda, H., Defain, M. V., Rodriguez, L., Mamone, L., MacRobert, A., Casas, A., Batlle, A. (2009). Comparation of liposomal formulations of ALA Undecanoyl ester for its use in photodynamic therapy. *Journal of Photochemistry and Photobiology B: Biology,* Vol.96, No.2-3, (August 2009), pp. 152-158, ISSN 1011-1344.

Watanabe, M., Kawano, K., Toma, K., Hattori, Y., Maitani, Y. (2008). In vivo antitumor activity of camptothecin incorporated in liposomes formulated with an artificial lipid and human serum albumin. *Journal of Controlled Release,* Vol.127, No.3, (May 2008), pp. 231-238, ISSN 0168-3659.

Williams, A. C., Barry, B. W. (2004). Penetration enhancers. *Advanced Drug Delivery Reviews,* Vol.56, No.5 (March 2004), pp. 603-618, ISSN 0169-409X.

Wong, H. L., Bendayan, R., Rauth, A. M., Li, Y., Wu, X. Y. (2007). Chemotherapy with anticancer drugs encapsulated in solid lipid nanoparticles. *Advanced Drug Delivery Reviews,* Vol.59, No.6, (July 2007), pp. 491-504, ISSN 0169-409X.

Zaafarany, G. M. E., Awad, G. A. S., Holyel, S. M., Mortada, N. D. (2010). Role of edge activators and surface charge in developing ultradeformable vesicles with enhanced skin delivery. *International Journal of Pharmaceutics,* Vol.397, No.1-2, (September 2010), pp.164-172, ISSN 0378-5173.